Essential Pharmacognosy

Essential Pharmacognosy

Editor: Arlo Snyder

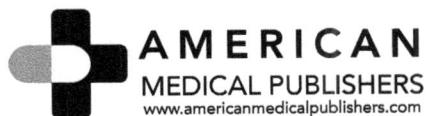

AMERICAN
MEDICAL PUBLISHERS
www.americanmedicalpublishers.com

AMERICAN
MEDICAL PUBLISHERS
www.americanmedicalpublishers.com

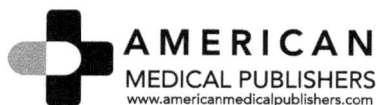

Cataloging-in-Publication Data

Essential pharmacognosy / edited by Arlo Snyder.
    p. cm.
Includes bibliographical references and index.
ISBN 978-1-63927-541-0
1. Pharmacognosy. 2. Pharmacy. 3. Drugs. 4. Materia medica. I. Snyder, Arlo.
RS160 .E87 2022
615.321--dc23

American Medical Publishers,
41 Flatbush Avenue,
1st Floor, New York,
NY 11217, USA

ISBN 978-1-63927-541-0 (Hardback)

Contents

Permissions

List of Contributors

Index

Preface

It is often said that books are a boon to mankind. They document every progress and pass on the knowledge from one generation to the other. They play a crucial role in our lives. Thus I was both excited and nervous while editing this book. I was pleased by the thought of being able to make a mark but I was also nervous to do it right because the future of students depends upon it. Hence, I took a few months to research further into the discipline, revise my knowledge and also explore some more aspects. Post this process, I begun with the editing of this book.

The study of plants and other natural sources in order to determine if they can be used to make drugs is known as pharmacognosy. It also includes the study of the physical, biochemical, chemical and biological properties of drugs along with its substances. It is mainly concerned with the analysis of natural product molecules that are useful for their medicinal, ecological and gustatory properties. It is a broad field that encompasses various biological subjects such as microbiology, marine biology, botany and herbal medicine. All plants produce phytochemicals during their normal metabolic activities. These chemicals are divided into primary and secondary metabolites. The primary metabolites include sugars and fats commonly found in all plants. The secondary metabolites are found in lesser number of plants and serve a more defined function. These can have therapeutic effects on humans, and can be refined to produce drugs such as quinine. This book contains some path-breaking studies in the field of pharmacognosy. It consists of contributions made by international experts. The book will serve as a valuable source of reference for graduate and post graduate students.

I thank my publisher with all my heart for considering me worthy of this unparalleled opportunity and for showing unwavering faith in my skills. I would also like to thank the editorial team who worked closely with me at every step and contributed immensely towards the successful completion of this book. Last but not the least, I wish to thank my friends and colleagues for their support.

Editor

Citrus Bioflavonoids Ameliorate Hyperoxaluria Induced Renal Injury and Calcium Oxalate Crystal Deposition in Wistar Rats

Sridharan Badrinathan[1], Micheal Thomas Shiju[1], Ramachandran Arya[1], Ganesh Nachiappa Rajesh[2], Pragasam Viswanathan[1]*

[1] Renal Research Lab, Centre for Bio Medical Research, School of Biosciences and Technology, VIT University, Vellore, Tamil Nadu, India.

[2] Department of Pathology, Jawaharlal Institute of Postgraduate Medical Education and Research (JIPMER), Dhanvantrinagar, Puducherry, India.

Article info

Keywords:
· Citrus bioflavonoids
· Urolithiasis
· Hyperoxaluria
· THP
· Inflammatory marker

Abstract

Purpose: Citrus is considered as a medically important plant from ancient times and the bioflavonoids of different variety of citrus fruits were well explored for their biological activities. The study aim was to explore the effect of citrus bioflavonoids (CB) to prevent and cure hyperoxaluria induced urolithiasis.

Methods: Twenty four Wistar rats were segregated into 4 Groups. Group 1: Control; Group 2: Urolithic (EG-0.75%); Group 3: Preventive study (EG+CB, day 1-50); Group 4: Curative study (EG+CB, day 30-50). Animals received CB orally (20mg/kg body weight) after performing a toxicity study.

Results: Urinary risk factors and serum renal function parameters were significantly reduced by CB administration in both preventive and curative study ($p<0.001$). Hematoxylin & Eosin and von Kossa staining demonstrated that renal protection was offered by CB against EG insult. Immunohistochemical analyses revealed over expression and abnormal localization of THP and NF-κB in urolithic rats, while it was effectively regulated by CB supplementation.

Conclusion: CB prevented and significantly controlled lithogenic factors and CaOx deposition in rats. We propose CB as a potential therapy in management of urolithiasis.

Introduction

Urolithiasis refers to formation of stones in urinary tract, predominantly calcium oxalate (CaOx) stones. Various inorganic and organic promoters of CaOx crystal aggregation were reported like oxalate, uric acid, calcium and phosphate, while inhibitors comprise of the urinary macromolecules like Tamm-Horsfall protein (THP), Osteopontin, Prothrombin fragment 1, and other urinary macromolecules in addition to citrate and magnesium.[1] Though hyperoxaluria and CaOx crystal aggregation are major processes in stone formation, crystal adhesion to the damage epithelium is an important step in urolithiasis, which actually drives the disease to an advanced stage.[2] Oxidative stress caused by CaOx crystals and high oxalate load, leads to interstitial inflammation that can be marked by increased expression of various pro-inflammatory cytokines like, NF-κB, p38-MAPK, etc.[3] Dietary supplements and edible plant products are acclaimed for health benefits offered by their micronutrients and phytochemical ingredients.[4] The diverse biological properties of herbal extracts attract medical experts and researchers to rely on plants for safer and prospective treatment for the kidney stone ailment.[5] Significant curative effect of plants was due to various flavonoids and other antioxidant compounds present in it.[6]

Studies had shown that supplementation of antioxidants provide cellular protection to the kidney, by inhibiting the over expression of inflammatory cytokines and improved the antioxidant status of the whole system.[7,8] Citrus fruit and their peels consist of a wide range of flavonoid compounds including Eriocitrin, Hesperidin, Naringin, Naringenin, which are known for its abilities to offer beneficial biological properties.[9] The major evident roles of citrus fruits in being a potential treatment for kidney stones were its ability to increase the urine pH and citrate content. Orange juice was the most favourable treatment that was reported from a number of clinical trials.[10,11] The study conducted by Touhami et al., (2007) found that administration of lemon juice significantly reduced the incidence of CaOx crystal deposition in the kidneys of experimental rats.[12] Citrus is one of the genuine choices for treatment of kidney stones, since they are one of the richest sources of polyphenolic agents, organic and inorganic enrichments.[13] Hence, in the present study we aimed to explore the preventive and curative effect of the commercially formulated citrus bioflavonoids in the management of hyperoxaluric animals progressing to calcium oxalate stone formation. We have also checked the expression and localization of THP in diseased and CB

Corresponding author: Pragasam Viswanathan, Email: pragasam.v@vit.ac.in

supplemented animals to exhibit the effective inhibition of crystal aggregation process by the flavonoids, which was primarily regulated by this anionic glycoprotein. On the other hand expression study of NF-κB, a proinflammatory cytokine also elaborates the role of CB in handling the renal oxidative and inflammatory insult.

Materials and Methods
Animals
Wistar rats of 8 weeks, weighing 200 – 250 g were used for the study. All animal experiments and maintenance were carried out according to the ethical guidelines suggested by the Institutional Animal Ethics Committee (Registration No – 1333/c/10/CPCSEA). Animals were housed in polypropylene cages and maintained under standard conditions of 12 hours dark/light cycle at 27±1°C. The rats were supplied with regular pellets and water *ad libitum*.

Acute oral toxicity
CB tablets were purchased from Health Aid Ltd, UK, and the composition of CB is given in Table 1. Citrus bioflavonoids tablet was orally administered to the female Wistar rats and the safe dose was calculated according to the OECD guidelines 423.[14] Animals were supplemented with CB at a dosage of 5000 mg/kg body weight. After administration the animals were monitored for 2 days to observe any immediate toxic effects. At the end of 14th day, the animals were sacrificed and blood was collected by cervical decapitation under anaesthetic condition. Blood collected with anticoagulant was used for haematological analyses while, blood without anticoagulant was centrifuged at 4000 rpm in 4°C to separate the serum for biochemical analyses.

Table 1. Composition of Citrus Bioflavonoids (CB) tablets

S. No	Content	Compounds*
1	Citrus Bioflavonoids	Flavonoids obtained from Citrus fruits
2	Bulking Agent	di-Calcium Phosphate
3	Binding Agent	Acacia gum
4	Anti-Caking Agent	Stearic acid and magnesium Stearate

* All the content are added at EC Recommended Daily Allowance

Anti-urolithic study
The anti-urolithic study includes 24 male rats segregated into 4 groups, which were used to demonstrate the preventive and curative effect of citrus bioflavonoid (CB). Group 1 consisted of normal animals while animals from group 2, 3 & 4 were challenged with 0.75% ethylene glycol (EG) for 50 days. Group 3 & 4 received CB (20 mg/kg of bodyweight) through oral administration. Group 3 animals received CB from day 1 to 50, whereas administration of CB was started from day 30 for group 4 animals and continued till end of the study.

Urine biochemical analyses
At the end of every 10th day rats were housed in metabolic cages and urine sample was collected under acidified conditions. The collected urine samples were centrifuged at 2,500 rpm (REMI, R24, India) for 5 min and the supernatant was used to estimate the amount of calcium, urea, creatinine and protein using commercially available kits. Oxalate was measured by the method of Hodgkinson & Williams (1972), phosphate by the method proposed by Goldenberg & Fernandez (1966).[15,16] The urinary urea level was expressed in g/24 hr urine and all other values are expressed as mg/24 hr urine.

Serum analyses
Serum analyses were performed on 50th day. The rats were anaesthetized and blood was collected from the retro-orbital region centrifuged at 10,000 rpm for 10 min, and the serum was separated. The serum was analysed for the presence of calcium, urea, phosphate, creatinine and protein and they are expressed as mg/dL. Calcium, urea, creatinine and protein were estimated using commercially available kits and phosphorus was measured using method proposed by Goldenberg & Fernandez (1966).[16]

Histopathological examinations
At the end of 50 days, the animals were euthanized under mild anaesthesia to avoid pain and stress. Kidneys were removed carefully and washed with phosphate buffered saline (PBS). The kidneys were fixed in 10% neutral buffered formalin and the fixed tissues were processed and embedded in paraffin. Sections were cut at a thickness of 4μm using Leica RM 2126 microtome and mounted on slides. The slides were stained by Haematoxylin & Eosin (H&E) and von Kossa for histopathological analyses. The sections were then photographed under microscope (Olympus BX51; Olympus optical, Tokyo, Japan) at a magnification of x400. H & E staining was used to study the tubular damage and crystal deposition while Von Kossa staining was performed to observe the intratubular calcium deposits.

Immunohistochemical analyses
Paraffin section (4 μm thick) were cut mounted on slides, dewaxed in xylene and rehydrated in graded alcohol. Endogenous peroxidase activity was blocked by incubation with 3% H_2O_2 for 15 min. Antigen retrieval was performed for NF-κB by heating the sections at 95°C for 10 min, citrate buffer (10mM, pH 6). After washing with PBS containing 0.1% Tween 20, the slides were incubated overnight with primary antibody for THP (1:200 dilutions) and NF-κB (1:200 dilutions) at 4°C. The immunoreactivity was performed using horseradish peroxidase conjugated with goat-anti-rabbit IgG antibody by incubating for 30 min at room temperature. The detection step was performed by treatment with 3, 3'-Diaminobenzidine (Dako) as chromogen. Slides were counter stained with Haematoxylin, rinsed with tap water, dehydrated, cleared in xylene and mounted. The sections were then photographed at a magnification of x400 (Olympus BX51; Olympus optical, Tokyo, Japan).

Statistical analysis

The data were analysed on Graph Pad Prism 5.01 software and expressed as mean ± SD (n=6). Statistical analysis was performed by One-way ANOVA followed by Dunnett's test to compare the diseased and the CB supplemented groups. At the same time, the statistical difference between the normal and experimental animals in toxicity study was analysed by Un-paired t-TEST. The results were considered statistically significant, if P<0.05.

Results

Acute oral toxicity

Animals were found to be normal and did not show any signs of toxicity for 14 days after administration of CB at a concentration of 5000 mg/kg body weight of animals. The serum and haematological parameters of the CB supplemented rats showed no significant changes when compared to the control rats (Table 2 & 3), except for serum triglycerides level and platelet count, which however is in normal physiological range. Hence, the results of the toxicity study clearly suggested that the LD_{50} cut off must be greater than 5000 mg/kg of body weight of animals and according to the Globally Harmonized Classification System (GHS), the CB falls under the category 5 or unclassified category of LD_{50} range. Hence, it is safer to use at a concentration below 5000mg/kg of body weight. Based on literature and the prescribed dosage from the company, 20 mg/kg body weight of CB was selected for kidney stone study.[17,18]

Table 2. Serum parameters of CB supplemented and control rats

Serum Parameter	Control	Citrus bioflavonoids (5000 mg/kg bodyweight)
Glucose[1]	83.5 ± 9	81.9 ± 8.1[NS]
Urea[1]	39.4 ± 6.1	40.7 ± 6.5[NS]
Creatinine[1]	0.99 ± 0.06	0.85 ± 0.1[NS]
Total Cholesetrol[1]	73.23 ± 2.5	75.49 ± 3.9[NS]
Triglyerides[1]	100 ± 3.8	121.9 ± 5.33*
Calcium[1]	11.05 ± 1.3	10.08 ± 0.8[NS]
Albumin[2]	4.57 ± 0.2	4.41 ± 0.5[NS]
Protein[2]	7.79 ± 0.4	7.55 ± 0.8[NS]
Alanine Transaminase[3]	26.62 ± 3.5	27.3 ± 0.8[NS]
Aspartate Transaminase[3]	47.52 ± 8.5	46.23 ± 3.6[NS]
Alkaline Phophatase[3]	48.89±16.3	47.39 ± 7.1[NS]

1 – mg/dL; 2 – g/dL; 3 – U/L. The values are expressed as mean ±SD (n=4). The study was carried out according to the OECD guidelines. 1 – mg/dL; 2 – g/dL; 3 – U/L. The values are expressed as mean ±SD (n=3). The results were statistically analysed by non-parametric student's t-test. The comparisons were made as 'Control Vs Citrus bioflavonoids supplemented rats'. *** p<0.001, ** p<0.01, * P<0.05, NS – Not Significant.

Urinary lithogenic factors

Urinary parameters after administration of EG showed drastic changes as a consequence of calcium oxalate crystal deposition in the kidneys. In our study we analysed the urinary parameters on every 10th day to observe the progression of hyperoxaluric state with prominent crystal deposition and to check the effect of CB.

The EG supplemented animals showed a significant elevation in both calcium and oxalate excretion relative to hyperoxaluric animals supplemented with CB (Figure 1a & 1b). The hyperoxaluric rats showed significant excretion of urinary calcium (4.3 mg/ 24 hr) compared to control rats (3 mg/ 24 hr), whereas the excretion of calcium was reduced significantly in hyperoxaluric rats supplemented with CB. Oxalate excretion was also found to be raised in 24 hr urine of hyperoxaluric rats (18 mg) when compared to the normal animals, which were excreting 2 mg/24 hr. CB was found to be equally good in preventing and curing the abnormal excretion of these two major risk factors of renal lithogenesis. CB supplemented to group 3 animals from day one had maintained calcium and oxalate excretion closer to normal and considerably interfered with the disease processes. The animals in group 4 had an initial phase of hyperoxaluria and crystallization for a period of 30 days and administration of CB at such an advanced stage of the disease was also observed to be stabilizing the level of both calcium and oxalate.

Inorganic phosphate is another important constituent in urine, which can lead to progression of urolithiasis when its excretion rate is beyond the renal threshold. EG supplementation in group 2, 3 & 4 resulted in raised urinary phosphate level. Hyperoxaluric rats (Group 2) showed the highest phosphate excretion in urine at the end of 50 days (7 mg/ 24 hr). Reduced level of urinary phosphate excretion was observed in animals supplemented with CB from the beginning of the study while, the phosphate level in 24 hr urine of group 4 animals showed an increase till day 30, since the supplementation of CB was not initiated. On the commencement of CB administration, we observed a significant reduction in the urinary inorganic phosphate excretion and at the end of the study it was maintained at 5.76 mg (Figure 1c).

Table 3. Haematological parameters of CB supplemented and control rats

Haematological Parameters	Control	Citrus bioflavonoids (5000 mg/kg bodyweight)
RBC[1]	6.39±0.1	6.46 ± 0.05[NS]
WBC[2]	4.1±0.2	3.93 ± 0.2[NS]
Platelet[3]	560±8.5	397 ± 11.1[***]
Hemoglobin[4]	12.5±0.3	12.72 ± 0.2[NS]
Hematocrit[5]	37.5±0.3	38 ± 0.4[NS]
Mean corpuscular Volume[6]	58.7±0.1	58.9 ± 0.1[NS]
Mean platelet Volume[6]	8.4±0.4	8.1 ± 0.3[NS]
Mean corpuscular Hemoglobin[7]	19.5±0.2	19.6 ± 0.08[NS]
Mean corpuscular Hemoglobin concentration[4]	33.3±0.1	36.5 ± 1.4[NS]

The study was carried out according to the OECD guidelines. 1 – x10[12]/µl; 2 – x10[3]/µl; 3 – x10[9]/µl; 4 – g/dL; 5 – %; 6 – Femtolitre (fL); 7 – Picogram (pg). The values are expressed as mean ±SD (n=3). The results were statistically analysed by unpaired student's t-test. The comparisons were made as 'Control Vs Citrus bioflavonoids supplemented rats'. *** p<0.001, ** p<0.01, * P<0.05, NS – Not Significant.

(A)

(B)

(C)

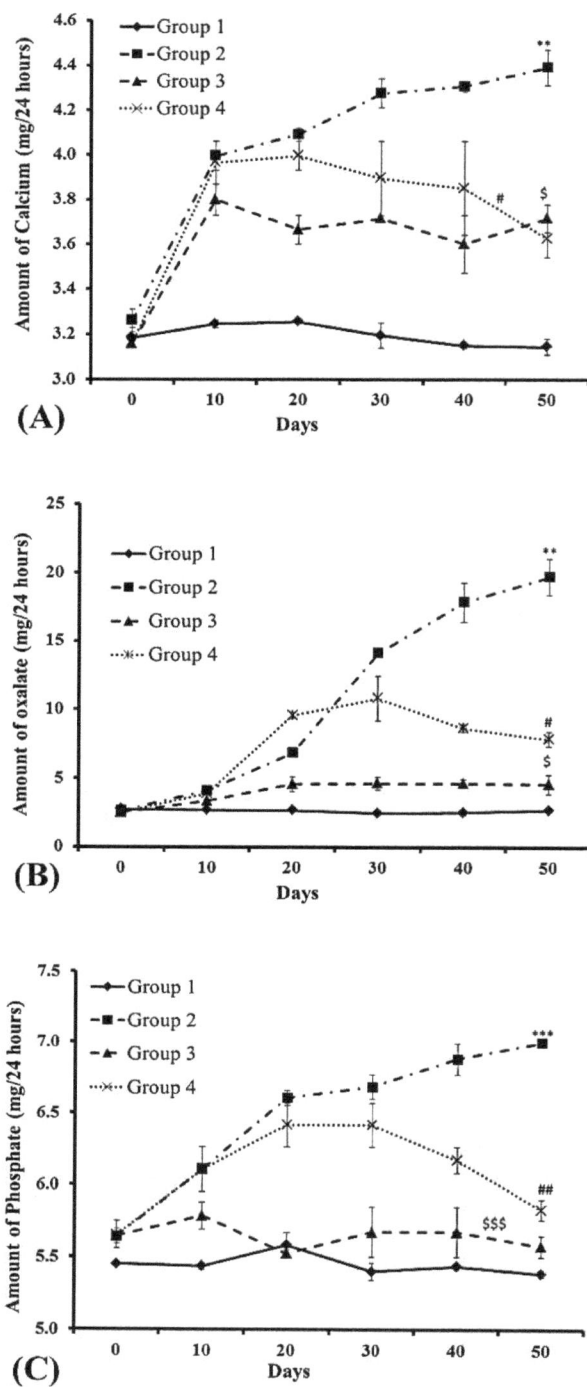

Figure 1. Effect of CB on urinary lithogenic factors
(a) Calcium; (b) Oxalate & (c) Phosphate. Results are statistically analysed by one way ANOVA with Dunnett's multiple comparison post test (n=6). The comparisons are made as follows: '*' – Control Vs Diseased; '#' – Diseased Vs Prevention; '$' – Diseased Vs Treatment. *** p<0.001, ** p<0.01, * P<0.05, NS – Not Significant.

Urinary renal damage markers

Urinary creatinine & urinary urea nitrogen are the scale of renal function in excretion of nitrogenous wastes from the system. EG challenged animals showed an abnormality in the excretion of creatinine and urea in 24

hr urine. The urolithic animals excreted a diminished amount of creatinine and urea of about 1 mg and 4 g /24 hr urine respectively (Figure 2a & 2b). CB was able to show protective effect on group 3 animals by alleviating these renal function parameters to near normal and it was also substantiated from the results obtained from group 4 animals, that the impaired renal function was also restored after supplementation of CB.

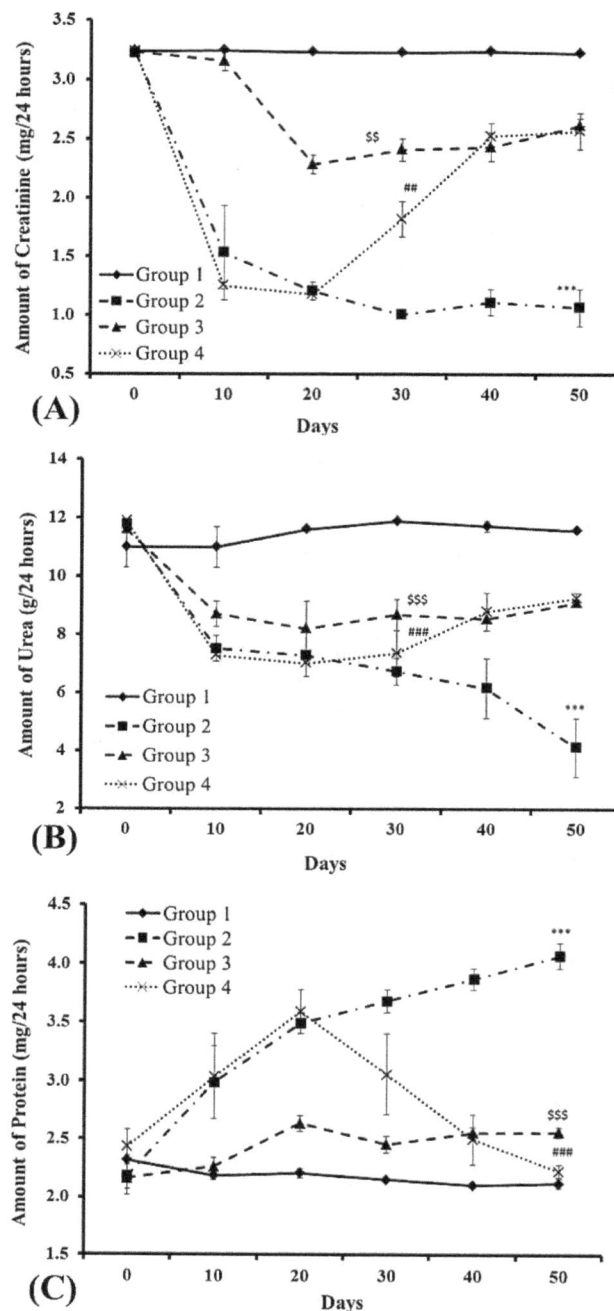

(A)

(B)

(C)

Figure 2. Effect of CB on urinary markers for renal damage
(a) Creatinine; (b) Urea & (c) Protein. Results are statistically analysed by one way ANOVA with Dunnett's multiple comparison post-test (n=6). The comparisons are made as follows: '*' – Control Vs Diseased; '#' – Diseased Vs Prevention; '$' – Diseased Vs Treatment. *** p<0.001, ** p<0.01, * P<0.05, NS – Not Significant.

Proteinuria, which was predominantly observed in the diseased animals, is a supportive observation of renal function. Citrus bioflavonoids had a constructive effect on protein excretion in both preventive and treatment strategies. As shown in the Figure 2c the excretion of protein in 24 hr urine of diseased animals showed as high as 4 mg, while CB supplemented animals had a check on excess protein excretion and maintained it close to the normal (2.5 mg/24 hr) excretion. This was observed in both group 3 & 4 animals, proving the ability of CB to protect and heal the damaged epithelium.

Serum parameters

Parameters like calcium, urea, creatinine and other lithogenic constituents were analysed in serum to show the effect of CB as an intervening substance in the genesis of CaOx stones and as a nephro-protectant. Serum parameters were analysed at the end of the study and the results are tabulated as shown (Table 4).

Increased urinary excretion of calcium and phosphate in EG supplemented rats had a reflection in the serum levels of these ions, which were correspondingly decreased. The results exhibit the positive effect of CB in sustaining the serum calcium & phosphate to 9.7 mg and 7.7 mg/ dL respectively (Table 4). Curative effect of CB also showed a significant observation in group 4 animals, where the initial reduction of calcium and phosphate in serum were restored close to normal.

The serum creatinine of EG challenged animals was found to be 2.9 mg/dL and blood urea nitrogen was 237 mg/dL (Table 4). Animals from group 3 were well protected from the CaOx and oxalate induced renal damage and this can be substantiated from the level of creatinine and blood urea nitrogen which was maintained at 1.8 mg and 82 mg in 100 ml of serum respectively. Whereas the accumulated nitrogenous wastes in serum of group 4 animals were cleared by the CB administration which started from day 30 and brought closer to normal level on 50th day (1.6 mg & 93 mg/dL). The reduction in the serum levels of urea and creatinine were concurrent to its increased urinary excretion.

Table 4. Effect of Citrus bioflavonoids on serum parameters on control and experimental groups

Parameter	Group 1	Group 2	Group 3	Group 4
Calcium	10.1±0.14	8.39±0.41^{a***}	9.7±0.25^{b*}	9.37±0.43^{cns}
Phosphorus	8.04±0.44	6.30±0.1^{a***}	7.76±0.1^{b*}	7.52±0.41^{c*}
Urea	91.9±3.2	236.9±7.2^{a***}	82.6±1.6^{b***}	93.0±4.2^{c***}
Creatinine	1.41±0.28	2.9±0.1^{a***}	1.82±0.1^{b***}	1.59±0.15^{c**}
Protein	1.16±0.06	1.54±0.08^{a***}	1.18±0.06^{b***}	1.21±0.07^{c*}

All the parameters were expressed as mg/dL.
The values are expressed as mean ± SD of four animals and results are statistically analysed by one way ANOVA with Dunnett's multiple comparison post test (n=6). The comparisons are made as follows
'a' – Control Vs Diseased
'b' – Diseased Vs Prevention
'c' – Diseased Vs Treatment
*** p<0.001, ** p<0.01, * P<0.05, NS – Not Significant.

Serum protein was slightly increased up to 1.5 mg/dL in the urolithic animals as a reflection of hepatotoxicity induced by EG, which was also ably prevented by CB in group 3 which showed a normal protein content, while in group 4 animals had a serum protein content of 1.21 mg/dL which was significantly lower than the diseased rats (Table 4).

Histology and immunohistochemistry

Urolithic rats are generally prone to crystal deposition in kidney after 30 days of ingestion with EG. The kidney sections of normal and experimental animals subjected to H & E and von Kossa staining (Figure 3). Significant deposition of crystals accompanied with tubular necrosis was observed in the kidney sections of the diseased rats. On the 50th day of the study, the animals supplemented with CB showed a prominent improvement in the kidney architecture. Rats from the preventive group showed near normal histology, since CB provided a strong membrane protection property; as a result of this a marked reduction in tubular necrosis and only a mild interstitial oedema were documented. The treatment group had a profound effect in repairing hyperoxaluria induced membrane damage which in turn helps in the expulsion of the deposited crystals. Kidney sections of group 4 rats showed tubular regeneration and moderate oedema. von Kossa staining of the kidney sections show dark intratubular aggregates, which confirm the presence of calcium containing stones. Dark spots observed in group 2 animals as a result of calcium deposition, were significantly reduced in CB administered rats. This substantiates the effectiveness of CB as an inhibitor of crystal aggregation and deposition process.

Expression of Tamm-Horsfall protein observed in animals from group 2 was found to be about 50 % greater than that of the control animals. THP, a secretory protein from nephron has been predominantly localized in distal tubule, was occasionally expressed in glomerulus of diseased kidney sections (Figure 4). Preventive therapy with CB showed a near normal expression of this protein without any abnormal localization. In group 4 animals we have detected a minimal elevation in the expression of this protein in the distal tubules which support the curative effect of CB. Nuclear Factor-κB is an important marker of the inflammatory process, whose expression was evidently increased in the lithogenic rats, as a result of oxalate and calcium oxalate crystal induced renal damage. This protein was mainly localized in the proximal and distal tubular regions (Figure 4). CB served from day one led to very low expression of this pro-inflammatory cytokine in preventive therapy and observed to be near normal, while an increased expression of NF-κB compared to control was seen in Group 4 animals, but significantly low compared to diseased animals. This shows that the physiological and biochemical events in the renal environment were brought to normal by CB.

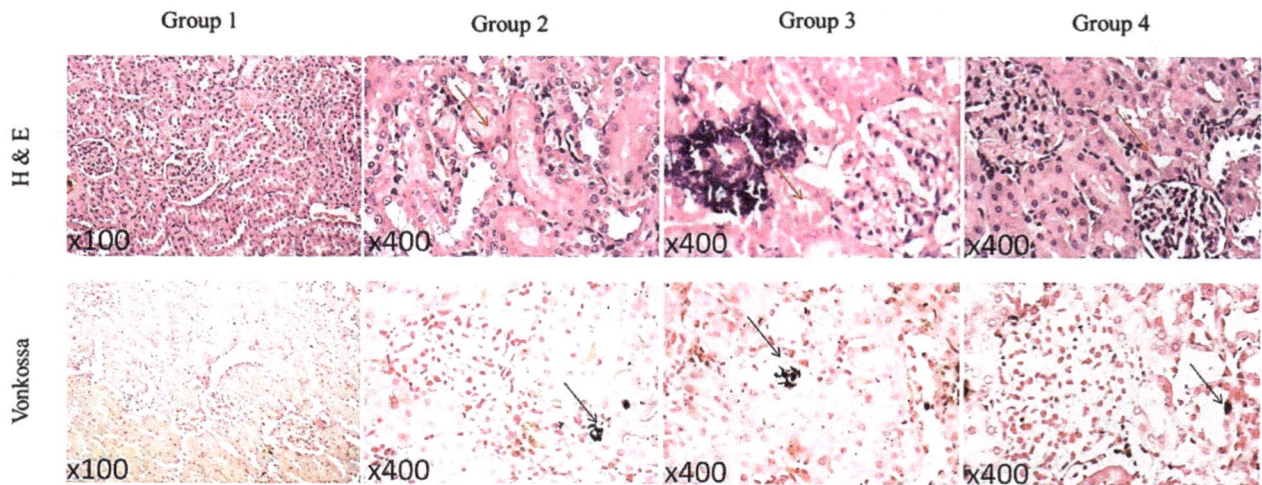

Figure 3. Histopathological staining of normal and experimental rats' kidney sections
Figure shows kidney sections of control and various experimental groups stained with Haematoxylin & Eosin and Von Kossa. Red arrows indicate the tubular changes and Black arrow shows the crystal deposition as brown spots

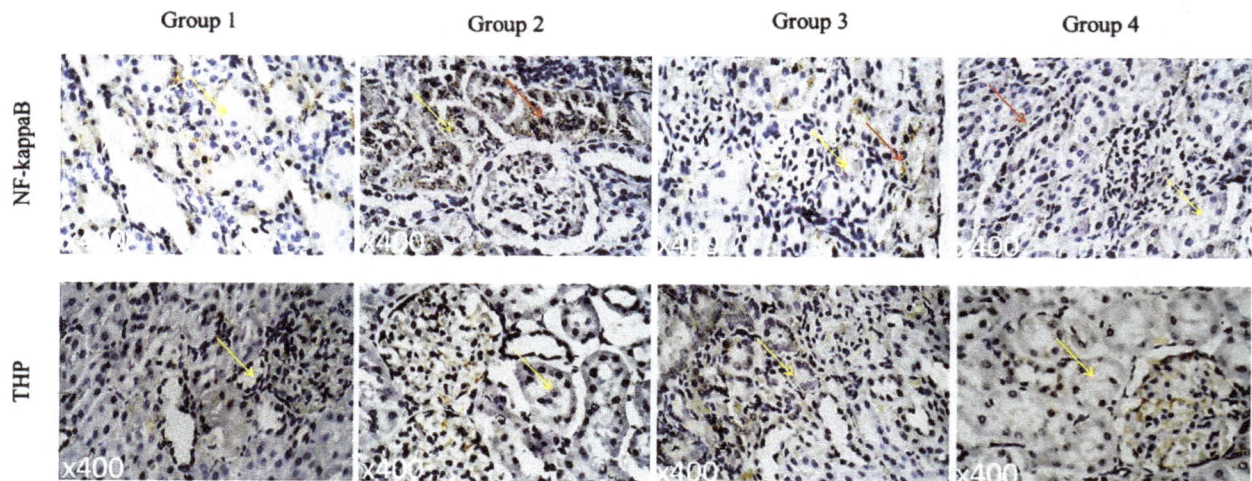

Figure 4. Immunohistochemical analyses of normal and experimental rats' kidney sections
Figure shows immunohistochemical expression of NF-κB and THP in control and various experimental groups. Red arrow indicate the proximal tubules and Yellow arrow indicate the distal tubules

Discussion

Herbal treatment in management of urolithiasis has become very popular among the researchers since it was found to be biocompatible and efficient. This can be solely attributed to the polyphenolic compounds present in those highly valuable plants and their parts which include flavonoids, alkaloids, triterpenes, and anthroquinones.[19] Studies have shown that citrus flavonoid as an effective nephroprotective agent and it was found to exert significant anti-inflammatory and analgesic properties.[20,21] In our investigation we proved that bioflavonoids obtained from this fruit also participate in the management of urolithiasis along with the indigenous citrate content. The study was designed in such a way to investigate the prophylactic and curative effect of citrus bioflavonoids. The CB formulation contains the essential bulking, binding and anti-caking agents. The major ingredients of this tablet are the bioflavonoids (1000 mg) obtained from citrus fruits like, hesperidin, eriocitrin, naringenin, neohesperidin etc. These are the flavonoids that are well-known for its biological properties. Apart from the flavonoids, the flavones and flavonols derivatives of the flavonoids from the fruits are also supplied in the tablets. The bioflavonoids and its derivatives from citrus origin are found to be effective in prevention and treatment of various metabolic, degenerative and infectious diseases.[5] Animals supplemented with EG showed first sign of the disease at the end of 20 days by excreting excess of oxalate and calcium, clinically represented as hyperoxaluria & hypercalciuria respectively. Increased oxalate metabolism in liver is responsible for hyperoxaluric condition in EG supplemented animals, while hypercalciuria has a multiple aetiological origin such as membrane damage, increased absorption of dietary calcium etc.[22,23] Our results evidently demonstrate the role of CB in maintaining the calcium and oxalate homeostasis, which can be an outcome of the renoprotective effect of bioflavonoids against the oxidative and nitrosative stress.[20] Heneghan et al., (2010) found that oxalate reabsorption is happening in the intestine through an anionic transporter mechanism, and we assume that this can also be ably targeted by the bioactive compounds in CB leading to dampen the increased rate of oxalate excretion in urine resulting in increased enteric excretion of oxalate.[24] Usually hypercalciuria will be accompanied by increased excretion of phosphorus in urine, designing a condition more favourable for stone formation and this condition was successfully reversed by CB administration in our study.[25] The observed urinary concentration of calcium and phosphorus coincides with the improvement in serum levels of the respective ions.

Reduction in glomerular filtration rate can be an outcome of crystals obstructing the renal passage.[26] This leads to accumulation of significant amount nitrogenous wastes like creatinine and urea. The obvious increase in serum creatinine and urea shows the renal dysfunction. This was well supported by the low level in the excretion of these nitrogenous wastes in urine of hyperoxaluric animals relative to normal animals. The flavonoids in commercial CB tablets were potent enough to maintain the normal renal function by protecting the membrane from crystal adhesion, which can lead to the obstruction anywhere in the urinary tract. Membrane protection offered by citrus flavonoids after supplementation, resulted in significant reduction of proteinuria compared to the EG administered animals which showed a high level of protein in urine as a result of oxidative stress exerted on the renal epithelium by calcium oxalate crystals and free oxalate. This can also be interpreted that the flavonoids can protect the renal cells by combating the ROS & RNS.[20]

The serum and urine biochemistry showed a significant change due to induction of the hyperoxaluric condition and reversal of these abnormal values to normal was observed upon CB ingestion. This was well supported by the Hematoxylin and Eosin staining, where observed acute tubular damage due to calcium oxalate crystallization in EG supplemented rats was found to be protected and treated by CB. Calcium deposits observed as brown spots distinguish the calcium oxalate nephrolithiasis from other type of stones. EG supplemented rats showed a prominent calcium deposition and animals fed with CB were found to have significantly reduced or no deposits (Figure 3).

Elevated expression of NF-κB was observed in kidney sections of hyperoxaluric animals as a result of inflammation mediated cellular damage due to EG challenge. Earlier studies were demonstrated that the inflammatory process in the epithelial cells was organized by NF-κB with the help of Renin – Angiotensin system (RAS) and researchers presume that inhibition of angiotensin converting enzyme (ACE) can diminish the calcium oxalate crystal mediated inflammation and epithelial degeneration.[27,28] In our study suppression of this pro-inflammatory cytokine to normal level is a consequence of antioxidant and anti-inflammatory effect exerted by the citrus flavonoids.[29] The ACE inhibitory activity of the flavonoids (in this case citrus flavonoids) can also be associated with the reduction in inflammatory response.[30] THP is one of the abundant proteins found in the urine and it was reported to be one of the important crystal inhibitory proteins and the expression of this particular protein was increased as expected in the EG challenged animals in order to meet up with the amount of crystal formed.[31] The reduction of this protein obviously shows the reduction in the crystal formation and deposition in the experimental animals supplemented with CB.

Conclusion

In conclusion, risk factors of stone disease were well managed by the administration of CB, which resulted in the cellular protection. Our results suggest bioflavonoids obtained from citrus fruits evade the urolithic risk factors like calcium, oxalate etc., and corresponding renal dysfunction (Urea, creatinine etc.). The major outcome in our study is the ability of CB to attenuate the expression of NF-κB, which initiate the renal epithelial damage. This shows that, CB is not only as an anti-urolithic agent but, it can also act as an efficient nephroprotectant. This shows effect of bioflavonoids from citrus fruit could be effective for management of calcium oxalate nephrolithiasis and restoration of the impaired kidney to normal. Further studies on various higher animal models and effective clinical trials may lead to a novel formulation for the management of urolithiasis and other renal diseases.

Acknowledgments

Shiju TM and Badrinathan S are thankful to Council of Scientific and Industrial Research and Indian Council of Medical Research respectively for providing fund in the form of Senior Research Fellowship. Authors are also thankful to VIT University for providing instrumentation and other resources to carry out the project.

Conflict of Interest

The authors declare that they have no conflict of interests.

References

1. Basavaraj DR, Biyani CS, Browning AJ, Cartledge JJ. The Role of Urinary Kidney Stone Inhibitors and Promoters in the Pathogenesis of Calcium Containing

Renal Stones. *EAU - EBU Update Series* 2007;5(3):126-36. doi: 10.1016/j.eeus.2007.03.002

2. Verkoelen CF. Crystal retention in renal stone disease: A crucial role for the glycosaminoglycan hyaluronan? *J Am Soc Nephrol* 2006;17(6):1673-87. doi: 10.1681/ASN.2006010088

3. Ilbey YO, Ozbek E, Simsek A, Cekmen M, Somay A, Tasci AI. Effects of pomegranate juice on hyperoxaluria-induced oxidative stress in the rat kidneys. *Ren Fail* 2009;31(6):522-31.

4. Yao C, Hao R, Pan S, Wang Y. Functional Foods Based on Traditional Chinese Medicine. In: Bouayed J, Bohn T, editors. *Nutrition, Well-Being and Health.* Luxembourg: In Tech; 2012.

5. Tripoli E, Guardia ML, Giammanco S, Majo DD, Giammanco M. Citrus flavonoids: Molecular structure, biological activity and nutritional properties: A review. *Food Chem* 2007;104(2):466-79. doi: 10.1016/j.foodchem.2006.11.054

6. Lin WC, Lai MT, Chen HY, Ho CY, Man KM, Shen JL, et al. Protective effect of flos carthami extract against ethylene glycol-induced urolithiasis in rats. *Urol Res* 2012;40(6):655-61. doi: 10.1007/s00240-012-0472-4

7. Thamilselvan S, Menon M. Vitamin e therapy prevents hyperoxaluria-induced calcium oxalate crystal deposition in the kidney by improving renal tissue antioxidant status. *BJU Int* 2005;96(1):117-26. doi: 10.1111/j.1464-410X.2005.05579.x

8. Selvam R. Calcium oxalate stone disease: Role of lipid peroxidation and antioxidants. *Urol Res* 2002;30(1):35-47.

9. Chinapongtitiwat V, Jongaroontaprangsee S, Chiewchan N, Devahastin S. Important flavonoids and limonin in selected Thai citrus residues. *J Funct Foods* 2013;5(3):1151-8. doi: 10.1016/j.jff.2013.03.012

10. Odvina CV. Comparative value of orange juice versus lemonade in reducing stone-forming risk. *Clin J Am Soc Nephrol* 2006;1(6):1269-74. doi: 10.2215/CJN.00800306

11. Wabner CL, Pak CY. Effect of orange juice consumption on urinary stone risk factors. *J Urol* 1993;149(6):1405-8.

12. Touhami M, Laroubi A, Elhabazi K, Loubna F, Zrara I, Eljahiri Y, et al. Lemon juice has protective activity in a rat urolithiasis model. *BMC Urol* 2007;7:18. doi: 10.1186/1471-2490-7-18

13. Turner T, Burri BJ. Potential nutritional benefits of current citrus consumption. *Agric* 2013;3(1):170-87. doi: 10.3390/agriculture3010170

14. Organisation for Economic Co-operation and Development (OECD) Guidelines for the Testing of Chemicals: 423. Acute Oral Toxicity - Acute toxic class method. Paris: Organisation for Economic Co-operation and Development; 2001.

15. Hodgkinson A, Williams A. An improved colorimetric procedure for urine oxalate. *Clin Chim Acta* 1972;36(1):127-32. doi: 10.1016/0009-8981(72)90167-2

16. Goldenberg H, Fernandez A. Simplified method for the estimation of inorganic phosphorus in body fluids. *Clin Chem* 1966;12(12):871-82.

17. Meyer OC. Safety and security of daflon 500 mg in venous insufficiency and in hemorrhoidal disease. *Angiology* 1994;45(6 Pt 2):579-84.

18. Citrus bioflavonoid tablets. HealthAid Ltd; Available from: http://www.healthaid.co.uk/shopexd.aspx?id=598.

19. Yao LH, Jiang YM, Shi J, Tomas-Barberan FA, Datta N, Singanusong R, et al. Flavonoids in food and their health benefits. *Plant Foods Hum Nutr* 2004;59(3):113-22. doi: 10.1007/s11130-004-0049-7

20. Singh D, Chander V, Chopra K. Protective effect of naringin, a bioflavonoid on glycerol-induced acute renal failure in rat kidney. *Toxicology* 2004;201(1-3):143-51. doi: 10.1016/j.tox.2004.04.018

21. Galati EM, Monforte MT, Kirjavainen S, Forestieri AM, Trovato A, Tripodo MM. Biological effects of hesperidin, a citrus flavonoid. (note i): Antiinflammatory and analgesic activity. *Farmaco* 1994;40(11):709-12.

22. Khan SR, Hackett RL. Hyperoxaluria, enzymuria and nephrolithiasis. *Contrib Nephrol* 1993;101:190-3.

23. Pragasam V, Kalaiselvi P, Sumitra K, Srinivasan S, Varalakshmi P. Oral l-arginine supplementation ameliorates urinary risk factors and kinetic modulation of tamm-horsfall glycoprotein in experimental hyperoxaluric rats. *Clin Chim Acta* 2005;360(1-2):141-50. doi: 10.1016/j.cccn.2005.04.016

24. Heneghan JF, Akhavein A, Salas MJ, Shmukler BE, Karniski LP, Vandorpe DH, et al. Regulated transport of sulfate and oxalate by slc26a2/dtdst. *Am J Physiol Cell Physiol* 2010;298(6):C1363-75. doi: 10.1152/ajpcell.00004.2010

25. Prie D, Ravery V, Boccon-Gibod L, Friedlander G. Frequency of renal phosphate leak among patients with calcium nephrolithiasis. *Kidney Int* 2001;60(1):272-6. doi: 10.1046/j.1523-1755.2001.00796.x

26. Bayir Y, Halici Z, Keles MS, Colak S, Cakir A, Kaya Y, et al. Helichrysum plicatum dc. Subsp. Plicatum extract as a preventive agent in experimentally induced urolithiasis model. *J Ethnopharmacol* 2011;138(2):408-14. doi: 10.1016/j.jep.2011.09.026

27. Toblli JE, Cao G, Casas G, Stella I, Inserra F, Angerosa M. Nf-kappab and chemokine-cytokine expression in renal tubulointerstitium in experimental hyperoxaluria. Role of the renin-angiotensin system. *Urol Res* 2005;33(5):358-67. doi: 10.1007/s00240-005-0484-4

28. Grande MT, Perez-Barriocanal F, Lopez-Novoa JM. Role of inflammation in tubulo-interstitial damage associated to obstructive nephropathy. *J Inflamm (Lond)* 2010;7:19. doi: 10.1186/1476-9255-7-19

29. Hadjzadeh MA, Rad AK, Rajaei Z, Tehranipour M, Monavar N. The preventive effect of n-butanol fraction of nigella sativa on ethylene glycol-induced kidney calculi in rats. *Pharmacogn Mag* 2011;7(28):338-43. doi: 10.4103/0973-1296.90416

30. Guerrero L, Castillo J, Quinones M, Garcia-Vallve S, Arola L, Pujadas G, et al. Inhibition of angiotensin-converting enzyme activity by flavonoids: Structure-activity relationship studies. *PLoS One* 2012;7(11):e49493. doi: 10.1371/journal.pone.0049493

31. Mo L, Huang HY, Zhu XH, Shapiro E, Hasty DL, Wu XR. Tamm-horsfall protein is a critical renal defense factor protecting against calcium oxalate crystal formation. *Kidney Int* 2004;66(3):1159-66. doi: 10.1111/j.1523-1755.2004.00867.x

Evaluation of Betulin Mutagenicity by *Salmonella*/Microsome Test

Edson Hideaki Yoshida[1], Natália Tribuiani[1], Giovana Sabadim[1], Débora Antunes Neto Moreno[1], Eliana Aparecida Varanda[2], Yoko Oshima-Franco[1]*

[1] *Post-Graduate Program in Pharmaceutical Sciences, University of Sorocaba (UNISO), Sorocaba, SP, Brazil.*
[2] *Pharmaceutical Sciences Faculty of Araraquara, São Paulo State University (UNESP), Rodovia Araraquara-Jau, Km 1, CEP 14801-902, Araraquara, São Paulo, Brazil.*

Article info

Keywords:
· Ames test
· Betulin
· Salmonella mutagenicity
· Triterpenoid

Abstract

Purpose: Betulin is a pentacyclic triterpene found in the outer barks of innumerous plants. This secondary metabolite is easily isolated from plants with the major interest in converting it to betulinic acid, which pharmacological properties were much more exploited than betulin. But, investments in the own betulin have been grown since no chemical step is necessary. In this study we focused the precursor betulin in order to evaluate its mutagenicity by *Salmonella*/microsome assay (Ames test).

Methods: The Ames test was carried out using a commercial betulin exposed to *Salmonella typhimurium* strains TA98, TA100, TA102, and TA97a, in experiments with (+S9) and without (-S9) metabolic activation.

Results: Betulin was unable to increase the number of revertants (+S9 and -S9 metabolic activation) showing the absence of any mutagenic effect by Ames test.

Conclusion: This study allowed attribute safety to betulin being important for exploiting its pharmacological uses.

Introduction

Betulin, betulinol, betuline, or betulinic alcohol (3-lup-20(29)-ene-3β,28-diol)[1] is an abundant pentacyclic lupane-type triterpenoid ubiquitously occurring in many plants as described by Ferraz et al.,[2] besides being a compound easily isolable, which gives to betulin a role as a precursor biomolecule to betulinic acid.

Betulinic acid is produced by plants in small amounts[3;4] justifying the conversion from betulin to betulinic acid, which the pharmacological activities have been more exploited than betulin.[1,5] However, a new reasoning to avoid this expensive chemical steps of conversion (betulin to betulinic acid) is simply addressing the pharmacological focus to betulin.

It is known that the oil from birch bark of *Betulae pix* has been used for some skin diseases, the eczema and psoriasis;[6] betulin also exerts an anticonvulsant action in mice, showing ability in penetrating the blood-brain barrier due its lipophilic property;[7] betulin has antibacterial, antifungal, and antiviral properties,[1] anticancer and chemopreventive potential;[8] betulin from *Dipteryx alata* protects against the neuromuscular effects of *Bothrops jararacussu* snake venom either *in vitro*[9] as *in vivo*.[2]

Advantages of betulin is its good bioavailability when administered intraperitoneally (i.p.) or subcutaneously (s.c.) described in a preliminary pharmacokinetic analysis, besides it did have no subchronic toxicity in rats (injected i.p.) or dogs (injected s.c.).[10]

In this study we evaluated the mutagenicity of a commercial betulin towards four *Salmonella typhimurium* strains (TA98, TA97a, TA100, and TA102) by Ames *Salmonella*/microsome assay, since does not exist toxicological studies concerning the safety of this biomolecule.

Materials and Methods
Betulin
Commercial betulin was purchased from Sigma Chemical Co. (St. Louis, MO, USA) and used throughout this study.

Preliminary toxicity assay
Before the Ames test evaluation is mandatory to know the toxicity of betulin to *Salmonella* strains. Here, the toxicity of betulin was firstly submitted to TA98 and TA 100, both being histidine dependent as all other *Salmonella* tester strains, both contain a deletion mutation through the *uvrB-bio* genes;[11] a mutation (*rfa*) in all strains that leads to a defective lipopolysaccharide (LPS) layer;[11] and presence of plasmid pKM101.[12] The reversion event caused to TA98 and TA100 are frameshift and base-pair substitution, respectively. Betulin (100 mg) from Sigma Chemical Co. (St. Louis, MO, USA) were dissolved in dimethyl sulfoxide by which 10.0, 7.5, 5.0, and 2.5 mg/plate were initially assayed using TA98 and TA100 strains. Toxicity was apparent either as a reduction in the number of His+

*Corresponding author: Yoko Oshima-Franco, Email: yoko.franco@prof.uniso.br

revertants or as an alteration in the auxotrophic background,[13] and were visualized in the two first concentration (10.0 and 7.5 mg/plate), which lead us to use betulin 5.0 mg/mL (the highest non-toxic dose) in a new set of assay, where 5.0, 3.75, 2.5, 1.25 and 0.63 mg/plate were selected for further Ames assay.

In vitro mutagenicity assay

Mutagenic activity was tested by the *Salmonella*/microsome assay, using the *S. typhimurium* tester strains TA98, TA100, TA102, and TA97a,[14] kindly provided by B.N. Ames (Berkeley, CA, USA), with and without metabolization by the preincubation method.[15] This assay was made as described by Yoshida et al.,[16] as following: the strains from frozen cultures were grown overnight for 12–14 h in Oxoid Nutrient Broth No. 2. The S9 fraction, prepared from livers of Sprague-Dawley rats treated with the polychlorinated biphenyl mixture Aroclor 1254 (500 mg/kg), was purchased from Molecular Toxicology Inc. (Boone, NC, USA) and freshly prepared before each test. The metabolic activation system consisted of 4% of S9 fraction, 1% of 0.4M $MgCl_2$, 1% of 1.65M KCl, 0.5% of 1M D-glucose-6-phosphate disodium and 4% of 0.1M nicotinamide adenine dinucleotide phosphate (NADP), 50% of 0.2M phosphate buffer and 39.5% sterile distilled water.[14] Defined the betulin concentrations by preliminary toxicity tests, in all subsequent assays were used the upper limit of the dose range tested was either the highest non-toxic dose or the lowest toxic dose. The concentrations varied from 0.63 to 5.0 mg/plate for betulin. The various concentrations of betulin to be tested were added to 0.5 mL of 0.2M sodium phosphate buffer (pH 7.4), or to 0.5 mL de 4% S9 mixture, with 0.1 mL of bacterial culture and then incubated at 37°C for 20 min. Next, 2 mL of top agar (0.6% agar, histidine and biotin 0.5 mM each, and 0.5% NaCl) was added and the mixture was poured on to a plate containing minimal glucose agar (1.5% Bacto-Difco agar and 2% glucose in Vogel-Bonner medium). The plates were incubated at 37°C for 48 h and the His(+) revertant colonies were counted manually. All experiments were carried out in triplicate. The standard mutagens used as positive controls in experiments without S9 mix were 4-nitro-*O*-phenylenediamine (10 µg/plate) for TA98 and TA97a, sodium azide (1.25 µg/plate) for TA100 and mitomycin (0.5 µg/plate) for TA102. 2-anthramine (1.25 µg/plate) was used with TA98, TA97a and TA100 and 2-aminofluorene (1.25 µg/plate) with TA102 in the experiments with metabolic activation. DMSO served as the negative (solvent) control (50 µL/plate). Figure 1 shows representatives His(+) revertant colonies (A) and positive control (B).

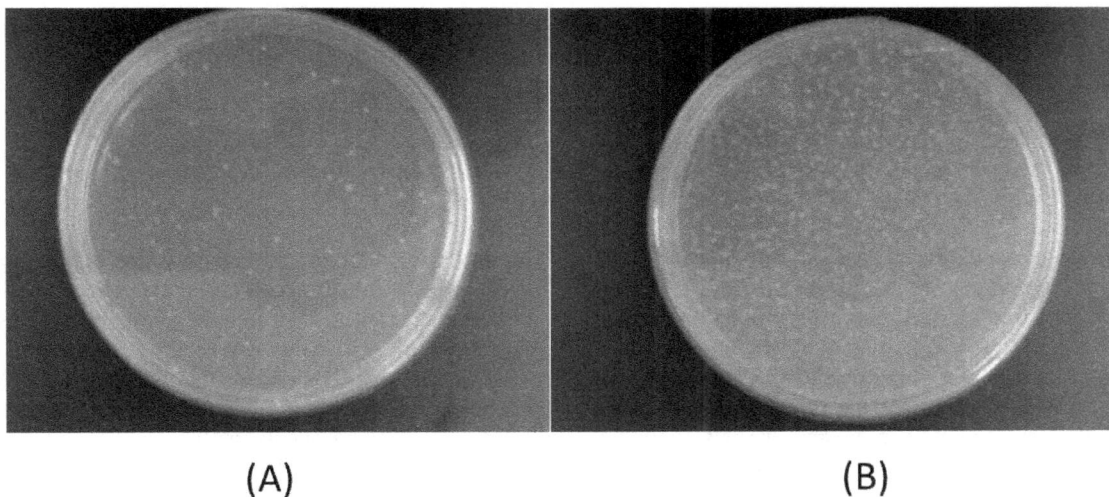

(A)   (B)

Figure 1. Photography of bacterial colonies grown in representative His(+) revertants (A) and positive control (B).

The mutagenic index (MI) was calculated for each concentration tested, this being the average number of revertants per plate with the test compound divided by the average number of revertants per plate with the negative (solvent) control. A sample was considered mutagenic when a dose-response relationship was detected and a two-fold increase in the number of mutants (MI ≥ 2) was observed with at least one concentration.[17]

Statistical analysis

The results of the mutagenicity tests were analyzed with the Salanal statistical software package (U.S. Environmental Protection Agency, Monitoring Systems Laboratory, Las Vegas, NV, version 1.0, from Research Triangle Institute, RTP, North Carolina, USA), adopting the Bernstein et al. model.[18] The data (revertants/plate) were assessed by analysis of variance (ANOVA), followed by linear regression.

Results and Discussion

Our experience with *Dipteryx alata* Vogel,[19] one of many betulin-plants,[2] showed an unexplained facilitatory effect on mouse nerve-muscle synapse,[9] besides it possesses antiophidian properties against the neuromuscular and myotoxicity, two known toxic effects of *Bothrops jararacussu*,[20] and *Crotalus durissus terrificus*[21] venoms (protection of betulin against the toxic effects of *Bothrops jararacussu* venom > *Crotalus durissus terrificus* venom). Aiming to confirm the antiophidian efficacy of betulin against *Bothrops jararacussu* venom, we further assayed it in *in vivo* experimental model, using rat external popliteal/sciatic nerve-tibialis anterior muscle (EPSTA) preparation.[2] Intraperitoneally (i.p.) injections of betulin were compared to intravenously (i.v.) commercial bothropic antivenom (CBA) injections, in venom-pretreated animals. No statistically difference was observed between betulin and CBA, showing a promising complementary therapeutical use for betulin, either in veterinary as in human area.

However, chemicals can induce damage in germ line causing fertility problems and leading to mutations in future generations, besides they also are capable of inducing cancer. Gene mutations can occur with only a single base changes (base-pair substitution mutants), or one or a few bases inserted or deleted (frameshift mutants), and are readily measured in bacteria and other cell systems.[22] Thus, the evaluation of betulin mutagenicity is an inevitable step in the safety assessment. Here, the Ames *Salmonella*/mutagenicity assay, a short-term bacterial assay, was chosen for testing betulin, since it is able in identifying substances that can produce genetic damage that leads to gene mutations. After preliminary test, five concentrations of betulin were submitted to Ames test: 0.63, 1.25, 2.5, 3.75, and 5.0 mg/plate.

Table 1 shows betulin at various concentrations exposed to *S. typhimurium* TA98, TA97a, TA100 and TA102 tester strains, without metabolic activation.

Table 1. Revertants/plate, standard deviation and mutagenicity index (in brackets) for the strains TA98, TA100, TA102 and TA97a of *S. typhimurium* after treatment with various doses of phytochemical Betulin without metabolic activation (−S9)

Treatments mg/plate	Number of revertants (M ± SD)/plate and MI			
	TA 98	TA 100	TA 102	TA 97a
	- S9	- S9	- S9	- S9
0.0[a]	19 ± 2	120 ± 15	341 ± 5	178 ± 12
0.63	19 ± 4 (1.0)	105 ± 2 (0.9)	338 ± 27 (1.1)	221 ± 27 (1.2)
1.25	21 ± 5 (1.1)	89 ± 1 (0.7)	367 ± 28 (1.1)	185 ± 33 (1.0)
2.50	19 ± 3 (1.0)	96 ± 10 (0.8)	299 ± 18 (0.9)	173 ± 16 (0.9)
3.75	20 ± 5 (1.1)	99 ± 22 (0.8)	314 ± 67 (0.9)	197 ± 12 (1.1)
5.00	18 ± 3 (1.0)	112 ± 10 (0.9)	350 ± 54 (1.0)	161 ± 52 (0.9)
Control +	1044 ± 56[b]	1161 ± 292[c]	968 ± 77[d]	1175 ± 43[b]

M ± SD = mean and standard deviation; MI = mutagenicity index; [a]Negative control: dimethylsulfoxide (DMSO - 50 µL/ plate); Control+ = Positive control - [b]4 -nitro-o-phenylenediamine (NOPD – 10.0 µg/ plate – TA98, TA97a); [c]sodium azide (1.25 µg/ plate – TA100); [d]mitomycin (0.5 µg/ plate – TA102), in the absence of S9 (−S9).

It is important to remark the DNA (deoxyribonucleic acid) sequences of the target mutations of *Salmonella* tester strains used in this study. The *hisD3052* mutation carried by TA98 is a -1 frameshift mutation which affects the reading frame of a nearby repetitive -C-G-C-G-C-G-C-G- sequence,[23] which reversion of the mutation back to the wild-type state by 2-nitrofluorene and various aromatic nitroso derivatives of amine carcinogens. In this study we used 4 -nitro-*o*-phenylenediamine as a positive control. Note in TA98 column that brackets expressing the MI are all < than 2.0, showing no mutagenicity in all tested concentrations.

The *hisG46* marker in TA100 strain results from the substitution of a leucine (GAG/CTC) by a proline (GGG/CCC),[24] that is reverted to the wild-type state by mutagens that cause base-pair substitution mutations primarily at one of the GC pairs, as that showed by sodium azide (positive control). In this study, no mutagenic activity was seen in any betulin concentrations when submitted to TA100.

TA102 strain contains AT base pairs at the *hisG428* mutant site, which mutation is carried on the multi-copy plasmid pAQ1 aiming to amplify the number of target sites, which in turn confers tetracycline resistance, a convenient marker to detect the presence of plasmid. In this strain, the *uvrB* gene was retained (differently of other *Salmonella* strains) making the bacterium DNA repair proficient, and enhancing the ability of this strain to detect DNA cross-linking agents, as those caused by bleomycin and mitomycin C (used here as positive control).[25] The *hisG428* mutation is an ochre mutation (TAA) in the *hisG* gene, which the reversion involves transitions and transversions events. In our study none concentrations of betulin caused mutagenicity when submitted to TA102.

The *hisD6610* mutation carried by TA97 is +1 frameshift mutation (cytosine) resulting in a run of 6 cytosines (-C-C-C-C-C-C-), which reversion of the mutation back to the wild-type state occurs by the same compounds as seen by TA98,[26] as 4 -nitro-*o*-phenylenediamine used here as positive control. Betulin in all concentrations used in this study caused no mutagenicity in TA97a strains.

Table 2 shows betulin at various concentrations exposed to *S. typhimurium* TA98, TA100, TA102, and TA97a tester strains, with metabolic activation (+S9).

Table 2. Revertants/plate, standard deviation and mutagenicity index (in brackets) for the strains TA98, TA100, TA102 and TA97a of *S. typhimurium* after treatment with various doses of phytochemical Betulin with (+S9) metabolic activation

Treatments (mg/plate)		Number of revertants (M ± SD)/plate and MI			
		TA 98	TA 100	TA 102	TA 97a
		+ S9	+ S9	+ S9	+ S9
Betulin	0.0[a]	24 ± 9	107 ± 20	205 ± 11	84 ± 16
	0.63	27 ± 4 (1.1)	117 ± 6 (1.1)	219 ± 19 (1.1)	102 ± 24 (1.2)
	1.25	27 ± 7 (1.1)	97 ± 5 (0.9)	199 ± 21 (1.0)	84 ± 6 (1.0)
	2.50	29 ± 3 (1.2)	105 ± 15 (1.0)	223 ± 38 (1.1)	80 ± 15 (0.9)
	3.75	27 ± 1 (1.1)	95 ± 17 (0.9)	240 ± 27 (1.2)	71 ± 16 (0.8)
	5.00	37 ± 5 (1.5)	94 ± 17 (0.9)	183 ± 21 (0.9)	74 ± 13 (0.9)
	Control +	1551 ± 81[e]	2627 ± 297[e]	1043 ± 39[f]	1252 ± 30[e]

M ± SD = mean and standard deviation; MI = mutagenicity index; [a]Negative control: dimethylsulfoxide (DMSO - 50 µL/ plate); Control+ = Positive control - [e]2-anthramine (1.25 µg/ plate – TA 97a, TA98, TA100); [f]2-aminofluorene (10.0 µg/ plate – TA102), in the presence of S9.

As some carcinogenic chemicals are biologically inactive unless they are metabolized to active forms by cytochrome P450 enzymes, an exogenous mammalian organ activation system needs to be added to the petri plate together with the chemical and the bacteria.[11] Here, we purchased a commercial metabolic activation system that consists of a 9000xg supernatant fraction of a rat liver homogenate (S9 microsomal fraction), that in presence of nicotinamide adenine dinucleotide (NADH) and cofactors for nicotinamide adenine dinucleotide phosphate (NADPH) (S9 mix), enzymes are delivered to the test system. Positive controls used in this metabolic activation step were 2-anthramine (TA 97a, TA98, TA100) and 2-aminofluorene (TA102), with visible grown of colonies in the histidine absence, showing the mutation ability of these mutagens. Even in the presence of metabolic activation all concentrations of betulin exposed to *S. typhimurium* strains were unable to cause any mutation.

The lack of mutagenicity for betulin, a triterpenoid with many pharmacological properties,[1,2,6-9] that has a good bioavailability but no subchronic toxicity (rats and dogs),[10] is very promising. Some positive correlation can be taken with the facilitatory nature of betulin on mouse nerve-muscle synapse[9] with its anticonvulsant action.[7] At the same mode, phenobarbital, a known anticonvulsant, also acts increasing the amplitude of contractile response in mouse phrenic nerve-diphragm preparation,[27] probably involving the glutamatergic regulation, since the role of glutamate as an acetylcholine co-transmitter in motoneurons was already established.[28,29]

Conclusion
In conclusion, betulin is a safety bioactive molecule (for intraperitoneal and subcutaneous administrations, limited by its solubility), with absence of mutagenicity by *Salmonella*/microsome assay.

Acknowledgments
This work was supported by São Paulo Research Foundation (FAPESP 2004/09705-8, 2007/53883-6, 2008/52643-4, 2008/11005-5, and 2012/08271-0) and FINEP (07/2010).

Conflict of Interest
The authors report no conflicts of interest in this work.

References
1. Alakurtti S, Makela T, Koskimies S, Yli-Kauhaluoma J. Pharmacological properties of the ubiquitous natural product betulin. *Eur J Pharm Sci* 2006;29(1):1-13. doi: 10.1016/j.ejps.2006.04.006
2. Ferraz MC, de Oliveira JL, de Oliveira Junior JR, Cogo JC, Dos Santos MG, Franco LM, et al. The triterpenoid betulin protects against the neuromuscular effects of bothrops jararacussu snake venom in vivo. *Evid Based Complement Alternat Med* 2015;2015:939523. doi: 10.1155/2015/939523
3. Kim DSHL, Chen Z, VanNguyen T, Pezzuto JM, Qiu S, Lu Z-Z. A concise semi-synthetic approach to betulinic acid from betulin. *Synth Commun* 1997;27(9):1607-12. doi: 10.1080/00397919708006099
4. Liu J, Fu ML, Chen QH. Biotransformation optimization of betulin into betulinic acid production catalysed by cultured armillaria luteo-virens sacc zjuqh100-6 cells. *J Appl Microbiol* 2011;110(1):90-7. doi: 10.1111/j.1365-2672.2010.04857.x
5. Santos RC, Salvador JA, Marin S, Cascante M. Novel semisynthetic derivatives of betulin and betulinic acid with cytotoxic activity. *Bioorg Med Chem* 2009;17(17):6241-50. doi: 10.1016/j.bmc.2009.07.050
6. Hänsel R, Keller K, Rimpler H, Schneider G. *Drogen A-D: Betula*. Berlin: Springer Verlag; 1992.
7. Muceniece R, Saleniece K, Rumaks J, Krigere L, Dzirkale Z, Mezhapuke R, et al. Betulin binds to gamma-aminobutyric acid receptors and exerts

anticonvulsant action in mice. *Pharmacol Biochem Behav* 2008;90(4):712-6. doi: 10.1016/j.pbb.2008.05.015

8. Krol SK, Kielbus M, Rivero-Muller A, Stepulak A. Comprehensive review on betulin as a potent anticancer agent. *Biomed Res Int* 2015;2015:584189. doi: 10.1155/2015/584189

9. Ferraz MC, Parrilha LAC, Moraes MSD, Amaral Filho J, Cogo JC, dos Santos MG, et al. The effect of lupane triterpenoids *(Dipteryx* alata Vogel) in the *in vitro* neuromusuclar blockade and myotoxicity of two snake venoms. *Curr Org Chem* 2012;16(22):2717-23. doi: 10.2174/138527212804004481

10. Jager S, Laszczyk MN, Scheffler A. A preliminary pharmacokinetic study of betulin, the main pentacyclic triterpene from extract of outer bark of birch (betulae alba cortex). *Molecules* 2008;13(12):3224-35. doi: 10.3390/molecules13123224

11. Ames BN, Lee FD, Durston WE. An improved bacterial test system for the detection and classification of mutagens and carcinogens. *Proc Natl Acad Sci U S A* 1973;70(3):782-6.

12. Ames BN, McCann J, Yamasaki E. Methods for detecting carcinogens and mutagens with the salmonella/mammalian-microsome mutagenicity test. *Mutat Res* 1975;31(6):347-64.

13. Resende FA, Vilegas W, Dos Santos LC, Varanda EA. Mutagenicity of flavonoids assayed by bacterial reverse mutation (ames) test. *Molecules* 2012;17(5):5255-68. doi: 10.3390/molecules17055255

14. OECD Guideline for Testing of Chemicals, Bacterial Reverse Mutation Test, 1997. http://www.oecd.org/chemicalsafety/risk-assessment/1948418.pdf Accessed 23 May 2016.

15. Maron DM, Ames BN. Revised methods for the salmonella mutagenicity test. *Mutat Res* 1983;113(3-4):173-215.

16. Yoshida EH, Ferraz MC, Tribuiani N, Tavares RVS, Cogo JC, dos Santos MG, et al. Evaluation of the safety of three phenolic compounds from *Dipteryx alata* Vogel with antiophidian potential. *Chin Med* 2015;6:1-12. doi: 10.4236/cm.2015.61001

17. Varella SD, Pozetti GL, Vilegas W, Varanda EA. Mutagenic activity of sweepings and pigments from a household-wax factory assayed with salmonella typhimurium. *Food Chem Toxicol* 2004;42(12):2029-35.

18. Bernstein L, Kaldor J, McCann J, Pike MC. An empirical approach to the statistical analysis of mutagenesis data from the salmonella test. *Mutat Res* 1982;97(4):267-81.

19. Puebla P, Oshima-Franco Y, Franco LM, Santos MG, Silva RV, Rubem-Mauro L, et al. Chemical constituents of the bark of dipteryx alata vogel, an active species against bothrops jararacussu venom. *Molecules* 2010;15(11):8193-204. doi: 10.3390/molecules15118193

20. Rodrigues-Simioni L, Borgese N, Ceccarelli B. The effects of bothrops jararacussu venom and its components on frog nerve-muscle preparation. *Neuroscience* 1983;10(2):475-89.

21. Oshima-Franco Y, Hyslop S, Prado-Franceschi J, Cruz-Hofling MA, Rodrigues-Simioni L. Neutralizing capacity of antisera raised in horses and rabbits against crotalus durissus terrificus (south american rattlesnake) venom and its main toxin, crotoxin. *Toxicon* 1999;37(10):1341-57.

22. Mortelmans K, Zeiger E. The ames salmonella/microsome mutagenicity assay. *Mutat Res* 2000;455(1-2):29-60.

23. Isono K, Yourno J. Chemical carcinogens as frameshift mutagens: Salmonella DNA sequence sensitive to mutagenesis by polycyclic carcinogens. *Proc Natl Acad Sci U S A* 1974;71(5):1612-7.

24. Barnes W, Tuley E, Eisenstadt E. Base-sequence analysis of His[+] revertants of the *hisG46* missense mutation in *Salmonella typhimurium*. *Environ Mutagen* 1982;4:297.

25. Levin DE, Hollstein M, Christman MF, Schwiers EA, Ames BN. A new salmonella tester strain (ta102) with a x t base pairs at the site of mutation detects oxidative mutagens. *Proc Natl Acad Sci U S A* 1982;79(23):7445-9.

26. Levin DE, Yamasaki E, Ames BN. A new Salmonella tester strain, TA97, for the detection of frameshift mutagens. A run of cytosines as a mutational hot-spot. *Mutat Res* 1982;94(2):315-30. doi: 10.1016/0027-5107(82)90294-9

27. Rubem-Mauro L, Rocha-Jr DS, Barcelos CC, Varca GH, Andreo-Filho N, Barberato-Filho S, et al. Phenobarbital pharmacological findings on the nerve-muscle basis. *Lat Am J Pharm* 2009;28(2):211-8.

28. Waerhaug O, Ottersen OP. Demonstration of glutamate-like immunoreactivity at rat neuromuscular junctions by quantitative electron microscopic immunocytochemistry. *Anat Embryol (Berl)* 1993;188(5):501-13.

29. Meister B, Arvidsson U, Zhang X, Jacobsson G, Villar MJ, Hokfelt T. Glutamate transporter mrna and glutamate-like immunoreactivity in spinal motoneurones. *Neuroreport* 1993;5(3):337-40.

3

Chromatographic Fingerprint Analysis of Marrubiin in *Marrubium vulgare* L. via HPTLC Technique

Keyvan Yousefi[1], Sanaz Hamedeyazdan[2], Mohammadali Torbati[3], Fatemeh Fathiazad[2]*

[1] Department of Pharmacology, Faculty of pharmacy, Tabriz University of Medical Sciences, Tabriz, Iran.
[2] Department of Pharmacognosy, Faculty of pharmacy, Tabriz University of Medical Sciences, Tabriz, Iran.
[3] Department of Traditional Pharmacy, Faculty of Traditional Medicine, Tabriz University of Medical Sciences, Tabriz, Iran.

Article info

Keywords:
· *Marrubium vulgare*
· Marrubiin
· Folin-Ciocalteau
· Free radicals
· TLC scanner
· Densitometry

Abstract

Purpose: In the present study we aimed to quantify marrubiin, as the major active compound, in the aerial parts of *Marrubium vulgare* from Iran using a HPTLC-densitometry technique.

Methods: Quantitative determination of marrubiin in *M. vulgare* methanol extract was performed by HPTLC analysis via a fully automated TLC scanner. Later on, the in vitro antioxidant activity of the *M. vulgare* methanol extract was determined using 1,1-diphenyl-2-picryl-hydrazil (DPPH) free radical scavenging assay. Furthermore, total phenolics and flavonoids contents of the methanol extract were quantified, spectrophotometrically.

Results: The amount of marrubiin was calculated as 156 mg/g of *M. vulgare* extract. The antioxidant assay revealed a strong radical scavenging activity for the *M. vulgare* methanol extract with RC_{50} value of 8.24µg/mL. Total phenolics and flavonoids contents for *M. vulgare* were determined as 60.4 mg gallic acid equivalent and 12.05 mg quercetin equivalent per each gram of the extract, correspondingly.

Conclusion: The presented fingerprint of marrubiin in *M. vulgare* extract developed by HPTLC densitometry afforded a detailed chemical profile, which might be useful in the identification as well as quality evaluation of herbal medications based on *M. vulgare*. Besides, the considerable antioxidant activity of *M. vulgare* was associated with the presence of marrubiin along with phenolics and flavonoids exerting a synergistic effect.

Introduction

Marrubium vulgare (Lamiaceae), known as horehound in English and Khanak in Persian, is a popular medicinal herb which has been used traditionally as a remedy for a wide range of diseases such as hypertension, infections, pain and etc.[1,2] *M. vulgare* shows strong antioxidant activity due to the presence of flavonoids, terpenes, and phenols.[3] The main active ingredient of *M. vulgare* was found to be marrubiin which has been identified in 1984 as the first diterpene isolated from leaves of this plant. Marrubiin is a furan labdane diterpenoid which is produced and accumulated only in the aerial parts of the plant.[1,4] It is important to mention that marrubiin is generated as an artifact from pre-marrubiin during the extraction procedure when heat is involved in the extraction or concentration procedure.[5] Marrubiin has been associated with the bitter principle of the horehound and lots of other medicinal plants of the family Lamiaceae. The broadly known diterpenoid lactone, marrubiin, has been marked with assorted types of biological activities such as analgesic, vasorelaxant, cardioprotective, gastroprotective, antidiabetic, antioxidant, antispasmodic, anti-hypertensive, anti-edematogenic and immunomodulating properties.[1,6-15] In a study conducted by Mnonopi *et al*, marrubiin which was isolated from *Leonotis leonurus* L. found to be a cardioprotective compound by inducing anticoagulant, antiplatelet and anti-inflammatory properties in obese rat models.[6] Our previously published paper on cardioprotective effect of the total methanolic extract of *M. vulgare,* containing marrubiin as the major ingredient of the extract, in an animal model with myocardial infarction was in consistence with the reported activity related to the compound marrubiin.[16] Furthermore, in a recent study gastroprotective activity of the methanolic extract of *M. vulgare* had been revealed due to the presence of marrubiin as evidenced by inhibitory effect of both marrubiin and the methanol extract of *M. vulgare* on the indomethacin-induced ulcers.[17] Generally, considering loads of published data over the past century on the chemical and biological aspects of marrubiin in the genus *Marrubium* (Lamiaceae), we could consider this compound as a biomarker within the plants of this genus.

In view of these facts, High Performance Thin Layer Chromatography (HPTLC) has been widely used as a rapid, precise and cost-effective method for

*Corresponding author: Fatemeh Fathiazad, Email: fathiazad@tbzmed.ac.ir

determination of biological compounds from medicinal plants; accordingly, in this study we adopted HPTLC as a promising technique for determination of marrubiin quantitatively within the *M. vulgare* extract.[18] It is of note to mention that HPTLC encompasses the use of chromatographic layers of utmost separation efficiency, utilization of instrumentation for all steps in the approach, defined sample applications, validated reproducible chromatogram developments and software controlled analysis. Nonetheless, adaptation on optimized new approaches would not be inevitable in displacement of existing methods but a supplement to already existing techniques. The standardized method might be useful in identification as well as quality evaluation of herbal medications based on a specific phytochemical. Following our previous work, in the present study a preliminary phytochemical screening of the methanol extract of *M. vulgare* from Iran was performed. Additionally, an HPTLC-densitometry assay was conducted for the purpose of quantitative determination of marrubiin content in the extract.

Materials and Methods
Materials
All the chemicals, including solvents, were of analytical grade from Merck Company Germany. 1,1-Diphenyl-2-picryl-hydrazyl (DPPH), quercetin, gallic acid, Folin-Ciocalteu reagent, and aluminum chloride from Sigma-Aldrich chemical company Madrid-Spain, potassium acetate, and silica gel 60 F_{254} HPTLC (20cm × 20cm) plates (Merck, Darmstadt, Germany) were used in this study.

Plant Material, Extraction and Preparation
The aerial parts of *M. vulgare* were collected in 2012 during flowering stage on June from Kiasar (Mazandaran Province, Iran). They were authenticated by Dr. M. Mazandarani (Department of Biology, Azad Islamic University, Gorgan, Iran). Voucher specimens (No. 712 Tbz-Fph) have been deposited at the herbarium of the Department of Pharmacognosy, Faculty of Pharmacy, Tabriz University of Medical Sciences, Tabriz, Iran. Air dried aerial parts (200g) were grounded and extracted with methanol (2L×4) by maceration at room temperature (25-30 °C). The obtained extract was concentrated to dryness under vacuum at 40 °C using a rotary evaporator. A greenish residue weighing 17.8 % (w/w) was obtained and kept in air tight bottle in a refrigerator until use. To identify the chemical constituents, the resultant methanol extract was subjected to preliminary phytochemical analysis.

Determination of Total Phenolic Content
Total phenolic content was determined by Folin-Ciocalteau method as described by Ghasemi *et al* and Ebrahimzadeh *et al*.[19,20] Briefly, 0.5 ml of the extract was mixed with Folin-Ciocalteau reagent (5 mL, 1:10 diluted with distilled water) for 5 min and aqueous Na_2CO_3 (4 mL, 1 M) was then added. The mixture was allowed to stand for 15 min where the phenolics were determined by colorimetry at 765 nm (Shimadzu 2100, Japan). The standard curve was prepared by 50, 100, 150, 200, and 250 mg/mL solutions of gallic acid in methanol: water (50:50, v/v). Total phenol values are expressed in terms of gallic acid equivalent (mg/g of the extract) by reference to calibration curve: y=0.0067x+0.0132, (R^2=0.987).

Determination of Total Flavonoids Content
In order to determine the total flavonoids content of the *M. vulgare* extract, the colorimetric aluminum chloride method was employed according to the method described by Ghasemi *et al* and Ebrahimzadeh *et al*.[19,20] Briefly, 0.5 mL solution of methanolic extract were mixed with 1.5 mL of methanol, 0.1 mL of 10% aluminum chloride, 0.1 mL of 1 M potassium acetate and 2.8 mL of distilled water, and were left at room temperature for 30 min. The absorbance of the reaction mixture was measured spectrophotometrically at 415 nm. Total flavonoids content were calculated as quercetin from a calibration curve prepared using 31.25-250 µg/mL solutions of quercetin in methanol as standard (y=0.008x-0.068, R^2=0.999).

Determination of In Vitro Antioxidant Activity
The free radical scavenging capacity of the extract was measured from the bleaching of the purple colored methanol solution of 1,1-diphenyl-2-picryl-hydrazil. The stock concentration 1 mg/ml of the methanol extract of the *M. vulgare* was prepared followed by dilution in order to obtain concentrations of $5×10^{-1}$, $2.5×10^{-1}$, $1.25×10^{-1}$, $6.25×10^{-2}$, $3.13×10^{-2}$ and $1.56×10^{-2}$ mg/mL. The obtained concentrations in equal volumes of 2 mL were added to 2 mL of a 0.004% of DPPH solution. After a 30 min of incubation period at 25 °C, the absorbance at 517 nm was determined against a blank. Tests were carried out in triplicate where the average absorption was noted for each concentration. Furthermore, as the positive control the same procedure was repeated with quercetin. The inhibition percentages of DPPH free radicals of by the samples were calculated following the equation:

R (%) = 100 × [(A blank – A sample) / A blank]

Hereon, "A blank" represents the absorbance value of the control reaction and "A sample" is the absorbance value for each sample. Besides, RC_{50} value, concentration of the extract reducing 50% of the DPPH free radicals, was calculated from the graph of inhibition percentages against concentrations of *M. vulgare* extract in mg/mL.

Quantitative Analysis of Marrubiin
Preliminary HPTLC analysis of the *M. vulgare* extract was performed on silica gel 60 F_{254} HPTLC plate with benzene-acetone (17:3) as the mobile phase. Later on, detection of the spots after spraying with anisaldehyde-sulfuric acid reagent revealed the presence of marrubiin at RF=0.82 as the major compound in the extract such as

expressed by Popa et al, in 1968. Following the preliminary qualitative analysis of HPTLC analysis of the *M. vulgare* extract, quantitative determination of marrubiin, as the major bioactive component in *M. vulgare*, was performed by photodensitometric method via a fully automated TLC scanner (CAMAG TLC scanner 3 coupled with Automatic TLC Sampler 4, Automatic Developing chamber 2 and a TLC Visualizer). In addition, winCATS (Planar chromatography manager) software was used for analyzing results of the plate scan.

As far as we know, automatic sample application is a key factor for productivity of the HPTLC laboratory evaluations, to this end; Automatic TLC Sampler 4 was used in spraying samples onto plates in the form of bands in the presence of nitrogen air. In this regard, samples were applied on the plate as 4 mm wide bands with constant application rate from 1 to $7\mu L$ s^{-1}, an automatic TLC sampler under a flow of N_2 gas, 20 mm from the bottom, 15 mm from the side, and spaces among the spots were 8 mm of the plate. In order to quantitative determine the content of marrubiin in the extract and obtain a standard curve, stock solution of marrubiin was prepared in methanol to achieve the concentration of 0.44 mg/ml. Samples of marrubiin on the HPTLC plate with volume of $1\mu l$ to $7\mu l$ were consequently spotted to afford 0.44, 0.88, 1.31, 1.75, 2.19, 2.63 and 3.06 μg marrubiin (spots number 1 to 7). Similarly, a stock solution of extract in methanol (10 mg/ml) was prepared and spotted with three volumes of 1, 2 and $3\mu l$ immediately after standard solutions' spots (spots number 8 to 10). Subsequently, the linear ascending development was carried out in a twin trough chamber, which was pre-saturated with 25 mL mobile phase with benzene-acetone (17:3) for 30 min, at room temperature (25 ± 2 °C) and 50 ± 5% relative humidity. The developing chamber of the HPTLC system automatically performed the development step minimizing environmental effects. Thus, the activity and preconditioning of the layer, chamber saturation, developing distance and final drying were completely pre-set and monitored during this step. When the Linomat is operated under software, plate dimensions, number and distance of tracks, designation, sample volumes and sequence are software controlled. All the operating data were automatically transferred to the densitometric processing evaluation step. Ultimately, the HPTLC plate was placed on a TLC Scanner and scanned under the UV 509 nm light (A 509-nm UV light was used to illuminate the plate).

Results

Phytochemical Screening of M. vulgare Extract

Preliminary phytochemical screening of *M. vulgare* extract indicated the presence of flavonoids and phenolic compounds in the plant extract. Regarding the absorbance values of the extract solutions, reacted with Folin-Ciocalteu and aluminum chloride reagents compared to the standard solutions as described in the methods section, the amount of total phenolic and flavonoids contents for *M. vulgare* were determined as 60.4 mg gallic acid equivalent/g extract and 12.05 mg quercetin equivalent/g of the extract, respectively.

In Vitro Antioxidant Activity of M. vulgare Extract

The free radical scavenging activity of *M. vulgare* extract was evaluated using the DPPH method in vitro. According to our results, the RC_{50} values for methanol extract of *M. vulgare* and quercetin were found to be 8.24 and 3μg/ml, correspondingly. Our results showed that the *M. vulgare* methanol extract has a considerable free radical scavenging activity comparable with the standard compound, quercetin.

Marrubiin Quantification

Preliminary HPTLC analysis of the extract revealed marrubiin with R_f value of 0.82 as a major compound present in the *M. vulgare* extract. The quantitative determination of marrubiin on the fluorescent HPTLC plate on TLC scanner yielded a 3D graph on the basis of optical density (densitogram). In Figure 1, densitograms 1 to 7 are the increasing concentrations of pure compound marrubiin. The calibration curve was calculated automatically according to the densitograms 1 to 7 that in this curve the Y axis is marrubiin concentration and the X axis is the peak height of the corresponding concentration (Figure 2). The densitograms 8 to 10 are three repeated samples of the methanol extract from aerial parts of *M. vulgare* where the mean value of the heights of these three points were used to quantify the marrubiin content in the extract. Eventually, the amount of Marrubiin was calculated as 156 mg/g of *M. vulgare* extract by reference to the standard curve: (y=0.335x-27.87, R^2= 0.999) (Figure 2).

Discussion

Our preliminary phytochemical findings in this study revealed the presence of phenolic compounds, flavonoids and marrubiin as the major diterpenoid in the methanolic extract of *M. vulgare*. It was found that the considerable radical scavenging activity of the extract against the DPPH free radicals was in line with the high phenolic and flavonoid contents of *M. vulgare* extract. The naturally occurring flavonoids and phenolics are believed to possess the ideal chemical structure for scavenging free radicals.[21,22]

Owing to the fact that free radicals are molecules with an odd, unpaired electron that these unpaired electrons make them unstable and highly reactive,[23] they could be extremely toxic to human cells attacking fatty acids, leading to lipid peroxidation of membranes, reacting with proteins, destruction and oxidation of amino acids, oxidation of sulfhydryl groups and polypeptide chain scission. Accordingly, these free radicals are the important factors in diseases related to oxidative stress conditions such as cardiovascular and neurodegenerative diseases.[24] The use of natural antioxidants, especially phenolics and flavonoids, might be very promising in treatment of these kinds of diseases. Hence, in recent years more investigations have been focused on the plants especially those with remarkable antioxidant activities.[22,25] Overall, here in this study it was suggested that the observed scavenging activity of the *M. vulgare*

methanol extract could be assigned to the hydrogen-donating capacity of the phenolic and flavonoid components, in cooperation with the presence of marrubiin in the extract.

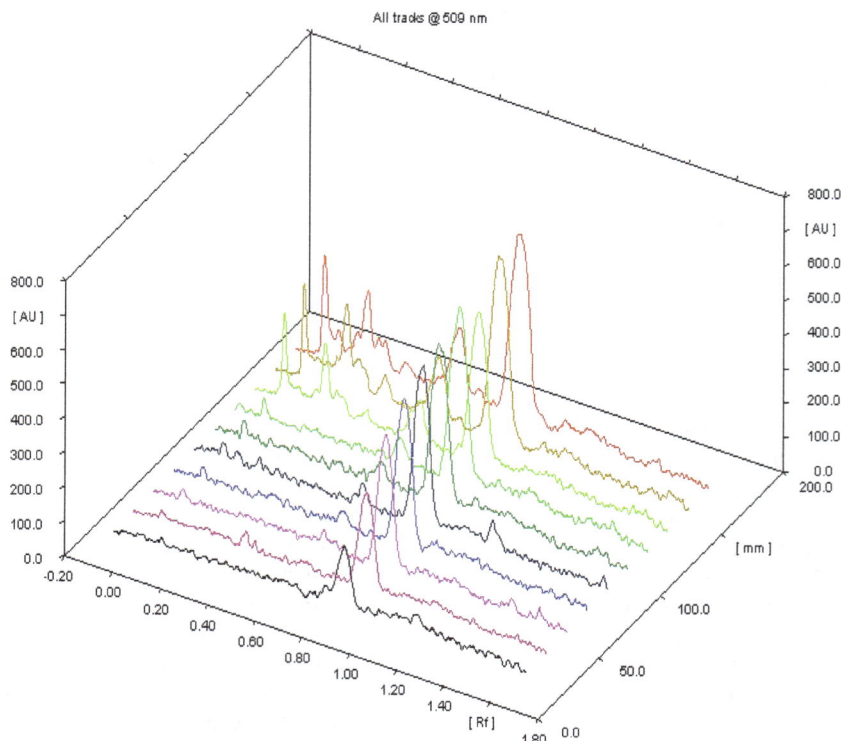

Figure 1. Photodensitogram of the fluorescent HPTLC plate of marrubiin (densitograms 1-7) and *M. vulgare* extract (densitograms from 8-10) depicted by TLC scanner 3 (CAMAG) in which the X, Y and Z axis represents RF of each detected spot, height of the peaks (Spot's density), and location on the plate, respectively.

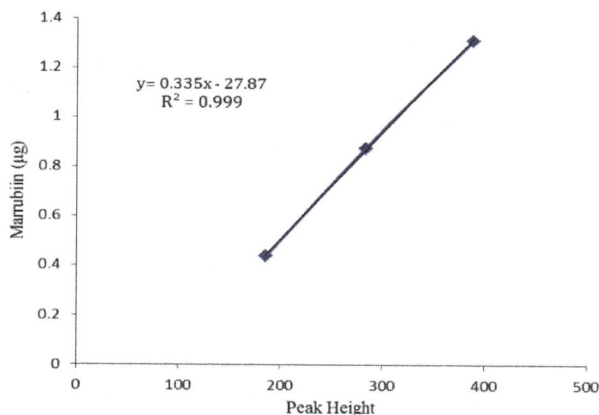

Figure 2. The calibration curve drawn automatically by TLC Scanner used to quantify marrubiin in the methanol extract of *M. vulgare*.

Formerly in a report by our team, the methanol extract of *M. vulgare* showed significant improvements to the hemodynamic, electrocardiographical and histopathological changes in a myocardial infarction model induced by isoproterenol.[16] However, our new findings in this paper provided sufficient evidence for the

presence of high quantities of a diterpenoid marrubiin along with flavonoids and phenolics corroborating the cardioprotective effect of *M. vulgare*. Furthermore, we can come to the conclusion that these compounds might have a synergistic antioxidant effect through which they induce protection against oxidative stress. Taken together, *M. vulgare* from Iran have the potential to be considered as a suitable applicant to be probed as a source of bioactive components in search of new efficient versatile phytomedicines for treating various ailments especially those caused by oxidative stress.

On the other hand, a high performance thin layer chromatography method coupled with densitometric analysis was developed in this study for the identification and quantification of marrubiin in *M. vulgare*. This method was considered to be precise, consistent, rapid and low-cost which can be used for quantitative determination of marrubin in the extracts from *Marrubium* species. According to the findings, the presented chemical fingerprint of *M. vulgare* extract that was developed using HPTLC densitometry afforded a detailed chemical profile which might be useful in the identification as well as quality evaluation of herbal medications based on *M. vulgare*. As follows, the developed fingerprint could be of value in preparation of a standardized herbal product with consistent biological activity. Likewise, providing these kinds of chemical fingerprints may also be helpful in differentiation of the plant from adulterants according to the simplicity, flexibility and cost efficiency of the HPTLC technique in both qualitative and quantitative aspect with minimal time requirement.

Conclusion

Regarding the phytochemical findings of the present study it can be concluded that the sizeable radical scavenging activity of *M. vulgare* methanol extract could be attributed, to some extent, to its remarkable flavonoids and phenolics content. Moreover, it was revealed that marrubiin was the main compound in the aerial parts of *M. vulgare* grown in Iran. The quantification of marrubiin could be performed using HPTLC technique which is a precise, simple and relatively inexpensive method. According to our knowledge, there is no report on this method for analyzing marrubiin in the genus *Marrubium* so far. Thereby, this method could be used simply and rapidly for the routine analysis and quality control of marrubiin in the *Marrubium* species.

Acknowledgments

The authors would like to thank Biotechnology Research Center of Tabriz University of Medical Sciences for their help in conducting the HPTLC analysis. Financial support of this work by the Research Vice-Chancellor of Tabriz University of Medical Sciences is faithfully acknowledged. Authors are also thankful to Dr. M. Mazandarani for authenticating the plant.

Conflict of Interest

The authors report no conflicts of interest.

References

1. Piccoli PN, Bottini R. Accumulation of the labdane diterpene marrubiin in glandular trichome cells along the ontogeny of *marrubium vulgare* plants. *Plant Growth Regul* 2008;56:71-6. doi: 10.1007/s10725-008-9286-3

2. Pukalskas A, Venskutonis PR, Salido S, Waard PD, van Beek TA. Isolation, identification and activity of natural antioxidants from horehound (*marrubium vulgare* L.) cultivated in lithuania. *Food Chem* 2012;130(3):695-701. doi: 10.1016/j.foodchem.2011.07.112

3. Vanderjagt TJ, Ghattas R, Vanderjagt DJ, Crossey M, Glew RH. Comparison of the total antioxidant content of 30 widely used medicinal plants of New Mexico. *Life Sci* 2002;70(9):1035-40. doi: 10.1016/S0024-3205(01)01481-3

4. Appleton RA, Fulke JWB, Henderson MS, McCrindle R. The stereochemistry of marrubiin. *J Chem Soc C* 1967:1943-8. doi: 10.1039/J39670001943

5. Henderson MS, McCrindle R. Premarrubiin. A diterpenoid from *Marrubium vulgare* L. *J Chem Soc C* 1969:2014-5. doi: 10.1039/J39690002014

6. Mnonopi N, Levendal RA, Davies-Coleman MT, Frost CL. The cardioprotective effects of marrubiin, a diterpenoid found in *Leonotis leonurus* extracts. *J Ethnopharmacol* 2011;138(1):67-75. doi: 10.1016/j.jep.2011.08.041

7. De Jesus RA, Cechinel-Filho V, Oliveira AE, Schlemper V. Analysis of the antinociceptive properties of marrubiin isolated from *Marrubium vulgare*. *Phytomedicine* 2000;7(2):111-5. doi: 10.1016/S0944-7113(00)80082-3

8. de Souza MM, de Jesus RA, Cechinel-Filho V, Schlemper V. Analgesic profile of hydroalcoholic extract obtained from *Marrubium vulgare*. *Phytomedicine* 1998;5(2):103-7. doi: 10.1016/S0944-7113(98)80005-6

9. El Bardai S, Morel N, Wibo M, Fabre N, Llabres G, Lyoussi B, et al. The vasorelaxant activity of marrubenol and marrubiin from *Marrubium vulgare*. *Planta Med* 2003;69(1):75-7. doi: 10.1055/s-2003-37042

10. Meyre-Silva C, Yunes RA, Schlemper V, Campos-Buzzi F, Cechinel-Filho V. Analgesic potential of marrubiin derivatives, a bioactive diterpene present in *Marrubium vulgare* (Lamiaceae). *Farmaco* 2005;60(4):321-6. doi: 10.1016/j.farmac.2005.01.003

11. Meyre-Silva C, Cechinel-Filho V. A review of the chemical and pharmacological aspects of the genus marrubium. *Curr Pharm Des* 2010;16(31):3503-18. doi: 10.1016/j.jep.2006.05.023

12. Schlemper V, Ribas A, Nicolau M, Cechinel Filho V. Antispasmodic effects of hydroalcoholic extract of *Marrubium vulgare* on isolated tissues. *Phytomedicine* 1996;3(2):211-6. doi: 10.1016/S0944-7113(96)80038-9

13. Mnonopi N, Levendal RA, Mzilikazi N, Frost CL. Marrubiin, a constituent of *Leonotis leonurus*, alleviates diabetic symptoms. *Phytomedicine* 2012;19(6):488-93. doi: 10.1016/j.phymed.2011.12.008

14. Karioti A, Skopeliti M, Tsitsilonis O, Heilmann J, Skaltsa H. Cytotoxicity and immunomodulating characteristics of labdane diterpenes from *Marrubium cylleneum* and *Marrubium velutinum*. *Phytochemistry* 2007;68(11):1587-94. doi: 10.1016/j.phytochem.2007.03.027

15. Stulzer HK, Tagliari MP, Zampirolo JA, Cechinel-Filho V, Schlemper V. Antioedematogenic effect of marrubiin obtained from *Marrubium vulgare*. *J Ethnopharmacol* 2006;108(3):379-84. doi: 10.1016/j.jep.2006.05.023

16. Yousefi K, Soraya H, Fathiazad F, Khorrami A, Hamedeyazdan S, Maleki-Dizaji N, et al. Cardioprotective effect of methanolic extract of

Marrubium vulgare L. On isoproterenol-induced acute myocardial infarction in rats. *Indian J Exp Biol* 2013;51(8):653-60.

17. de Oliveira AP, Santin JR, Lemos M, Klein Júnior LC, Couto AG, da Silva Bittencourt CM, et al. Gastroprotective activity of methanol extract and marrubiin obtained from leaves of *Marrubium vulgare* L. (Lamiaceae). *J Pharm Pharmacol* 2011;63(9):1230-7. doi: 10.1111/j.2042-7158.2011.01321.x

18. Prasanth KG, Anandbabu A, Venkatanarayanan R, Dineshkumar B, Sankar V. HPTLC technique: Determination of flavonoid from *Clerodendrum viscosum vent* roots. *Der Pharma Chemica* 2012;4(3):926-9.

19. Ghasemi K, Ghasemi Y, Ebrahimzadeh MA. Antioxidant activity, phenol and flavonoid contents of 13 citrus species peels and tissues. *Pak J Pharm Sci* 2009;22(3):277-81.

20. Ebrahimzadeh MA, Nabavi SM, Nabavi SF, Dehpour AA. Antioxidant activity of hydroalcholic extract of *Ferula gummosa* boiss roots. *Eur Rev Med Pharmacol Sci* 2011;15(6):658-64.

21. Choi CW, Kim SC, Hwang SS, Choi BK, Ahn HJ, Lee MY, et al. Antioxidant activity and free radical scavenging capacity between korean medicinal plants and flavonoids by assay-guided comparison. *Plant Sci* 2002;163(6):1161-8. doi: 10.1016/S0168-9452(02)00332-1

22. Skerget M, Kotnik P, Hadolin M, Hras AR, Simonic M, Knez Z. Phenols, proanthocyanidins, flavones and flavonols in some plant materials and their antioxidant activities. *Food Chem* 2005;89(2):191-8. doi: 10.1016/j.foodchem.2004.02.025

23. Burton KP, McCord JM, Ghai G. Myocardial alterations due to free-radical generation. *Am J Physiol* 1984;246 (6 Pt 2):H776-83.

24. Burton KP. Evidence of direct toxic effects of free radicals on the myocardium. *Free Radic Biol Med* 1988;4(1):15-24.

25. Fugh-Berman A. Herbs and dietary supplements in the prevention and treatment of cardiovascular disease. *Prev Cardiol* 2000;3(1):24-32. doi: 10.1111/j.1520-037X.2000.80355.x

4

Qualitative and Quantitative Content Determination of Macro-Minor Elements in *Bryonia Alba* L. Roots using Flame Atomic Absorption Spectroscopy Technique

Uliana Vladimirovna Karpiuk[1]*[§], Khaldun Mohammad Al Azzam[2]*[§], Zead Helmi Mahmoud Abudayeh[3], Viktoria Kislichenko[4], Ahmad Naddaf[3], Irina Cholak[1], Oksana Yemelianova[1]

[1] *Bogomolets National Medical University, Kiev, Ukraine.*
[2] *Department of Pharmaceutical Chemistry, Pharmacy Program, Batterjee Medical College for Sciences and Technology (BMC), 21442 Jeddah, Kingdom of Saudi Arabia.*
[3] *Faculty of Pharmacy, Isra University, 11622 Amman, Jordan.*
[4] *National University of Pharmacy, Kharkiv, Ukraine.*

Article info

Keywords:
· *Bryonia alba* L.
· Roots
· Atomic absorption spectrometry
· Elements
· Dry ashing

Abstract

Purpose: To determine the elements in *Bryonia alba* L. roots, collected from the Crimean Peninsula region in Ukraine.

Methods: Dry ashing was used as a flexible method and all elements were determined using atomic absorption spectrometry (AAS) equipped with flame and graphite furnace.

Results: The average concentrations of the determined elements, expressed as mg/100 g dry weight of the sample, were as follow: 13.000 for Fe, 78.000 for Si, 88.000 for P, 7.800 for Al, 0.130 for Mn, 105.000 for Mg, 0.030 for Pb, 0.052 for Ni, 0.030 for Mo, 210.000 for Ca, 0.130 for Cu, 5.200 for Zn, 13.000 for Na, 1170.000 for K, 0.780 for Sr, 0.030 for Co, 0.010 for Cd, 0.010 for As, and 0.010 for Hg. Toxic elements such as Cd and Pb were also found but at very low concentration. Among the analyzed elements, K was the most abundant followed by Ca, Mg, P, Si, Fe, Na, and Zn, whereas Hg, As, Cd, Co, Mo, and Pb were found in low concentration.

Conclusion: The results suggest that the roots of *Bryonia alba* L. plant has potential medicinal property through their high element contents present. Moreover, it showed that the AAS method is a simple, fast, and reliable for the determination of elements in plant materials. The obtained results of the current study provide justification for the usage of such fruit in daily diet for nutrition and for medicinal usage in the treatment of various diseases.

Introduction

Bryonia alba L., is one of the smallest genus in the family cucurbitaceae, consists of 12 species distributed throughout the Europe and West Asia.[1,2] It has been traditionally used in the treatment of different diseases such as cough, frontal pain, inflammation of serous tissues, peritonitis, pneumonia, jaundice, typhoid, rheumatism, brain disorders with serous exudation and as a heart tonic.[2]

Nowadays, the interest in chemical composition analysis of medicinal herb products is growing owing to the continuing developments in nutrition and in biochemical surveying and mineral prospecting.[3,4] Additionally, the studies related to therapeutic plants not only aim to characterize the active components found in plants, but also for scientific support of its therapeutic properties.[5]

Macro, micro and trace elements are known to play a vital role in biological functions in plants and in human metabolic reactions. Moreover, trace elements play an important role in the formation of bioactive chemical constituents in medicinal herb plants and thus are responsible for their medicinal and toxic properties accordingly.[6,7]

Several number of techniques such as voltammetery, atomic absorption spectrometry (AAS),[8] inductively coupled plasma atomic optical emission spectrometry (ICP-OES),[9] X- ray fluorescence (XRF),[10] differential pulse cathode stripping voltamperometry (DPCSV)[11] and instrumental neutron activation analysis (INAA)[12] are normally used for the determination of trace elements in medicinal herbal plants. Because of its specificity, sensitivity, high precision, simplicity, rapid analysis, low cost, low detection limit, and wide linear range, AAS is the most widely recommended instrument used in analytical procedures for the trace metal analysis found in complex biological samples.[3] AAS methods are considered as direct aspiration determinations where they are accomplished as single element analysis and are relatively free of interelement spectral interferences. In other words, the use of special light sources produced by the cathode lamp is emitted from excited atoms of the same element of interest and specific spectrum selection allows the quantitative determination of individual components of a multielement mixture.[13] AAS as an accurate and rapid technique was chosen for the present work. The most commonly used methods for the sample preparation of plant species are dry ashing, wet ashing and microwave assisted treatment.[14]

In the present work, nineteen minor and trace nutrient elements (Fe, Si, P, Al, Mn, Mg, Pb, Ni, Mo, Ca, Cu, Zn, Na, K, Sr, Co, Cd, As, and Hg) in *Bryonia alba* L. roots growing in Ukraine were determined by AAS coupled with dry ashing method.

Material and Methods
Reagents and solutions
Standard stock solutions with a concentration (1000 mg L^{-1}) of the individual metal element were used to prepare the requested concentrations by dilution using a 1% (v/v) nitric acid solution. The diluted standard solutions were used to build the calibration curves. Metal element standards were purchased from Sigma-Aldrich (St Louis, MO, USA). An analytical reagents grade of concentrated nitric acid (70%) and hydrogen peroxide (30%) were purchased from Sigma-Aldrich (St Louis, MO, USA). In all experiments carried out, the glass /plastic containers were cleaned by soaking in10%, v/v HNO$_3$ for at least 24 h and rinsing with distilled water prior to use. All other chemicals used were of analytical grade. The ultrapure deionized water obtained from a Milli-Q water purification system (Millipore, Bedford, MA, USA) was used for preparing the solutions and for all dilutions.

Instrumentation
An AAS instrument (Perkin Elmer AAnalyst 700 model AAS) with deuterium background corrector was used for the determination of Fe, Si, P, Al, Mn, Mg, Pb, Ni, Mo, Ca, Cu, Zn, Na, K, Sr, Co, Cd, As, and Hg. Pb, Cd, and Ni were determined by HGA graphite furnace using high purity argon while other measurements were carried out in an air/acetylene flame. The operating parameters for working elements were set according to the recommendations of the manufacturer.

Plant materials
Fresh roots of *Bryonia alba* L. were collected from the Crimean Peninsula region, which is located south of the Ukrainian region of Kherson and west of the Russian region of Kuban. The collection has been done in autumn during 2014 – 2015. The temperature recorded at harvesting time ranged between 15 – 20°C. Botanical identification/authentication was performed at Bogomolets National Medical University, Kiev, Ukraine.

Macroscopic techniques for identification/authentication of Bryonia alba L.
It is well known that authentication/identification of raw material is the essential starting point in developing a botanical product. However, inherent chemical variability will certainly be observed with any botanical. Additionally, each step of harvest, storage, processing, and formulation may significantly change the quality and uniformity of the final product, whether by preserving the desired marker components or by eliminating unwanted contaminants.[15] Therefore, methods to assure quality control in manufacturing and storage are required tools not only to ensure optimal efficacy but also safety of these products. Additionally, such controls are important for the evaluation of toxicological, pharmacological, or clinical studies involving botanical dietary supplements.[16]

Macroscopic study
The macroscopic study of the morphological description of the plant parts was conducted by our naked eye and with the aid of magnifying lens.

Sample preparation
The collected roots were washed thoroughly with tap water followed by deionized water and then allowed to dry in an oven at 50 – 60 °C. The sample was dried to constant weight (0.0005 g). One gram sample was accurately weighed and ground with the aid of a food processor Power Plus 1300 (Braun, Germany) for 3 min (instead of using mortar and pestle for better homogeneity as it allows for faster decomposition, thus more precise results). Then it was sieved through a 0.5 mm diameter sieve. The obtained powder of the plant material was stored in a dry and dark place at room temperature in the polyethylene bags till used.

Dry ashing procedure
One gram of sample was transferred into a porcelain crucible. The muffle furnace temperature was gradually increased from room temperature to 450°C in 1 h. The sample was redried for 1h in the oven, cooled, and reweighed. The steps were repeated at 1h drying intervals until the differences in the variations in the released water were less than 0.05%. The obtained sample was ashed for about 8 h until a gray or white ash residue was obtained. The residue was dissolved in 5 mL of HNO$_3$ (25%, v/v) and, if necessary, the mixture was heated slowly to dissolve the residue. Then the digestion solution was heated up using an electric hot plate at 150°C until evaporated to near dryness. The residue was filtered through Whatman filter paper and transferred into a volumetric flask and made up to 25 mL with 3% HNO$_3$. The blank digestion experiment was also prepared in the same way. This procedure was adopted from the work of Soylak *et al.*[17]

Analytical procedure
AAS is a widely used technique for determining a large number of metals. In AAS, an aqueous sample containing the metal analyte of interest is aspirated into an air-acetylene flame, causing evaporation of the solvent as well as vaporization of the free metal atoms (atomization). Fe, Si, P, Al, Mn, Mg, Pb, Ni, Mo, Ca, Cu, Zn, Na, K, Sr, Co,

Cd, As, and Hg in *Bryonia alba* L. root sample was analyzed using AAS equipped with flame and graphite furnace. Graphite furnace was used for the determination of trace and ultra-trace concentrations (Pb, Ni, Mo, Co, Cd, As, Hg). The following solutions (La(III) ions when determining Mg or Ca, and CsCl solutions were used as an ionization buffer in measurements of K, Mg and Na and were added to both sample and standard solutions in order to overcome chemical interferences in the flame upon determination.[18] The operation conditions used to operate AAS instrument were as recommended by the manufacturer. Data were rounded off properly based on the value of standard deviation from measurement conducted in triplicate.

Results and Discussion

Some of the trace elements known to be essential to our body such as As, Co, Cu, Fe, Mn, Ni, Si, Zn and the other essential major elements are Ca, K, Na, and Mg. So, different trace elements in the different medicinal plants will have their definite role in the functioning of our body. The roles of the detected elements are given below.

In our preliminary trials we examined the accuracy of the current work by analyzing the spiked samples at three level concentrations (low, medium and high), which were taken from stock solution of each metal and spiked in a 100 mL Erlenmeyer flask containing 1g sample. The recoveries of all metals in the spiked samples were ranged from 90 to 101 %.

The average results of elemental analysis obtained by the AAS technique for the analysis of *Bryonia alba* L. roots are shown in Table 1 in mg /100 g dry weight of the sample. It is to be noted that each result is an average of three independent triplicate measurements. As can be seen in this table, K, Ca, Mg, P, and Si are the most abundant elements in roots presenting concentrations ranging from 78 to 1170 mg/100 g dry weight of the sample levels.

Table 1. The content of macro-minor elements of *Bryonia alba* L. roots using flame atomic absorption spectrophotometry (n = 3).

Elements found in B. alba L.	Content, mg/ 100 g dry weight of the sample (Mean ± SD)
Fe	13 ± 0.12
Si	78 ± 1.21
P	88 ± 2.31
Al	7.8 ± 0.91
Mn	0.13 ± 0.020
Mg	105 ± 2.31
Pb	<0.03 ± 0.011
Ni	0.052 ± 0.0033
Mo	<0.03 ± 0.0023
Ca	210 ± 2.52
Cu	0.13 ± 0.02
Zn	5.2 ± 0.34
Na	13 ± 0.21
K	1170 ± 4.20
Sr	0.78 ± 0.07
Co	<0.03 ± 0.097
Cd	<0.01 ± 0.015
As	<0.01 ± 0.092
Hg	<0.01 ± 0.015

The concentrations of trace elements Fe, Al, Zn, and Na were found in the medium range of 5.2 to 13 mg/100 g dry weight of the sample. Ni, Cd and Pb are toxic elements which occur naturally in plants as a result of uptake, generally in places with high concentration caused by atmospheric and industrial fallout.[3] These are found in <0.01 to 0.0052 mg /100 g dry weight of the sample. Other elements such as Mo, Co, As, Hg, Mn, Cu, and Sr were found in the range 0.01 to 0.13 mg/100 g dry weight of the sample.

Iron (Fe)

Iron (Fe) is considered an essential element necessary for human body. It is the main component of myoglobin, hemoglobin, and a number of enzymes that play an important role in the oxygenation of red blood cells. It is needed for a healthy immune system as well as for energy production. It has been reported that iron severe deficiency results in anemia, which ranges from a fall in plasma ferritin to the strict iron deficiency that characterized by small red blood cells and low hemoglobin concentration level.[3,19] The daily requirement of Fe for a child is 10 mg/day, whereas for an adult is 20 mg/day. The Fe concentration in *Bryonia alba* L. roots sample analyzed was found 13 mg /100 g dry weight of the sample.

Manganese (Mn)

As known pyruvate carboxylase and superoxide dismutase are enzymes which contain manganese.[19] The manganese content found in *Bryonia alba* L. roots sample was 0.13 mg /100 g dry weight of the sample.

Magnesium (Mg)

It has been reported that magnesium (Mg) is considered the most imperative mineral for stress relief,[3] and as a non-essential element for living organisms.[20] *Bryonia alba* L. roots sample was found to contain 105 mg /100 g dry weight of the sample. The concentrations of this element upon analysis the roots of four medicinal samples by Dafalla, 2014 ranged from 1.42 to 42 ppm.[20]

Lead (Pb), Cadmium (Cd), and Nickel (Ni)

Bryonia alba L. roots sample contains Pb <0.03, Cd <0.01, and Ni 0.052 mg /100 g dry weight of the sample. These elements are considered to be toxic in nature, and thus their presence at trace level in various medicinal plant samples analyzed may be due to the pollution occurring from industrial activities and automobile.[19] Cadmium is considered a very hazardous to human health. Additionally, it causes high blood pressure, damages kidneys and liver.[21] The permissible limits set by WHO[22] are 0.2 to 0.81 ppm and from 0.1 to 10 ppm for cadmium and lead, respectively. Thus the concentrations of cadmium and lead found in *Bryonia alba* L. roots were within the limits. In the work of Dafalla, 2014,[20] who studied the roots of four medicinal plants, Cd concentrations varied from 1.8 to 14.4 ppm compared to the obtained results.

Calcium (Ca)

Calcium (Ca) plays a vital role in the absorption of dietary vitamin B, also for the activation of enzymes like the pancreatic lypase, and for the synthesis of the neurotransmitter acetylcholine. The recommended daily allowance for taking Ca is 800 mg for adults and for children 500 - 1000 mg. Therefore, in order to attain a Ca level of practically one percent of the total diet would be difficult.[3] The concentration of Ca found in *Bryonia alba* L. roots sample was 210 mg /100 g dry weight of the sample.

Sodium (Na) and Potassium (K)

The concentration of sodium (Na) and potassium (K) in *Bryonia alba* L. roots sample was found to be 13, and 1170 mg /100 g dry weight of the sample, respectively. Potassium is considered the richest element among all elements found. Usually, plants absorb potassium and sodium from the soil in the form of K and Na ions. Moreover, it is very important for enzyme activation, photosynthesis, water use efficiency, starch formation and protein synthesis.[21] The obtained data in our study indicate that the *Bryonia alba* L. roots sample is not deficient in potassium. Therefore, it is useful to be used as a food source, rich in K, for humans as it might help in the case of potassium deficiency.[3] The high concentration of K was found as well in the roots of the four medicinal plants studied by Dafalla, 2014 where the concentrations ranged from 400 - 842 ppm.[21]

Zinc (Zn)

Zinc is considered as one of the main components of over 200 enzymes having both catalytic and structural roles including the alcohol dehydrogenase, ribonucleic polymerases, alkaline phosphatase, and carbonic anhydrase.[23] Scientific studies conducted on animals have shown that zinc deficiency occurred during pregnancy may cause developmental disorders in the offspring.[24] Low intake of zinc may cause coronary artery disease. The concentration of zinc in *Bryonia alba* L. roots sample was 5.2 mg/ 100 g dry weight of the sample.

Copper (Cu)

Following zinc and iron, copper is considered the third most abundant trace element in the body. It has also been reported that it is an important catalyst for iron absorption. Its deficiency may be a risk factor for cardiovascular disease. When obvious copper deficiency occurs, symptoms such as neuropenia, cardiac disorders, osteoporosis and anemia may occur.[25]

In *Bryonia alba* L. roots sample, copper was found to be 0.13 mg/ 100 g dry weight of the sample. Excess copper is toxic. Normal daily intake of copper is 2-5 mg per day. In edible plants permissible limit set by FAO/WHO[26] in 1984 was 3.00 ppm. Thus, in *Bryonia alba* L. roots copper is less than the permissible limit.[21]

Cobalt (Co)

Cobalt is one of the most important essential components for the B12 vitamin and thyroid metabolism.[3] It is necessary in very small amounts in all mammals. It is used to treat different types of cancer in humans anemia treatment. The intake of high amount can cause heart diseases.[13] Cobalt is present in *Bryonia alba* L. roots sample at very low concentration of about <0.03 mg/ 100 g dry weight of the sample.

Silicon (Si)

Silicon (Si) is one of the most abundant elements found in the earth's crust and is commonly distributed in nature in different forms. It is well known that Si is associated to bone structure and its strength (Osteoporosis), reducing the risk of developing Alzheimer's disease, and preventing collagen metabolism abnormalities.[27] The concentration of silicon in *Bryonia alba* L. roots sample was 78 mg/ 100 g dry weight of the sample.

Phosphorus (P)

Phosphorus (P) is the constituent of more than 240 enzymes. Its deficiency in the organism is accompanied by multisystem dysfunction. Moreover, P is responsible for fetus development, sperm manufacture, and suitable function of the immune response.[20,28] The concentration of P in *Bryonia alba* L. roots sample was 88 mg/ 100 g dry weight of the sample. According to Dafalla work,[20] P concentrations were from 2.61 to 14.24 ppm.

Aluminum (Al)

Aluminum (Al) ions are considered toxic to most plants. It has negative results in being suppressed root growth and causing a series of abnormal metabolic effects.[29] Being an important herbal plant in the world, *Bryonia alba* L. roots also contain a concentration of Al of about 7.8 mg/ 100 g dry weight of the sample, and can be considered an important source of dietary Al.

Molybdenum (Mo)

Molybdenum (Mo) concentration found in *Bryonia alba* L. roots sample was <0.03 mg/ 100 g dry weight of the sample. Although Mo is required in trace amounts for the body as it is mostly present in the pancreas and plays a significant role in the production of insulin. Deficiency of Mo results in the disorder of the liver, and the daily intake should not exceed 1.0 mg. Beyond this level is toxic.[30] When analyzed in the roots of four medicinal plants namely; Ocimum basilicum, Poupulus nigra, Taraxacum officinale, and Convallaria maialis, its concentration varied from 0.82 to 9.2 ppm as most samples usually have concentrations between 0.51 and 0.72 ppm are considered the highest Mo concentration.[20]

Strontium (Sr)

Strontium (Sr) is an element which can be found in the environment in a large concentration ranges. The transfer of such a contaminant from the environment to plants will lead to contamination of the food pathway and finally into the human body. Then it deposits in bones and teeth and can cause bone and renal diseases accordingly.[31] It has been reported by Brambilla et al.[32] that plants can be contaminated by three main pathways namely; leaf uptake, root uptake, and deposition of contaminant on plant aerial parts.[33] Additionally, it is also affected by the properties of soil such as organic matter content, ionic composition, and pH.[34] The concentration of strontium in *Bryonia alba* L. roots sample was 0.78 mg/ 100 g dry weight of the sample.

Arsenic (As)

Arsenic (As) is a toxic pollutant in the environment, which results from anthropogenic and natural sources. It has been reported that plants growing in As contaminated soils accumulate As in their biomass.[35] Additionally, As may accumulate in soils and sediments owing to the use of arsenical pesticides, fertilizers, irrigation, and oxidation of volatile arsine in air disposal of industrial, municipal and animal waste.[36] Once a plant is contaminated with arsenic, it causes toxicity such as leaf chlorosis and necrosis, and also reduces growth. Different As species in plants show different toxicity, so it is important to quantify As in plants to better understand their metabolism. The concentration of arsenic in *Bryonia alba* L. roots sample was <0.01 mg/ 100 g dry weight of the sample.

Mercury (Hg)

Mercury (Hg) is extremely toxic trace metal pollutant. Bio-accumulation of Hg in plants and then its entry into the food chain results in long term health hazards.[37] The toxicity of Hg depends on its chemical state. Some forms of Hg are relatively non-toxic and have been used as medicines, e.g., for the treatment of syphilis. Speciation of mercury at trace and ultra-trace levels is a matter of current interest. The concentration of Hg in *Bryonia alba* L. roots sample was <0.01 mg/ 100 g dry weight of the sample.

In this study, the concentration of K, Ca, Mg, P, and Si were found to be the highest followed by the remaining elements in trace levels. Referring to the elemental concentration in Table 1, we can use the particular medicinal plant as requested by knowing the functional values of each element. Extra attention must be paid not to take those medicinal plants containing a large concentration of the above elements for a long time daily. For toxicity, the presence of arsenic in *Bryonia alba* L. roots sample will not lead to any undesirable effect because its concentration is very low as indicated by the World Health Organization Maximum Tolerable Daily Intake (WHO-MTDI, 2008)[38] value (2μg/day/ kg body weight). The low level observed for Pb and Cd leads to the conclusion that the plant is grown in the pollution free soil as elemental uptake by the plant mainly depends on regional soil as well as climate conditions and thus could be used as a medicinal plant.

Conclusion

The different concentrations of elements present in *Bryonia alba* L. roots leads to the conclusion that these roots will have different specific roles in the treatment of different diseases. The results obtained from the present study provide vital data on the availability of diverse essential elements, which can be useful to provide dietary information for designing value –added foods and for food bio fortification. This study provides a comprehensive investigation of the contents of 19 trace elements in *Bryonia alba* L. roots sample growing in Ukraine. The dry ashing method coupled with atomic absorption spectrometry was used for the determination of trace elements in *Bryonia alba* L. roots. The results indicated that *Bryonia alba* L. roots had a high content of K, Ca, Mg, P, and Si. The contents of the toxic heavy trace elements Cd and Pb were very low (<0.03 mg/ 100 g dry weight of the sample) and could not cause any threat to the consuming population. This technique is considered reliable for routine analysis elements determination in a wide range of botanicals and dietary supplements.

Conflict of Interest

The authors declare no conflict of interests.

References

1. Bailey LH. The Standard Cyclopedia of Horticulture. New York: The MacMillian Company;1950.
2. Manvi M, Garg GP. Evaluation of Pharmacognostical parameters and Hepatoprotective activity in *Bryonia alba* Linn. *J Chem Pharm Res* 2011;3:99-109.
3. Niamat R, Khan MA, Khan KY, Ahmad M, Ali B, Mazari P, et al. Element Content of Some Ethnomedicinal Ziziphus Linn. Species Using Atomic Absorption Spectroscopy Technique. *J Appl Pharm Sci* 2012;2:96-100.
4. Rodushkin I, Ruth T, Huhtasaari A. Comparison of two digestion methods for elemental determinations in plant material by ICP techniques. *Anal Chim Acta* 1999; 378: 191-200. doi: 10.1016/S0003-2670(98)00635-7
5. Lapa AJ, Souccar C, Lima-Landman MTR, Castro MSA, Lima TCM. Métodos de avaliação da atividade farmacológica de plantas medicinais. Brazil: Sociedade Brasileira de Plantas Medicinais; 2003.
6. Rajurkar NS, Damame MM. Mineral content of medicinal plants used in the treatment of diseases resulting from urinary tract disorders. *Appl Radiat Isot* 1998;49(7):773-6.
7. Zhang X, Ding W, Li J, Liu F, Zhou X, Tian S. Multi-elemental analysis of *Ziziphora clinopodioides* from different regions, periods and parts using atomic absorption spectrometry and chemometric approaches. *Rev Bras de Farmacogn* 2015;25(5):465-72. doi: 10.1016/j.bjp.2015.07.021
8. Wang HW, Liu YQ. Evaluation of trace and toxic element concentrations in Paris polyphylla from China with empirical and chemometric approaches. *Food Chem* 2010;121(3):887-92. doi: 10.1016/j.foodchem.2010.01.012

9. Liu F, Liu WX, Ding WH, Lv GY, Zhou XY. Trace elements analysis by ICP-OES after microwave digestion of *Medicago sativa* L. seeds from differentlocations in Xinjiang. *China Asian J Chem* 2014;26(12):3522-6. doi: 10.14233/ajchem.2014.16163

10. Kierdorf U, Stoffels D, Kierdorf H. Element concentrations and element ratios in antler and pedicle bone of yearling red deer (cervus elaphus) stags-a quantitative x-ray fluorescence study. *Biol Trace Elem Res* 2014;162(1-3):124-33. doi: 10.1007/s12011-014-0154-x

11. Daiane D, do Nascimento PC, Jost CL, Denise B, de Carvalho LM, Andrea K. Voltammetric determination of lowmolecular- weight sulfur compounds in hydrothermal vent fluids - studies with hydrogen sulfide, methanethiol, ethanethiol and propanethiol. *Electroanal* 2010;22(10):1066-71. doi: 10.1002/elan.200900472

12. Njinga RL, Moyo MN, Abdulmaliq SY. Analysis of essential elements for plants growth using instrumental neutron activation analysis. *Int J Agr* 2013:1-9. doi: 10.1155/2013/156520

13. Khan KY, Khan MA, Niamat R, Munir M, Fazal H, Mazari P, et al. Element content analysis of plants of genus Ficus using atomic absorption spectrometer. *Afr J Pharm Pharmaco* 2011;5(3):317-21. doi: 10.5897/AJPP10.339

14. Belay K, Tadesse A, Kebede T. Validation of a method for determining heavy metals in some ethiopian spices by dry ashing using atomic absorption spectroscopy. *Int J Innov Appl Stud* 2014;5(4):327-2.

15. Smillie TJ, Khan IA. A comprehensive approach to identifying and authenticating botanical products. *Clin Pharmacol Ther* 2010;87(2):175-86. doi: 10.1038/clpt.2009.287

16. Abudayeh ZHM, Al Azzam KM, Karpiuk UV, Hassouneh LK, Abuirmeileh A. Isolation, identificationand quantification of lectin protein contents in *Chamerion Angustifolium* L. dried raw material and the study of its activity using ratuserytroagglutination. *Int J Pharm Pharm Sci* 2016;8(2):150-3.

17. Soylak M, Tuzen M, Hayatisari IN. Comparison of microwave, dry and wet digestion procedures for the determination of trace metal contents in spice samples produced in Turkey. *J Food Drug Anal* 2004;12(3):254-8.

18. Pohl P, Dzimitrowicz A, Jedryczko D, Szymczycha-Madeja A, Welna M, Jamroz P. The determination of elements in herbal teas and medicinal plant formulations and their tisanes. *J Pharm Biomed Anal* 2016;S0731-7085(16)30042-5. doi:10.1016/j.jpba.2016.01.042

19. National Academy of Sciences (NAS). Food and Nutrition Board, Commission on Life Sciences, National Research Council, Recommended Dietary Allowances. 10 th ed. Washington DC: National Academy Press; 1989.

20. Dafalla A, Abdalla H. Determination the minerals contents of the roots of four medicinal plants as Asaudian indigenous plants using flame atomic absorption spectroscopy (FAAS). *J Chem Pharm Res* 2014;6(11):101-4.

21. Gupta J, Gupta A, Gupta AK. Determination of trace metals in the stem bark of *Moringa oleifera Lam. Int J Chem Stud* 2014;2(4):39-42.

22. World Health Organization. Consultation on Tolerable Daily Intake from Food of PCDDs and PCDFs. Bilthoven: World Health Organization, Regional Office for Europe; 1991.

23. Institute of Medicine. Dietary reference intakes for vitamin A, vitamin K, arsenic, boron, chromium, copper, iodine, iron, manganese, molybdenum, nickel, silicon, vanadium, and zinc. Washington DC: National Academy Press; 2001.

24. Hurley IS, Baley DI. The effects of zinc deficiency during pregnancy. In: Prasad AS, editor. Clinical, biochemical, and nutritional aspects of trace elements. Current topics in nutrition and disease. New York: Alan R. Liss, Manhattan Publisher;1982.

25. Klevay IM. The role of copper, zinc, and other chemical elements in ischemic heart disease. In: Rennert OM, Chan WY, editors. Metabolism of Trace Elements in Man, Developmental Aspects. Boca Raton: CRC Press; 1984.

26. FAO/WHO. Evaluation of certain food additives and contaminants: fifty-seventh report of the Joint FAO/WHO Expert Committee on Food Additives. Geneva: World Health Organization, (WHO Technical Report Series, No. 909); 2002.

27. Boschetti W, Dalagnol LMG, Dullius M, Zmozinski AV, Becker EM, Vale MGR, et al. Determination of silicon in plant materials using direct solid sample analysis with high-resolution continuum source graphite furnace atomic absorption spectrometry. *Microchem J* 2016;124:380-5. doi: 10.1016/j.microc.2015.09.017

28. Aisha AA, Nassar ZD, Siddiqui MJ, Abu-Salah KM, Alrokayanm SA, Ismail Z. Evaluation of antiangiogenic, cytotoxic and antioxidant effects of *Syzygium aromaticum* L. extracts. *Asian J Biol Sci* 2002;4(3):282-90. doi: 10.3923/ajbs.2011.282.290

29. Ruan J, Wong MH. Aluminium absorption by intact roots of the Al-accumulating plant *Camellia sinensis* L. *Agron* 2004;24(3):137-42. doi: 10.1051/agro:2004012

30. Chaturvedi A, Bhawani G, Agarwal PK, Goel S, Singh A, Goel RK. Ulcer healing properties of ethanolic extract of eugenia jambolana seed in diabetic rats: Study on gastric mucosal defensive factors. *Indian J Physiol Pharmacol* 2009;53(1):16-24.

31. Cohen-Solal M. Strontium overload and toxicity: Impact on renal osteodystrophy. *Nephrol Dial Transplant* 2002;17 Suppl 2:30-4.

32. Brambilla M, Fortunati P, Carini F. Foliar and root uptake of 134cs, 85sr and 65zn in processing tomato plants (lycopersicon esculentum mill.). *J Environ Radioact* 2002;60(3):351-63.

33. Sasmaz A, Sasmaz M. The phytoremediation potential for strontium of indigenous plants growing in a mining area. *Environ Exp Bot* 2009;67(1):139-44. doi: 10.1016/j.envexpbot.2009.06.014

34. Tsialtas JT, Matsi T, Barbayiannis N, Sdrakas A, Veresoglou DS. Strontium absorption by two Trifolium species as influenced by soil characteristics and liming. *Water Air Soil Poll* 2003;144:363-73. doi: 10.1023/A:1022965100636

35. Zhao D, Li HB, Xu JY, Luo J, Ma LQ. Arsenic extraction and speciation in plants: Method comparison and development. *Sci Total Environ* 2015;523:138-45. doi: 10.1016/j.scitotenv.2015.03.051

36. Narayana B, Cherian T, Mathew M, Pasha C. Spectrophotometric determination of arsenic in environmentsal and biological samples. *Indian J Chem Techn* 2006;13(1):36-40.

37. Ahmed MJ, Alam MS. A rapid spectrophotometric method for the determination of mercury in environmental, biological, soil and plant samples using diphenylthiocarbazone. *J Spec* 2003;17(1):45-52. doi: 10.1155/2003/250927

38. Pal A, Chowdhury UK, Mondal D, Das B, Nayak B, Ghosh A, et al. Arsenic burden from cooked rice in the populations of arsenic affected and nonaffected areas and kolkata city in west-bengal, india. *Environ Sci Technol* 2009;43(9):3349-55.

5

Design, Formulation and Evaluation of an Oral Gel from *Punica Granatum Flower* Extract for the Treatment of Recurrent Aphthous Stomatitis

Abolfazl Aslani[1]*, Behzad Zolfaghari[2], Fatemeh Davoodvandi[3]

[1] *Department of Pharmaceutics, School of Pharmacy and Novel Drug Delivery Systems Research Center, Isfahan University of Medical Sciences, Isfahan, Iran.*
[2] *Department of Pharmacognosy, School of Pharmacy and Isfahan Pharmaceutical Sciences Research Center, Isfahan University of Medical Sciences, Isfahan, Iran.*
[3] *Novel Drug Delivery Systems Research Center, Isfahan University of Medical Sciences, Isfahan, Iran.*

Article info

Keywords:
· Aphthous stomatitis
· Pomegranate flower
· Gallic acid
· Oral mucoadhesive gel

Abstract

Purpose: Recurrent aphthous stomatitis is a disease with unknown etiology that's mostly treated symptomatically and has no definite cure. Pomegranate (*Punica granatum)* flowers have been used as medicinal herb that due to its antimicrobial, antioxidant, anti-inflammatory, analgesic and healing effects, has been useful in treatment of oral aphthous. Therefore, we decided to formulate a mucoadhesive gel with pomegranate flower extract to reduce the need for corticosteroid therapy in patients.

Methods: Pomegranate flowers are extracted by percolation method. Several formulations with different amounts of carbomer 934, sodium carboxymethylcellulose (SCMC) and hydroxypropyl methylcellulose K_4M were prepared and the condensed extract was dispersed in polyethyleneglycol (PEG) 400 and added to gel bases. Then the formulations underwent macroscopic and microscopic studies. The formulations that passed these tests successfully were studied through assay tests using spectrophotometry in 765 nm, drug release from mucoadhesive gel using cell diffusion method, viscosity test, mucoadhesion test and accelerated stability test.

Results: The phenolic content of pomegranate flower dried extract was found to be 212.3 ± 1.4 mg/g in dried extract. The F_4–F_6 formulations contains carbomer 934, SCMC, pomegranate flower extract, PEG 400, potassium sorbate and purified water passed all above tests.

Conclusion: The F_4 formulation had higher viscosity and mucoadhesion values due to its higher carbomer 934 and SCMC content. Since F_4, F_5 and F_6 had no significant variation in drug release, the F_4 formulation was chosen as the superior formulation because of proper appearance and uniformity, acceptable viscosity, mucoadhesion and stability in different temperatures.

Introduction

Recurrent aphtous stomatitis is a rather common disease with unknown etiology that's identified by one or more sore ulcers with red margins on the mucous membrane of mouth and is self-limiting in one or two weeks but can reoccur monthly or a few times a year. Since this disease has an unknown cause, its diagnosis is based on clinical signs.[1] Aphthous patients can be categorized into three groups based on clinical status: minor, major and herpetifom; the most common of which is the minor type. The disease prevalence was reported differently in studies; for example in some surveys its prevalence in the general population was reported to be between 5 and 50 % and in specific populations such as students and military soldiers was said to be about 50 to 60 % because of daily stressful tasks like exams, etc.[2]

There is no definite etiology and pathology known for aphthous; although some factors are considered important such as topical trauma, bacterial and viral infections, genetics, nutrition, immunological, hormonal and psychological factors, allergies, medications and etc. Triamcinolone paste (Triadent), Irsha mouthwash, Persica and chlorhexidine mouthwash are medications for aphthous treatment in Iranian pharmaceutical market. Some generally suggested aphthous treatments are: antibiotics and antiseptics, herbal treatments, local analgesics, immunological mediators, both steroidal and non-steroidal anti-inflammatory drugs.[1,2]

Because of higher compatibility of herbal treatments with biological systems, these treatments are considered to have fewer side effects compared to synthetic

---
Corresponding author: Abolfazl Aslani, Email: aslani@pharm.mui.ac.ir

medications. Many herbal compounds have been found in the past to be effective in buccal diseases. A preliminary study has demonstrated that a 5% solution of *Myrtus communis* and *Melissa officinalis* extracts can treat the sore and lead to elimination of ulcer.[2] It has been shown in another study that a 2% mouth wash of *Zataria mutiflora* has a significant effect on minor aphthous compared to placebo.[3] *Anthemis nobelis* is another herbal treatment suggested to be effective in aphthous ulcer improvement.[4] The *Hypericum perforatum* extract used as a mouth wash may also reduce pain and shorten disease period in minor aphthous.[5]

Another suggested herb is pomegranate flowers of (*Punica granatum* L.) from the punicacea family. This plant grows as a 2 to 5 m tall tree or shrub that is indigenous to Iran, Afghanistan, China and Indian subcontinent.[6] Pomegranate is found abundantly in parts of Iran with semi-warm climate. Different parts of pomegranate tree have had several applications in Iranian folk and traditional medicine. Pomegranate flowers have been used as for oral and anal ulcers, intra-nasal ulcers, peptic ulcer, sores between toes and ear pain. In Iranian medicine pomegranate flower is believed to have strengthening effect on gums and can be useful for loose teeth. Applying it to scrape or wounds can rapidly heal them.[7]

Tanins are the major compounds in pomegranate flowers. Tannins are a great group of natural compounds with complex phenolic structures. Hydrolysable tannins like Ellagic acid, Gallic acid and Punicalagin are the most important tannins in different parts of pomegranate plant.[6] These compounds have an astringent effect on live tissues and can be used as digestive system astringent and treatment of burns and wounds. In burns and wounds, tissue proteins are precipitated by tannins and form a protective anti septic coating. Under this coating, new cells can grow and heal the wound.[8]

Free radicals have lately been suggested to play an important role in the etiology of aphthous. An increase in production of free radicals or the weakening of anti-oxidative defense systems causes a condition called the oxidative stress that can lead to tissue injury.[9] Due to the established role of oxidative stress in inflammation and the inflammatory nature of recurrent aphthous stomatitis, this oxidative stress seems to be one of the factors causing this condition.[10] According to this finding, the use of anti-oxidants might be effective in aphthous healing. The pomegranate flower seems to have a positive effect on treatment of aphthous symptoms due to its high antioxidant content.[11] Pomegranate has an antimicrobial effect too. Machado et al. have studied the effects of pomegranate fruits on a bacterial species and have found most of the anti-bacterial properties to be due to Ellagitannin and Punicallagin in the fruit.[12] Also in another study, antimicrobial effects of different extracts in methanol, water, chloroform and petroleum were analyzed. All extracts had anti-microbial properties which was significant in methanol extracts.[13]

Studies on effect of pomegranate flower extract on wound healing demonstrated positive effects on shortening the healing period.[8] Pomegranate flower may also act as an analgesic to ameliorate aphthous symptoms.[14]

Since antioxidant and immune system activity disturbances are considered important factors in aphthous etiology and because this disease is accompanied by inflammation and pain, pomegranate flower can be used for exoneration of symptoms and decreasing disease period due to antioxidative, antimicrobial, antiinflammatory, analgesic and wound healing properties. Moreover, the existing tannins form a protective layer by precipitating proteins and preventing the ulcer from getting infected or exacerbated.[8]

Ointments, creams, pastes, emulsions and gels are topical formulations for diseases such as aphtous. Patient compliance and acceptance is extremely important for oral topical products. Ointments, creams and some emulsions are rarely used for oral topical treatment while the patients have lower acceptance for application of ointments in mouth. Formulation base must have acceptable mucoadhesion so that the medication remains on the spot of application for a longer time. Emulsions have low mucoadhesion and are rapidly washed away by saliva. Pastes and gels allow longer adhesion and allow both the protection of lesion and release of drug. Pomegranate flower extract seems to be more compatible with hydrogels because of its hydroalcoholic phase. Gel bases have high water content and low surface friction and have better application on mucous membranes and burned or injured tissues.

Topical steroid such as triamcinolone and prednisolone are the most important medication for aphthous treatment, but these medications have many side effects like adrenal suppression, immune suppress, osteoporosis, digestive disturbances, blood glucose elevation, etc.[15] Considering these side effects and based on preliminary studies on pomegranate flower effectiveness on aphthous ulcers.[16] We prepare a stable mucoadhesive formulation of pomegranate flower that can be used as an alternative treatment for aphthous stomatitis.

Materials and Methods

Punica granatum flowers were collected in Isfahan in May and June 2013 and underwent a validation process by Pharmacognosy specialists in department of pharmacognosy; then the flowers were dried at room temperature in shade. The flowers were then powdered and prepared for extracting.

In this study Carbomer 934, Sodium carboxymethylcellulose (SCMC), Hydroxypropyl methylcellulose (HPMC), potassium sorbate, Triethanolamine, polyethylen glycol 400 (PEG 400), ethanol, gallic acid, sodium carbonate were prepared from Merck Company (Germany) and Folin- ciocalteu's indicator was purchased from Sigma Aldrich Company (Germany).

Extracting

Percolation method was used for extracting. 500 grams flower powder was soaked in ethanol 70% (as solvent) for 2 hours. The extraction was completed by letting the percolator drip 4 to 6 drops per minute (for every 100 grams of powder) for 48 hours. The remaining solvent was added on top of the powder so that rate of input and output drops are equal.[17] After finishing extraction process, the extract was condensed by rotary evaporator (Heidolph VV 2000) with 70 rpm and 50°C to achieve sufficient viscosity.

pH determination

The pH of extract was measured by digital pH meter (Metrohm 827, Switzerland) right after extracting, in 48 hours, 1 week, 2 weeks, 1 month, 3 months and 6 months. The pH meter was calibrated with standard buffers before measurement and each time the measuring was repeated 3 times and the mean was calculated.

Determination of dried extract

One gram of the condensed extract was heated to 40°C in vacuum oven and weighted daily till its weight was stabilized for 3 consecutive days. To find the weight percentage of dried extract, the container weight was subtracted and then the percentage of dried extract weight to total weight of the extract of calculated three times and the mean was chosen.[18]

Determination of total polyphenols

We used folin-ciocalteu's method and gallic acid as standard. To prepare gallic acid stock solution, 0.5 gram gallic acid was dissolved in 10 ml ethanol 96% in a 100 ml volumetric flask and then filled to the etched line with water. Then volumes of 1, 2, 3, 5 and 10 ml of this stock solution were diluted with water in 100 ml volumetric flasks. These solutions had phenolic contents of 50, 100, 150, 250 and 500 mg/l of gallic acid. To prepare sample solution, 5 g of concentrated pomegranate flower extract was weighted and mixed with 10 ml of ethanol 96% and then diluted to 100 ml by water. 5 ml of this sample was then diluted to 100 ml by water in a volumetric flask.

20 µl of each of the samples, blank (purified water) and calibration solutions were added to 1.58 ml of purified water in test tubes. Then 100 µl of folin-ciocalteu's indicator was added and the test tubes were shaken till mixed. After 30 sec to 8 minutes, 300 µl of 20% w/v sodium carbonate solution was added to test tubes and again mixed by shaking. At last the UV absorbance of solutions was measured against the blank sample by spectrophotometry (UV mini 1240) and standard curve of gallic acid absorption was prepared. Using this standard diagram, concentration the test sample was found.[19]

Gel preparation methods

For different gels, the concentrated pomegranate flower extract as the active ingredient and carbomer 934, SCMC and HPMC K4M were used as gelling polymers. Table 1 demonstrates each formulation and their contents.

Table 1. Composition of gel formulations with different polymers (Carbomer 934, SCMC and HPMC K₄M)

Ingredients (g)	Formulations									
	F_1	F_2	F_3	F_4	F_5	F_6	F_7	F_8	F_9	F_{10}
Carbomer 934	0.5	1	-	1	0.5	0.75	0.5	0.75	-	-
Sodium CMC	-	-	3	3	3	2	2	1	-	-
HPMC K₄M	-	-	-	-	-	-	-	-	2	3
Golnar extract	12	12	12	12	12	12	12	12	12	12
PEG 400	13	13	13	13	13	13	13	13	13	13
Potassium Sorbate	0.1	0.1	0.1	0.1	0.1	0.1	0.1	0.1	0.1	0.1
Triethanolamin	qs	qs	-	-	-	-	-	-	-	-
Purified water to	100	100	100	100	100	100	100	100	100	100

Preparation of carbomer 934 gel

Using the amounts on Table 1, first potassium sorbate (as preservative) was dissolved in 40°C purified water and then a specific amount of carbomer 934 was mixed with it till homogenous using a magnetic stirrer with 1200 rpm for 30 minutes. A determined amount of concentrated punica extract was weighed and mixed well with PEG 400. This mixture was slowly added to the gel and mixed to achieve a uniform gel. While

monitoring the pH, triethanolamine was added to the gel for it to reach a pH of about 6.[20]

Preparation of SCMC gel

Pottasium sorbate was dissolved in 50°C purified water. Then an exact amount of SCMC was slowly added to it while being mixed with magnetic stirrer in 1200 rpm for 30 minutes till it was completely homogenous. Concentrated punica extract was weighted and added to

PEG 400. The extract was added slowly to the gel and mixed till uniform.[20]

Preparation of HPMC gel

Potassium sorbate was dissolved in about one third of the formulation's water heated to 80°C and then a specific amount of HPMC was slowly added and mixed using magnetic stirrer in 1200 rpm. The remaining water was cooled and slowly added and mixed till a uniform gel was achieved. The gel remained in refrigerator overnight (hot/cold technique). Then an exact amount of concentrated pomegranate flower extract was separately added to PEG 400 and mixed and then gradually added to the gel.[20]

Preparation of carbomer 934 and SCMC gel

For each of these formulations, the listed powders were separately made into transparent gels as said above and then gels were added to each other and mixed well. Finally the extract was dispersed in PEG 400 and added to the gel.[20]

Determination of polyphenols in formulations

48 hours after preparation of the formulations, 1 grams of each gel were diluted to 10 ml with water. The polyphenol contents were determined by folin-ciocalteu's method using gallic acid standard curve.

Evaluation of physicochemical properties

These tests are used to study the formulation physicochemical properties and their stability in a long period of time. During formulations' stability tests, they are undergone abnormal stress conditions and if these conditions are tolerated for a short time, this is an indicator of stability in normal conditions for a longer time. These tests include: microscopic and macroscopic appearance uniformity tests, centrifuge test, temperature change test, cooling and heating test, melting and freezing test, pH test, release test, viscosity determination and mucoadhesion tests.[20]

Macroscopic and microscopic tests

The formulations were studied 48 hours after preparation for macroscopic (lumps, color and transparency) and microscopic (by optic microscope with magnification of 10 and 40 for uniformity, gel texture and bubbles.[20]

Centrifuge test

Each of the chosen formulations were separately centrifuged in a test tube of 10 cm long and 1 cm width for 5, 15, 30 and 60 minutes with 2000 rpm (Hettich Universal Centrifuge) and then studied for sedimentation and gel stability.[20]

Temperature change test

To control the formulation stability in different seasons and different temperature conditions, tubes containing formulations were put in temperatures of 2-8°, 25°C and 40-45°C and then their appearance quality was controlled after 48 hours, 1 week, 2 weeks, 1 month, 3 months and 6 months.[20]

Melting, freezing, cooling and heating tests

The goal of this test is to study the formulation stability in extreme temperatures. Two sets of formulation test tubes were prepared. One set underwent 6 consecutive periods of temperature changes each including 48 hours in -8°C and 48 hours in 25°C (freezing and melting). The second set underwent 6 periods of temperature changes too but this time each period included 48 hours in 45°C and then 48 hours in 4°C (heating and cooling). After these 6 periods, the formulations' qualities were analyzed.[20]

pH determination test

1 gram of each formulation was dispersed in 10 ml purified water. pH was measured after 48 hours, 1 week, 2 weeks, 1 month, 3 months and 6 months after preparation and each time three repeats were done.[20]

Viscosity test

Viscosities were measured by Brookfield (DV-III) viscometer. Each gel was poured into the container and the proper spindle (number 74) was attached. Then the viscosities were measured in 25°C and 50-250 rpm.[20]

Release test

This test is done with cell diffusion and synthetic membrane. 1g of the sample was spread over the membrane and the membrane was fixed on top of the cell. The receiving phase of the cell was filled with 37°C purified water and constantly stirred. For 6 hours, every 30 minutes a sampling of 1 ml was done and each time 1 ml purified water of 37°C was added to keep the volume constant. UV absorption of each sample was measured and the concentrations were found using the foline-ciocalteu's method. To calculate the actual concentration of the sample, the following equation was used:[20]

$$Cn = C + \frac{(C_{n-1})V}{V_t} \qquad eq.1$$

Cn: Actual concentration of drug in sample n
C: Pseudo-concentration of drug in sample n
C_{n-1}: Actual concentration of drug in sample n-1
V_t: Total volume
V: Sample volume

Release of the active ingredient from each formulation has its own specific kinetics which is the rate of release based on the time variation. To study the release kinetics, three models of zero order, first order and Higuchi model were studied and their constants were calculated.

Mucoadhesion test

The tensiometer (fisher) was calibrated and then the gel came in contact with sodium alginate (substitute for mucin) for 5 minutes. Then the required force to detach the gels from solution surface (speed of 0.2 inch/min) were determined in dyne/cm^2. This test was done 6 times for each formulation.[20,21]

Results

51.2 grams concentrated extract was obtained from every 100 g of dried flower powder, 81% of which is dried extract and the rest is water. According to the standard curve and the dilution factor, phenolic content of Pomegranate flower dried extract was found to be 212.3 ± 1.4 mg/g in dried extract.

The pH of Pomegranate flower extract was about 3.7 and constant throughout 6 months. The results of extracts pH are demonstrated in Table 2.

Table 2. Determination of extracts pH

Time	pH (mean ± SD)
24 h after preparation	3.75 ±0.01
48 h later	3.76 ± 0.02
1 week	3.78 ± 0.01
2 weeks	3.77 ± 0.01
1 month	3.75 ± 0.00
3 months	3.71 ± 0.01
6 months	3.70 ± 0.02

48 hours after preparation, the formulations were studied for macroscopic and microscopic properties and appearance. The F_9 and F_{10} formulations with HPMC lost uniform gel characteristics right after the addition of extract. F_1 and F_2 formulations had darkened. F_3, F_7 and F_8 did not have proper thickness and viscosity. Other formulations (F_4, F_5 and F_6) were completely uniform with no bubbles and no lumps when touched. These three formulations underwent further tests.

The results for polyphenol assays 48 hours after preparation are shown in Table 3.

Table 3. Determination of total polyphenols (mean ± SD) according to mg GAE/g in formulations F_4-F_6

Formulations	Total polyphenols (mg GAE/g)
F_4	21.2 ± 0.2
F_5	20.0 ± 0.1
F_6	22.1 ± 0.1

There were no observable sediment in centrifuge tests and the gels kept their uniformity.

In temperature change test (heating, cooling, melting and freezing), there were no appearance changes observed.

pH of formulations were fairly constant and about 4-5 in 6 months. The results of pH measurements are shown in Table 4.

Table 4. Determination of formulations pH after preparation of formulations F_4-F_6

Time	pH (mean ± SD)		
	F_4	F_5	F_6
24 h after	4.43 ± 0.01	4.50 ± 0.02	4.56 ± 0.00
48 h after	4.40 ± 0.00	4.60 ± 0.01	4.71 ± 0.02
1 week	4.48 ± 0.00	4.56 ± 0.00	4.67 ± 0.03
2 weeks	4.40 ± 0.00	4.48 ± 0.02	4.74 ± 0.00
1 month	4.33 ± 0.02	4.45 ± 0.02	4.64 ± 0.01
3 months	4.31 ± 0.00	4.55 ± 0.02	4.51 ± 0.01
6 months	4.39 ± 0.02	4.45 ± 0.03	4.59 ± 0.01

Viscosities of the three best formulations were measured by Brookfield viscometer (DV-III). Figure 1 demonstrates the viscosity changes against rounds per minute of rotation. The faster the rotation, the more the increase in formulation viscosities. According to this figure, F_4 viscosity is the highest.

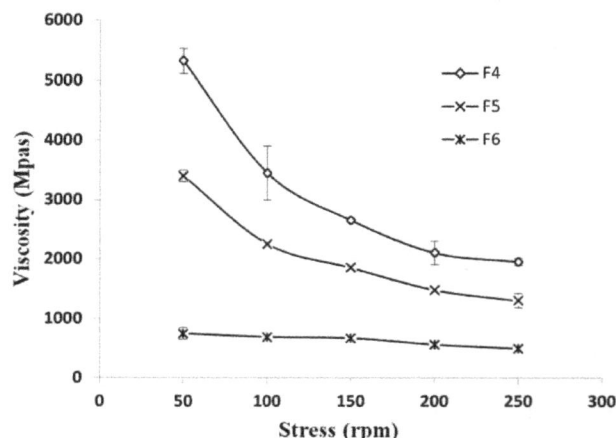

Figure 1. The viscosity changes against rpm, at 25°C

Results from mucoadhesion studies by tensiometery method are shown in Table 5. The F_4 formulation has the highest mucoadhesion.

Table 5. Mucoadhesive strength (mean ± SD) of formulations F_4-F_7 according to tensiometry method

Formulations	Mucoadhesive strength (dyne/cm^2)
F_4	54.6 ± 3.2
F_5	24.3 ± 3.8
F_6	31.3 ± 3.4
F_7	22.2 ± 3.6

The results of active ingredient release by cell diffusion method are displayed in Figure 2 as a curve of cumulative percentage of release in time.

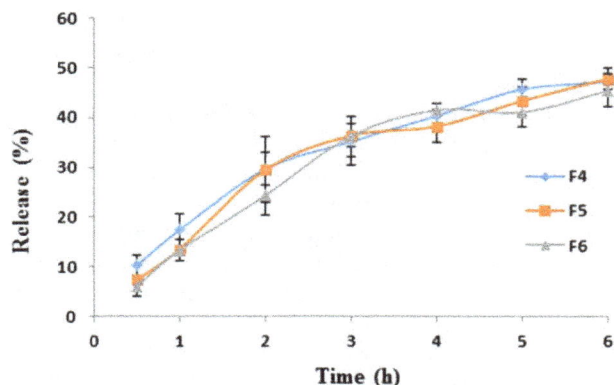

Figure 2. Percentage of cumulative drug release of formulations F_4, F_5 and F_6 in Franz diffusion cell through a cellulose acetate membrance, at 37°C, during 6 h

To study the kinetic of release from synthetic membrane, the zero order, first order and Higuchi models were controlled. To study the zero order model, a diagram was prepared for percentage of released ingredient in time. For first order kinetic, the diagram for logarithm of remaining drug percentage in time; and for Higuchi model, the percentage of released drug was drawn against square root of time. Table 6 demonstrates the cumulative percentage of polyphenol release and the equation constants for zero order (K_0), first order (K_1) and Higuchi (K_h). In these equations, Q_t is the percentage of release in time of t and Q_0 is the percent of remaining drug.

$$Q_t = K_0 t \qquad \text{eq. 2}$$

$$\ln Q_t = \ln Q_0 - K_1 \qquad \text{eq. 3}$$

$$Q_t = K_h t^{1/2} \qquad \text{eq. 4}$$

Discussion

Aphthous is an oral disease characterized by one or several recurrent ulcers on oral mucosa. The etiology of the disease is unknown and it is mostly symptomatically treated and the aim of the treatment is to decrease the period of the ulcers. The most frequently used drugs for treatment of aphthous are topical steroid which can cause several side effects on continuous application. The herbal medications have been widely used for different oral diseases. Due to its anti-microbial, anti-oxidant, analgesic and healing properties, the pomegranate flower can improve aphthous symptoms and because of the high amount of tannins, it can form a protective layer on the ulcers by precipitating proteins and hence accelerate the healing process. Considering these pharmacological effects of pomegranate flower extract and the preliminary studies indicating effectiveness of pomegranate flower extract on aphthous ulcers.[16] We decided to utilize these effects and design a suitable, stable and easily accessible formulation of this herb.

The folin-ciocalteu's method was used to indicate the amount of poly-phenols in dried extract. This determination can be done by the linear correlation between the concentration and absorbance of gallic acid after finding its standard curve using gallic acid standard solution. In this study, the poly-phenol content was about 212.3 ± 1.4 mg per gram of dried extract. In a study done by Mortezaei et al. in Iran's Chahar-Mahal-e-Bakhtiari, this was reported to be 480.6 mg per gram of dried extract.[22] The found difference might be due to the different drying and extracting methods, solvents and assay methods.

In this study the pomegranate flower extract was prepared as a mucoadhesive gel formulation. Considering the ease of application, good distribution and ability of adhesion and remaining on oral mucosa for a long enough time to release its drug, this formulation can be well accepted for treatment of oral ulcers and diseases such as aphthous.

To prepare a mucoadhesive gel, polymers like carbomer 934, SCMC and HPMC were used. These polyemers are all water soluble and useful in pharmaceutical industries.[20] Many gels, specially the water-based ones are susceptible to microbial growth and hence the use of a suitable preservative decreases the chance of microbial contamination and the change in formulation properties[21] In this study, potassium sorbate was applied as preservative agent. Sorbates are safe and effective against mold, yeast and bacteria. These materials are used to decrease the chance of contamination to a minimum.[23]

Formulations were prepared by different proportions of polymers and after 48 hours, the ones with superior microscopic and macroscopic properties were selected to undergo stability tests. The F_9 and F_{10} formulations with HPMC base didn't have suitable uniformity and physical properties, i.e. the gel base lost its homogenous texture right after the addition of extract. This may be because of pomegranate flower extract incompatibility with HPMC base. F_1 and F_2 formulations with Carbomer 934 base changed color after 48 hours. When only Carbomer is used to prepare the gel, we need to increase the pH and neutralize the mixture by triethanolamine so that the gel can swell and remain clear. Incompatibility of the extract with triethanolamine or its instability in neutral or basic pH can be the reason for its change of color. The F_3, F_7 and F_8 formulations did not have sufficient thickness. This is due to lower amounts of polymer in these formulations compared to F_4, F_5 and F_6 formulations. So it was made clear that polymers enhance thickness and the formulations with fewer polymers will not have a sufficient firmness. The F_4, F_5 and F_6 formulations had acceptable macroscopic and microscopic properties and underwent further tests. A study was conducted on the same formulation which confirms these results.[20]

Generally the formulation pH must be constant during storage time and its fluctuations can indicate complications such as microbial growth, ingredient incompatibilities or decomposition of some ingredients.[20] The F_4, F_5 and F_6 formulations had a rather constant pH throughout a 6 months duration and could be accepted as stable. The condensed extract also has a pH between 3.6 and 3.7 in 6 months which is almost constant and this might be a reason for extract stability for a long period of time.

The phenolic compounds assay was operated by the folin-ciocalteu's method and standard curve of gallic acid and the results show homogenous and uniform distribution of polyphenols in gel formulations.

The heat stress tests are applied to determine the formulation half-life. If the formulation can withstand 2 to 3 months of high temperature or 3 to 4 heat cycles, it is deemed to have an adequate half-life.[20] Our formulations showed no change in visual quality after stability tests such as temperature change, heating and cooling, melting and freezing tests. Hence, the results indicate that the formulations can endure 6 months of undesirable temperature conditions. A study conducted by Tavakoli et al also noted that if the formulation accomplishes the stability studies (such as changes in temperature and pH) without any changes, thus a 2-years shelf life can be suggested for it.[21]

According to Figure 1, the F_4 and F_5 formulations have higher viscosities. This might be due to higher proportions of Carbomer to SCMC in these formulations. Gels with mucoadhesion and proper viscosity have a longer adhesion time and better durability on site. Studies by Mortazavi et al. demonstrated that carbomers specially carbomer 934 have the highest mucoadhesion

and remain longer on mucous surface.[24] This study confirms our findings concerning mucoadhesion of formulations.

In release studies with Franz cell diffusion method, as it is demonstrated on Table 6, there is little difference in release percentage from different formulation and these small differences are minor and non-significant. This might be because of the similar polymer proportions in remaining formulations since the ones with considerably diverse proportions were omitted on the primary screenings. Also water is used as the release environment, so the release is possibly different in oral pH and due to the buffer nature of saliva, the active ingredient might have an increased release profile. To determine the amount of released drug, the folin-ciocalteu's method is used as a standard way to estimate the phenolic content. This method is based on reduction of folin-ciocalteu's indicator by phenolic compounds in basic environment and formation of a blue complex with maximum absorbance in 765 nm.[25] It was not possible to measure the amount of released extract in-vitro in a buffer environment. This may be due to the interaction between phosphate buffer and the folin-ciocalteu's reagent and preventing the basic environment needed for the reaction. This is why we used only water as the receiving phase.

Table 6. Drug release percent and drug release kinetics of gel formulations (F_4, F_5 and F_6)

Zero-order release		First-order release		Higuchi equation		Cumulative drug release (%)	Formulations
R^2	K_h	R^2	K_1	R^2	K_0		
22.15	0.982	0.102	0.825	6.621	0.936	47.72 ± 4.2 (6 h)	F_4
22.40	0.959	0.057	0.740	3.323	0.899	47.98 ± 2.5 (6 h)	F_5
23.24	0.949	0.062	0.755	3.449	0.891	45.57 ± 1.7 (6 h)	F_6

The release kinetics were studied by zero order, first order and Higuchi model and the kinetic was found to be following the Higuchi model in all formulations. So it is logical to conclude that the release kinetic in formulations is not independent from formulation base (cream, ointment, etc).

Conclusion

The ideal formulation for treatment of aphthous must have high mucoadhesion and suitable durability. The results showed that an increase in the amount of polymer in gel can increase mucoadhesion and lead to a longer durability in mouth. Hence, the F_4 formulation has the highest mucoadhesion and viscosity because of its higher polymer content and it is able to remain on mucous surface long enough to release its active ingredient. So because of uniformity, proper appearance, stability and acceptable viscosity and mucoadhesion the F_4 formulation was chosen as the superior formulation.

We suggest that the effectiveness of the superior formulation is determined through clinical studies.

Acknowledgments

We appreciate Isfahan University of Medical Science Vice Chancellery for Research that supported us financially through research project number 393066.

Conflict of Interest

The authors report no conflicts of interest in this work.

References

1. Rad F, Yaghmaee R, MehdiAbadi P, Khatibi R. A comparative clinical trial of topical triamcinolone (adcortyle) and a herbal solution for the treatment of minor aphthous stomatitis. *Armaghane-danesh* 2010;15(3):191-8.
2. Eslami Raveshty SS, Eslami Raveshty SB. The effect of combining essences of *Myrtus Communis* and *Melissa Officinalis* in the treatment of minor aphta. *J Zanjan Univ Med Sci* 2011;19(76):76-83.

3. Mansoori P, Hadji Akhoondi A, Ghavami R, Shafiei A. Clinical evaluation of *Zataria multiflora* essential oil mouthwash in the management of recurrent aphthous stomatitis. *DARU J Pharm Sci* 2002;10(2):74-7.

4. Jafari S, Amanlou M, Borhan-Mojabi K, Farsam H. Comparartive study of *Zataria multiflora* and *Anthemis nobelis* extracts with *Myrthus communis* preparation in the treatment of recurrent aphthous stomatitis. *DARU J Pharm Sci* 2003;11(1):23-7.

5. Motallebnejad M, Moghadamnia A, Talei M. The efficacy of *Hypericum perforatum* extract on recurrent aphthous ulcers. *J Med Sci* 2008;8(1):39-43. doi: 10.3923/jms.2008.39.43

6. Ismail T, Sestili P, Akhtar S. Pomegranate peel and fruit extracts: A review of potential anti-inflammatory and anti-infective effects. *J Ethnopharmacol* 2012;143(2):397-405. doi: 10.1016/j.jep.2012.07.004

7. Al-rhazes (Rhazes) M. Persian translation by Afsharipour S. Tehran: Academy of medical sciences publication; 2005.

8. Pirbalouti AG, Koohpayeh A, Karimi I. The wound healing activity of flower extracts of punica granatum and achillea kellalensis in wistar rats. *Acta Pol Pharm* 2010;67(1):107-10.

9. Najafi SM, Mohammadzadeh M, Monsef Esfahani HR, Meighani Gh, Rezaei N. The effect of Purslane in the treatment of recurrent aphthous stomatitis. *Tehran Univ Med J* 2013;71(2):102-8.

10. Caglayan F, Miloglu O, Altun O, Erel O, Yilmaz AB. Oxidative stress and myeloperoxidase levels in saliva of patients with recurrent aphthous stomatitis. *Oral Dis* 2008;14(8):700-4. doi: 10.1111/j.1601-0825.2008.01466.x

11. Celik I, Temur A, Isik I. Hepatoprotective role and antioxidant capacity of pomegranate (punica granatum) flowers infusion against trichloroacetic acid-exposed in rats. *Food Chem Toxicol* 2009;47(1):145-9. doi: 10.1016/j.fct.2008.10.020

12. Machado TdB, Leal ICR, Amaral ACF, Santos KRN, Silva MG, Kuster RM. Antimicrobial ellagitannin of *Punica granatum* fruits. *J Braz Chem Soc* 2002;13(5):606-10.

13. Prashanth D, Asha MK, Amit A. Antibacterial activity of punica granatum. *Fitoterapia* 2001;72(2):171-3.

14. Chakraborthy GS. Analgesic activity of various extracts of *Punica granatum* (Linn) flowers. *Int J Green Pharm* 2008;2(3):145. doi: 10.4103/0973-8258.42730

15. Katzung BG, Masters SB, Trevor AG. Basic and clinical pharmacology. 12th ed. London: McGraw-Hill Education; 2012.

16. Ghalayani P, Zolfaghary B, Farhad AR, Tavangar A, Soleymani B. The efficacy of punica granatum extract in the management of recurrent aphthous stomatitis. *J Res Pharm Pract* 2013;2(2):88-92. doi: 10.4103/2279-042X.117389

17. Aslani A, Emami SMH, Ghannadi A, Ajdari M. Formulation and physicochemical evaluation of an herbal antihemorrhoid ointment from Quercus, Black cumin and Fenugreek for the treatment of internal anal hemorrhoids. *Pharmaceut Sci* 2009;14(4):247-57.

18. Mohagheghi Samarin A, Poorazarang H, Akhlaghi H, Elhami Rad A, Hematyar N. Antioxidant activity of potato (Solanum tuberosum, raja) peel extracts. *Iran J Nutr Sci Food Technol* 2008;3(3):23-32.

19. Mena P, Garcia-Viguera C, Navarro-Rico J, Moreno DA, Bartual J, Saura D, et al. Phytochemical characterisation for industrial use of pomegranate (punica granatum l.) cultivars grown in spain. *J Sci Food Agric* 2011;91(10):1893-906. doi: 10.1002/jsfa.4411

20. Aslani A, Ghannadi A, Najafi H. Design, formulation and evaluation of a mucoadhesive gel from quercus brantii l. And coriandrum sativum l. As periodontal drug delivery. *Adv Biomed Res* 2013;2:21. doi: 10.4103/2277-9175.108007

21. Tavakoli N, Minaiyan M, Saghaei E. Preparation of diltiazem topical gel for the treatment of anal fissure and In-vitro, Ex-vivo drug release evaluations. *J Kerman Univ Med Sci* 2007;14(3):163-75.

22. Mortazaei S, Rafieian M, Ansary Samani R, Shahinfard N. Comparison of phenolic compounds concentrations and antioxidant activity of eight medicinal plants. *J Rafsanjan Univ Med Sci* 2013;12(7):519-30.

23. Barzegar H, Azizi MH, Barzegar M, Hamidi Z. Preparation and evaluation of active starch-clay nanocomposite film containing cinnamon oil and potassium sorbate. *J Res Innov Food Sci Technol* 2013;2(2):167-78.

24. Mortazavi A, Salehi A. In vitro assessment of the efficacy of various mucosa-adhesive materials for the preparation of a buccal mucosa-adhesive gel. *Hakim Res J* 2002;4(1):31-8.

25. Salmanian SH, Sadeghi Mahoonak AR, Alami M, Ghorbani M. Evaluation of total phenolic, flavonoid, anthocyanin compounds, antibacterial and antioxidant activity of hawthorn (*Crataegus Elbursensis*) fruit acetonic extract. *J Rafsanjan Univ Med Sci* 2014;13(1):53-66.

6

Effects of Pomegranate *(Punica Granatum* L.) Seed and Peel Methanolic Extracts on Oxidative Stress and Lipid Profile Changes Induced by Methotrexate in Rats

Farideh Doostan[1], Roxana Vafafar[2], Parvin Zakeri-Milani[3], Aliasghar Pouri[3], Rogayeh Amini Afshar[4], Mehran Mesgari Abbasi[5]*

[1] *Physiology Research Center, Kerman University of Medical Sciences, Kerman, Iran.*
[2] *Department of Biology, Faculty of Science, Islamic Azad University, Ahar Branch, Ahar, Iran.*
[3] *Liver and Gastrointestinal Diseases Research Center, Tabriz University of Medical Sciences, Tabriz, Iran.*
[4] *Faculty of Sciences, Urmia University, Urmia, Iran.*
[5] *Student Research Committee, Drug Applied Research Center, Tabriz University of Medical Sciences, Tabriz, Iran.*

Article info

Keywords:
· Methotrexate
· Oxidative stress
· Pomegranate
· Rats

Abstract

Purpose: Methotrexate (MTX) is prescribed in many diseases and can result in oxidative stress (OS) followed by injuries in some tissues. Antioxidants administration are effective in reducing OS. Pomegranate exhibits high anti-oxidant capacities. This study investigated whether pomegranate seed and peel methanolic extracts (PSE and PPE) could protect against MTX-induced OS and lipid profile changes in rats.

Methods: Forty-eight rats were randomly divided into 6 groups: control group (normal salin), PSE group (500 mg/kg, orally), PPE group (500 mg/kg, orally), MTX group (10 mg/kg, IM), MTX and PSE group, and MTX and PPE group. Blood samples were taken for analysis in the end of the procedure.

Results: The findings showed a significant reduction in Glutathione peroxidase (GPx) and Superoxide dismutase (SOD), and an enhancement in malondialdehyde (MDA) values after MTX treatment ($p < 0.05$). SOD and GPx levels reached the levels of the control group in MTX+SPE and MTX+PPE groups. No significant differences were observed in catalase (CAT) and total antioxidant capacity (TAC) levels between groups. The results showed a significant decrease in total cholesterol (TC), low density lipoprotein (LDL), and high density lipoprotein (HDL) in the MTX treated group ($p < 0.01$). The values of TC, HDL, and LDL became elevated to the normal control levels in the MTX+PSE and MTX+PPE treated groups.

Conclusion: The results showed the OS induced by MTX and the protective effects of PSE and PPE against MTX-induced serum oxidative stress and lipid profile changes in rats.

Introduction

The presence of active oxygen species in excess of the tissue's available antioxidant buffering capacity, results in oxidative stress. Reactive oxygen species (ROS) may damage DNA, proteins, lipids, and/or carbohydrates disturbing the cells or tissues structure and function. Tissue damage and sometimes chronic human diseases may occur following enzyme and non-enzyme-mediated biochemical reactions, which produce free radicals that are extremely reactive intermediate compounds. All body tissues are exposed chronically to oxidants from endogenous and/or exogenous sources.[1,2]

Methotrexate (MTX), which has inhibitory effect on di-hydrofolatereductase, is routinely prescribed in many diseases such as cancers and autoimmune diseases. MTX suppresses DNA synthesis and adversely influences several tissues particularly the liver. The long term application of MTX causes hepatic fibrosis or cirrhosis and increases cardiovascular risk.[3,4] MTX may affect the balance of pro-oxidants and antioxidants, which can result in the enhancement of oxidative stress, followed by injuries in some tissues. Antioxidants can be considered to reduce the OS during MTX treatment.[5,6]

Pomegranate (*Punica granatum L.*) represents a phyto-chemical reservoir that has been extensively referenced in medical folklore. This fruit has been used for centuries to treat common ailments such as microbial and parasitic infections, stomach ache, ulcers, diarrhea and dysentery. The fruit is composed of two parts: [1] the aril, that is the edible part, constitutes 52% of the total fruit (w/w), contains 78% juice and 22% seeds, and [2] the non-edible part or the peel, have been traditionally used in folk medicine. A large number of phyto-chemicals have been identified in the two parts of pomegranate, including poly-phenolics like hydrolysable tannins (ellagic and gallagic acids) and anthocyanin in the peel. The main benefit of PG has been attributed to its unique polyphenols composition, which has been shown to exhibit high anti-oxidant and anti-inflammatory capacities. The health benefits of PG consumption in preventing cardiovascular diseases and cancers have been widely investigated in both laboratory and clinical studies.[1,7-9]

This study investigated whether pomegranate seed and peel methanolic extracts (PSE and PPE) could protect against MTX-induced oxidative stress in rat blood serum.

Materials and Methods
Extraction
The pomegranates (*P. granatum* L.) were provided from Tabriz suburbs (East Azarbaijan, Iran). The fresh fruits (Post-Ghermez variety, 5-64-WS)[10] were manually washed and peeled. The peels and seeds were separated and air dried in an oven (40°C, 24 h). After that, using a blender the dried materials turned into a powder. Thereafter, 500 g of pomegranate seed and pomegranate peel powders were separately extracted in methanol (Merck, Germany) (1:10 w/v) at 25°C for 24 and 96 h, respectively. The mixture of each was then filtered throw 0.45 μ pore size filters. The methanol was completely evaporated (rotary vacuum evaporator, Heidolph, Germany) at 40°C. The PSE and the PPE were stored in a deep freezer (-70°C) until use.[10]

Animals
Forty-eight male Wistar rats, weighing 200 ± 20 g, were placed in a ventilated temperature-controlled room (22 ± 2°C) in standard cages (polycarbonate) under 12/12 h light/dark cycles. The animals were provided with clean drinking water and a standard rat diet *ad libitum*.

The animals were divided into 6 groups (n=8):
- Group I: placebo control, daily received normal saline (orally, for 18 days).
- Group II: daily received 500 mg/kg PSE (orally, for 18 days).
- Group III: daily received 500 mg/kg PPE (orally, for 18 days).
- Group IV: daily received 10 mg/kg MTX (IM, for three days beginning from the 10th day).
- Group V: daily received 500 mg/kg PSE (orally, for 18 days) and also 10 mg/kg MTX (IM, for three days beginning from the 10th day).
- Group VI: daily received 500 mg/kg PPE (orally, for 18 days) and also 10 mg/kg MTX (IM, for three days beginning from the 10th day).

After the intervention, blood samples were obtained using cardiac puncturing method under anesthetic condition and were centrifuged at 2000 g and 4°C for 10 min. The blood serum samples were placed at a temperature of -70°C in a freezer.

Biochemical tests
Commercial kits (Randox, Italy) were used for determining TAC, GPX, and SOD of samples. TC,

triglyceride (TG), LDL, and HDL were assayed using commercial kits (Pars Azmun, Karaj, Iran). Malondialdehyde (MDA) contents of samples were analyzed using barbituric acid method.[10] The automated biochemistry analyzer (Alcyon 300, Abbott, USA) was used for biochemical analysis after calibration and validation. Cayman kit (USA) was used for assaying the CAT activities of the samples.

Analyses of PSE and PPE
The antioxidant capacity of the extracts (PSE and PPE) were assayed using DPPH assay method.[10] The quercetin RC50 (control material) was 0.004 mg/ml. Folin-Ciocalteu reagent was used for determining the total phenolic equivalent (mg of gallic acid equivalent per gram of extract, GAE/ gram extract).[11] A spectrophotometric method was used for assaying total flavonoids.[10,12]

Statistical Analysis
SPSS (13) for Windows (SPSS Inc., Chicago, USA) was used for statistical analyses. The normality was surveyed by using Kolmogorov–Smirnov test and Q-Q chart. For comparing between groups, we used ANOVA (One-way analysis of variance) for normally distributed data. Tukey post-hoc test was used for multiple comparisons. The data were stated as mean ± SD (standard deviation). The median ± interquartile and Wilcoxon test were used for non-normally distributed data. P-values less than 0.01 and 0.05 were statistically considered significant.

Results and Discussion
Analysis of PSE and PPE
Total phenolic, flavonoid compounds, and antioxidant activity of PSE and PPE were assayed and the results are shown in Table1.

Table 1. Composition of pomegranate seed extract (PSE) and pomegranate peel extract (PPE).

Sample (n = 3)	Antioxidant activity (RC50; μg/ml)	Total phenolic content (mg GAE/g extract)	Total Flavonoid (%)
PSE	510.7 ± 2.5	41.1 ± 0.2	0.42 ± 0.01
PPE	27 ± 0.3	147.2 ± 0.2	1.17 ± 0.04

The results are expressed as means ± 1SD.

Lipid profile contents of the samples
The TC, TG, HDL, and LDL of the blood serum samples were determined. The results are shown in Table 2. As shown in the table, MTX administration decreased TC, LDL (p<0.01), and HDL (p<0.05) levels significantly. While, the administration of SPE and MTX caused an enhancement in TG and LDL levels (p<0.01). PPE together with MTX decreased the blood serum HDL content significantly (p<0.05).

Table 2. Effects of pomegranate seed extract (PSE) and pomegranate peel extract (PPE) on blood serum lipid profile in rats following methotrexate (MTX) treatment.

Parameter	Control	PSE	PPE	MTX	SPE + MTX	PPE + MTX
Cholesterol (mg/dl)	97.7 ± 11.9	89.8 ± 5.6	89.6 ± 5.6	54.3 ± 13.0[**]	109.2 ± 11.8	90.7 ± 9.9
Triglyceride (mg/dl)	42.0 ± 6.3	42.8 ± 5.8	41.8 ± 4.1	39.7 ± 5.6	86.8 ± 14.8[**]	49.5 ± 9.9
HDL (mg/dl)	31.5 ± 3	27.5 ± 2.9	30.6 ± 2.5	21.0 ± 5.1[*]	31.8 ± 6.7	20.5 ± 4.3*
LDL (mg/dl)	37.5 ± 1.6	35.0 ± 6.7	31.4 ± 3.1	16.4 ± 4.0[**]	70.5 ± 5.2**	45.3 ± 5.2

The results are expressed as means ± 1SD. * and ** significantly different when compared with the control group (p < 0.05 and p < 0.01, respectively).

Changes in antioxidant enzymes following MTX, PSE, and PPE administrations

SOD, GPx, CAT, TAC, and MDA levels were assayed in the blood serum samples following MTX, PSE, and PPE administrations and the results are shown in Figures 1–5, respectively. SOD and GPx levels were significantly decreased while MDA was increased in the MTX group following MTX administration as compared with the control group (p<0.05) (Figures 1, 2, and 5). The GPx level was significantly decreased in the PSE group (Figure 2). The MDA levels showed a significant enhancement in MTX (p<0.05), PSE, MTX + PSE, and MTX + PPE (p<0.01) groups as compared with the control group (Figure 5). Other differences between MTX and extract administered groups and the control group were not statistically significant (p > 0.05).

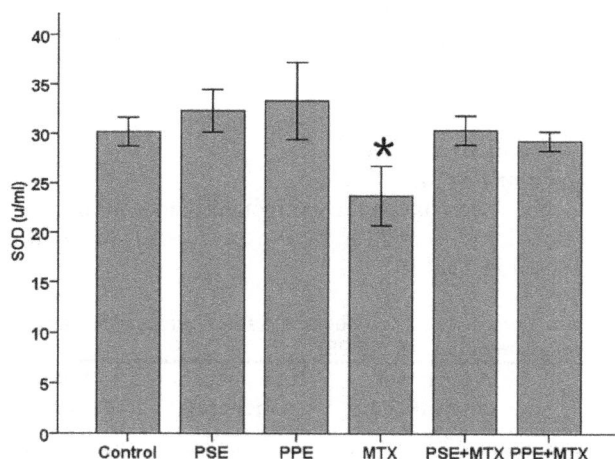

Figure 1. Effects of pomegranate seed extract (PSE) and pomegranate peel extract (PPE) on blood serum superoxide dismutase (SOD) content in rats following MTX treatment. The values are expressed as means ± 1SD. * significantly different at (p<0.05) when compared with the control group.

Endogenous enzymatic and non-enzymatic antioxidants affects the unwanted effects of oxidative agents. SOD, GPx, and CAT are water-soluble antioxidants. ROS and reactive nitrogen species (RNS) may be removed by antioxidant enzymes such as SOD, GPx, and CAT. SOD is in the first anti-oxidant defense line and results in dismutation of oxygen to H_2O_2. GPx reduces organic peroxides including H_2O_2 to H_2O and O_2, that requires glutathione (hydrogen donor and scavenger for H_2O_2,

hydroxyl radical and chlorinated oxidants). CAT reduces H_2O_2 to water.[13,14] Evaluation of the status and the aactivity of enzymatic antioxidants, such as SOD, GPx, and CAT, can be used to assess OS. Reduction in the antioxidant defense capacity can be measured by SOD, GPx, TAC, and CAT in the serum. Decreased levels of plasma SOD, GPx, and TAC activity have been reported in some oxidative stress conditions.[13]

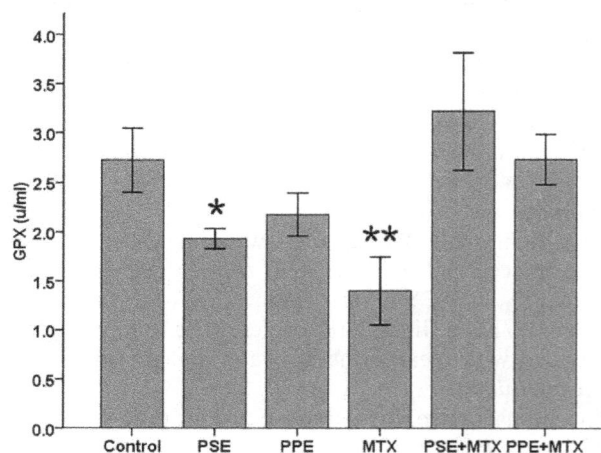

Figure 2. Effects of pomegranate seed extract (PSE) and pomegranate peel extract (PPE) on blood serum glutathione peroxidase (GPx) content in rats following MTX treatment. The values are expressed as means ± 1SD. * and ** significantly different when compared with the control group (p<0.05 and p<0.01, respectively).

Malondialdehyde (MDA) is considered the important lipopolysaccharide oxidative stress marker. DNA damage and tissue injury may result in excessive MDA. MDA can react with proteins free amino-groups and form MDA-modified protein adducts.[15] Aldehydic products, such as MDA, have relatively longer half-lives as compared with ROS. The products can diffuse to other intra- and extra-cellular places and amplify the effects of oxidative stress. ROS may damage poly-unsaturated fatty acids and cause cell organelle and membrane lipid peroxidation resulting in producing the above mentioned products.[14]

The results of this study indicated that oxidative stress was induced by MTX. The present findings showed a significant reduction in rat serum SOD (Figure 1) and GPx (Figure 2), and an enhancement in MDA values

(Figure 5) after MTX treatment ($p < 0.05$). The findings of this study also showed that the levels of SOD and GPx reached the control group levels when MTX was administered alongside PSE or PPE, suggesting the protective property of PSE and PPE against changes induced by MTX (Figures 1 and 2). There were no significant differences in CAT and TAC levels between the treated and control groups (Figure 3 and 4).

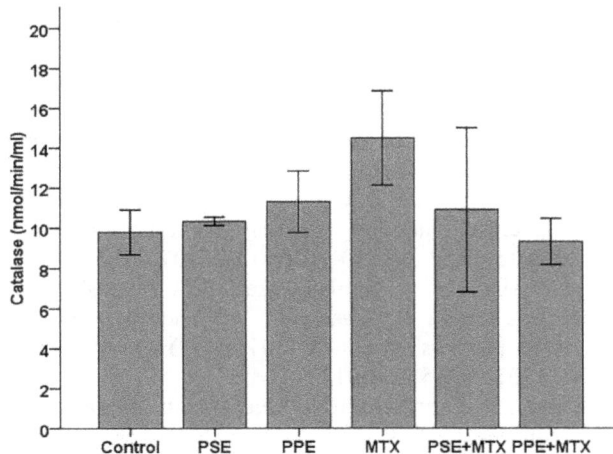

Figure 3. Effects of pomegranate seed extract (PSE) and pomegranate peel extract (PPE) on blood serum CAT content in rats following MTX treatment. The values are expressed as means ± 1SD.* significantly different at ($p < 0.05$) when compared with the control group.

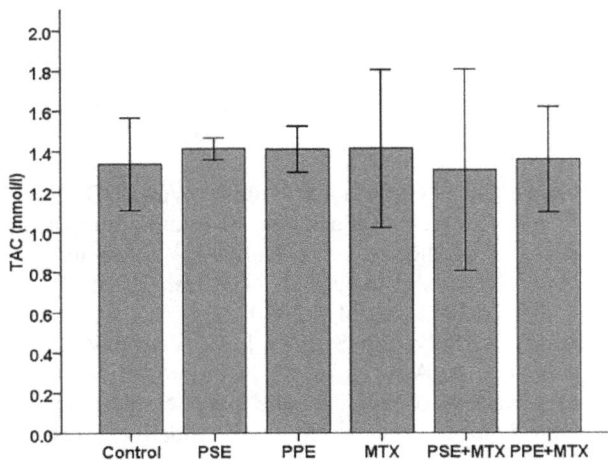

Figure 4. Effects of pomegranate seed extract (PSE) and pomegranate peel extract (PPE) on blood serum total antioxidant capacity (TAC) in rats following MTX treatment. The values are expressed as means ± 1SD. * significantly different at ($p < 0.05$) when compared with control group.

Oxidative stress induced by MTX has also been demonstrated in some previous studies. The findings of most previous investigations are in agreement with the findings of the present study. In a study by Elango et al.,[16] plasma MDA was significantly increased ($p < 0.001$) and the activities of plasma SOD, TAC, and serum CAT levels decreased (but not significant) after MTX treatment in psoriasis patients. WANG et al.,[7] in their

study, demonstrated that PPE and black bean peel extract, particularly a combination of both can inhibit the pancreas damage due to OS resulting in ameliorating hyperglycemia. Kumar et al.[17] demonstrated that PPE administration can enhance the antioxidant defense against oxidative stress induced by mercuric chloride. In another study, SOD and GPX values were significantly higher, but TAC was significantly lower in MTX-treated animals as compared with the controls ($p < 0.05$).[18] Further, Shema-Didi et al.[19] showed that one-year pomegranate juice (PJ) intake decreased oxidative stress and inflammation in hemodialysis patients. While Faria et al.[20] demonstrated the protective effect of PJ against systemic oxidative stress in mice. In their study, SOD, GPx, and CAT activities were found to be decreased by PJ treatment.

In the present study, the administration of MTX with PSE or PPE, surprisingly, increased the serum MDA levels as compared with MTX alone and control group (Figure 5). On the other hand, PSE (but not PPE) administration significantly decreased serum GPx and increased MDA levels as compared with the control group. This indicates that PSE may induce oxidative stress alone.

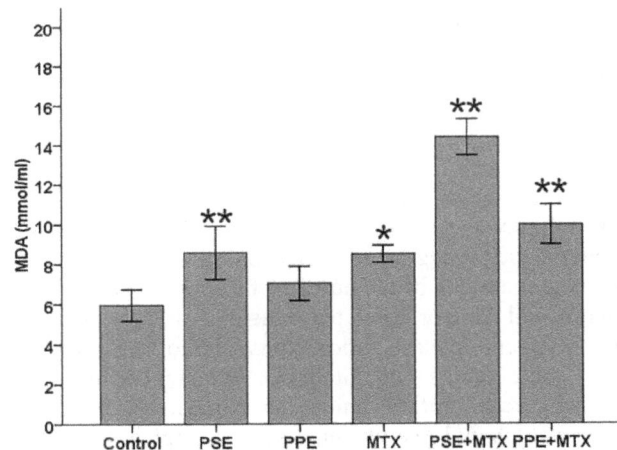

Figure 5. Effects of pomegranate seed extract (PSE) and pomegranate peel extract (PPE) on blood serum malondialdehyde (MDA) in rats following MTX treatment. The values are expressed as means ± 1SD. * and ** significantly different when compared with the control group ($p < 0.05$ and $p < 0.01$, respectively).

On the other hand, the present findings showed a significant decrease in TC, HDL, and LDL in the MTX treated group as compared with the control group. TC, HDL, and LDL levels elevated to normal control levels and more after treatment with MTX+PSE or MTX+PPE. Unpredictably, MTX+SPE treatment caused significant enhancement in serum TG and LDL levels ($p < 0.01$), and MTX+PPE treatment caused significant decrease in serum HDL level ($p < 0.05$) as compared with the control group (Table 2).

The results of this study are in accordance with reports of some previous studies, but some contradict our findings regarding serum lipid profile. In line with the findings of this study, Kilic et al.[21] showed that the serum concentrations of TC, HDL, and LDL decreased significantly after MTX treatment. In a study performed by Chen et al.,[22] no significant differences in lipid profiles and blood lipids were observed between MTX treated and non-treated subjects. Shema-Didi et al.[19] found no significant difference in TC, LDL, HDL, and triglycerides between the PJ and the placebo groups of hemodialysis patients. However, as reported by Navarro-Millán et al.,[23] the TC, the mean HDL, and mean LDL levels were increased in MTX-treated rheumatoid arthritis patients as compared with the baseline, but the ratio of TC to HDL-cholesterol was decreased. Saiki et al.,[24] in their study, found that TC and TG levels were elevated after MTX treatment. Some previous studies have demonstrated that pomegranate fights cardiovascular disease by different mechanisms such as reducing oxidative stress, inhibiting the oxidation of potentially harmful LDL, and quenching free radicals.[1]

Our findings of PSE and PPE analysis showed considerable antioxidant activity, total phenolic, and total flavonoid contents (Table 1). Poly-phenols are the major class of phytochemicals in pomegranate fruit and reportedly have antioxidant activity in vivo and in vitro. The antioxidant activity of dietary polyphenols include reactive species scavenging, enzyme modulation to interfere with cell signaling, and oxidative stability.[1] PJ is a major source of soluble polyphenols such as gallic acid, ellagic acid, punicalagin and quercetin.[25] Further, a research has demonstrated that polyphenols possess powerful antioxidant properties, which represent the most likely mechanism responsible for the protective benefits of pomegranate.[8] The antioxidant capacity of pomegranate has been shown to be 3 times higher than that of red wine or green tea infusion.[26] PPE is also rich in polyphenolic class antioxidants, including flavonoids like gallotannins, ellagitannins, ellagic, ferulic and gallagic acids, anthocyanins, quercetins, and catechins. The polyphenols show important biological activities including oxidation inhibition, free radical elimination, and reducing the risks of cardio-vascular diseases.[7] It seems that ellagitannins may be responsible for the anti-mutagenic and the promising antioxidant activities of PPE. PPE exhibits strong antioxidant activities.[7]

Conclusion
The results of this study showed the protective effects of PSE and PPE against MTX-induced serum oxidative stress (SOD and GPx) and lipid profile (TC, HDL, and LDL) changes in rats. The findings of this study also showed considerable antioxidant activity, total phenolic, and total flavonoid contents of PSE and PPE. However, further studies are needed to investigate the mechanisms of oxidative stress induction and protection, some un-expected results, and the controversies associated with previous studies.

Acknowledgments
The authors appreciate the members of the Drug Applied Research Center and Student Research Committee of Tabriz University of Medical Sciences (Tabriz, Iran) for their instrumental and financial support.

Conflict of Interest
The authors declare no conflict of interests.

References
1. Gouda M, Moustafa A, Hussein L, Hamza M. Three week dietary intervention using apricots, pomegranate juice or/and fermented sour sobya and impact on biomarkers of antioxidative activity, oxidative stress and erythrocytic glutathione transferase activity among adults. Nutr J 2016;15(1):52. doi: 10.1186/s12937-016-0173-x
2. Czerska M, Mikolajewska K, Zielinski M, Gromadzinska J, Wasowicz W. Today's oxidative stress markers. Med Pr 2015;66(3):393-405. doi: 10.13075/mp.5893.00137
3. Chan ES, Cronstein BN. Mechanisms of action of methotrexate. Bull Hosp Jt Dis 2013;71 Suppl 1:S5-8.
4. Braun J, Rau R. An update on methotrexate. Curr Opin Rheumatol 2009;21(3):216-23. doi: 10.1097/BOR.0b013e328329c79d
5. Jahovic N, Cevik H, Sehirli AO, Yegen BC, Sener G. Melatonin prevents methotrexate-induced hepatorenal oxidative injury in rats. J Pineal Res 2003;34(4):282-7.
6. Coomes E, Chan ES, Reiss AB. Methotrexate in atherogenesis and cholesterol metabolism. Cholesterol 2011;2011:503028. doi: 10.1155/2011/503028
7. Wang JY, Zhu C, Qian TW, Guo H, Wang DD, Zhang F, et al. Extracts of black bean peel and pomegranate peel ameliorate oxidative stress-induced hyperglycemia in mice. Exp Ther Med 2015;9(1):43-8. doi: 10.3892/etm.2014.2040
8. Braidy N, Selvaraju S, Essa MM, Vaishnav R, Al-Adawi S, Al-Asmi A, et al. Neuroprotective effects of a variety of pomegranate juice extracts against mptp-induced cytotoxicity and oxidative stress in human primary neurons. Oxid Med Cell Longev 2013;2013:685909. doi: 10.1155/2013/685909
9. Spilmont M, Leotoing L, Davicco MJ, Lebecque P, Mercier S, Miot-Noirault E, et al. Pomegranate and its derivatives can improve bone health through decreased inflammation and oxidative stress in an animal model of postmenopausal osteoporosis. Eur J Nutr 2014;53(5):1155-64. doi: 10.1007/s00394-013-0615-6
10. Mesgari Abbasi M, Heidari R, Amini afshari R, Zakeri milani P, Ghamarzad Shishavan N. Effects of pomegranate seed methanolic extract on

methotrexate-induced changes in rat liver antioxidant compounds. *Curr Top Nutraceutr* 2015;13(3):153-9.

11. Ghasemi Pirbalouti A, Siahpoosh A, Setayesh M, Craker L. Antioxidant activity, total phenolic and flavonoid contents of some medicinal and aromatic plants used as herbal teas and condiments in iran. *J Med Food* 2014;17(10):1151-7. doi: 10.1089/jmf.2013.0057

12. Vador N, Vador B, Hole R. Simple spectrophotometric methods for standardizing ayurvedic formulation. *Indian J Pharm Sci* 2012;74(2):161-3. doi: 10.4103/0250-474X.103852

13. Modaresi A, Nafar M, Sahraei Z. Oxidative stress in chronic kidney disease. *Iran J Kidney Dis* 2015;9(3):165-79.

14. de Andrade KQ, Moura FA, dos Santos JM, de Araujo OR, de Farias Santos JC, Goulart MO. Oxidative stress and inflammation in hepatic diseases: Therapeutic possibilities of n-acetylcysteine. *Int J Mol Sci* 2015;16(12):30269-308. doi: 10.3390/ijms161226225

15. Otunctemur A, Ozbek E, Cakir SS, Polat EC, Dursun M, Cekmen M, et al. Pomegranate extract attenuates unilateral ureteral obstruction-induced renal damage by reducing oxidative stress. *Urol Ann* 2015;7(2):166-71. doi: 10.4103/0974-7796.150488

16. Elango T, Dayalan H, Gnanaraj P, Malligarjunan H, Subramanian S. Impact of methotrexate on oxidative stress and apoptosis markers in psoriatic patients. *Clin Exp Med* 2014;14(4):431-7. doi: 10.1007/s10238-013-0252-7

17. Kumar D, Singh S, Singh AK, Rizvi SI. Pomegranate (punica granatum) peel extract provides protection against mercuric chloride-induced oxidative stress in wistar strain rats. *Pharm Biol* 2013;51(4):441-6. doi: 10.3109/13880209.2012.738333

18. Al-Saleh E, Al-Harmi J, Nandakumaran M, Al-Shammari M, Al-Jassar W. Effect of methotrexate administration on status of some essential trace elements and antioxidant enzymes in pregnant rats in late gestation. *Gynecol Endocrinol* 2009;25(12):816-22. doi: 10.3109/09513590903056811

19. Shema-Didi L, Kristal B, Ore L, Shapiro G, Geron R, Sela S. Pomegranate juice intake attenuates the increase in oxidative stress induced by intravenous iron during hemodialysis. *Nutr Res* 2013;33(6):442-6. doi: 10.1016/j.nutres.2013.04.004

20. Faria A, Monteiro R, Mateus N, Azevedo I, Calhau C. Effect of pomegranate (punica granatum) juice intake on hepatic oxidative stress. *Eur J Nutr* 2007;46(5):271-8. doi: 10.1007/s00394-007-0661-z

21. Kilic S, Emre S, Metin A, Isikoglu S, Erel O. Effect of the systemic use of methotrexate on the oxidative stress and paraoxonase enzyme in psoriasis patients. *Arch Dermatol Res* 2013;305(6):495-500. doi: 10.1007/s00403-013-1366-1

22. Chen DY, Chih HM, Lan JL, Chang HY, Chen WW, Chiang EP. Blood lipid profiles and peripheral blood mononuclear cell cholesterol metabolism gene expression in patients with and without methotrexate treatment. *BMC Med* 2011;9:4. doi: 10.1186/1741-7015-9-4

23. Navarro-Millan I, Charles-Schoeman C, Yang S, Bathon JM, Bridges SL, Jr., Chen L, et al. Changes in lipoproteins associated with methotrexate or combination therapy in early rheumatoid arthritis: Results from the treatment of early rheumatoid arthritis trial. *Arthritis Rheum* 2013;65(6):1430-8. doi: 10.1002/art.37916

24. Saiki O, Takao R, Naruse Y, Kuhara M, Imai S, Uda H. Infliximab but not methotrexate induces extra-high levels of vldl-triglyceride in patients with rheumatoid arthritis. *J Rheumatol* 2007;34(10):1997-2004.

25. Rom O, Volkova N, Nandi S, Jelinek R, Aviram M. Pomegranate juice polyphenols induce macrophage death via apoptosis as opposed to necrosis induced by free radical generation: A central role for oxidative stress. *J Cardiovasc Pharmacol* 2016;68(2):106-14. doi: 10.1097/FJC.0000000000000391

26. Tapias V, Cannon JR, Greenamyre JT. Pomegranate juice exacerbates oxidative stress and nigrostriatal degeneration in parkinson's disease. *Neurobiol Aging* 2014;35(5):1162-76. doi: 10.1016/j.neurobiolaging.2013.10.077

Evaluation of the Effect of Psyllium on the Viability of *Lactobacillus Acidophilus* in Alginate-Polyl Lysine Beads

Jaleh Esmaeilzadeh[1], Hossein Nazemiyeh[1], Maryam Maghsoodi[1]*, Farzaneh Lotfipour[1,2]*

[1] *Faculty of Pharmacy, Tabriz University of Medical Sciences, Tabriz, Iran.*
[2] *Gastrointestinal and Liver Disease Research Center, Tabriz University of Medical Sciences, Tabriz, Iran.*

Article info

Keywords:
· Lactobacillus acidophilus
· Alginate
· Psyllium
· Poly-L-Lysine
· Coating

Abstract

Purpose: Psyllium seeds are used in traditional herbal medicine to treat various disorders. Moreover, as a soluble fiber, psyllium has potential to stimulate bacterial growth in digestive system. We aimed to substitute alkali-extractable polysaccharides of psyllium for alginate in beads with second coat of poly-l-lysine to coat *Lactobacillus acidophilus*.

Methods: Beads were prepared using extrusion technique. Poly-l-lysine as second coat was incorporated on optimum alginate/psyllium beads using immersion technique. Beads were characterized in terms of size, encapsulation efficiency, integrity and bacterial survival in harsh conditions.

Results: Beads with narrow size distribution ranging from 1.85 ± 0.05 to 2.40 ± 0.18 mm with encapsulation efficiency higher than 96% were achieved. Psyllium concentrations in beads did not produce constant trend in bead sizes. Surface topography by SEM showed that substitution of psyllium enhanced integrity of obtained beads. Psyllium successfully protected the bacteria against acidic condition and lyophilization equal to alginate in the beads. Better survivability with beads of alginate/psyllium-poly-l-lysine was achieved with around 2 log rise in bacterial count in acid condition compared to the corresponding single coat beads.

Conclusion: Alginate/psyllium (1:2) beads with narrow size distribution and high encapsulation efficiency of the bacteria have been achieved. Presence of psyllium produced a much smoother and integrated surface texture for the beads with sufficient protection of the bacteria against acidic condition as much as alginate. Considering the health benefits of psyllium and its prebiotic activity, psyllium can be beneficially replaced in part for alginate in probiotic coating.

Introduction

Probiotics are defined as live microorganisms, which when administrated in sufficient dosage give one or more specific health benefits for the host.[1] The most significant role of probiotics in health system can be their function to maintain normal intestinal microflora and defense against enteropathogen infections. Furthermore beneficial microorganisms have been shown to control the cholesterol levels of serum, improve utilization of lactose in lactose maldigesters, and have anticarcinogenic and antimutagenic activities.[2] However, probiotics to show their potential abilities need to survive in the challenging conditions of gastrointestinal tract colonize and multiply on the epithelium of colon in appropriate population (more than 10^7 cfu/g of finished product). To improve viability and stability of probiotics and efficient delivery of the cells to their active sites, a number of techniques have been utilized including encapsulation of probiotics in a variety of polymers.[3] Alginate, a commonly used polymer to encapsulate probiotics, is a natural, biocompatible and biodegradable

linear anionic polysaccharide. Alginate beads encapsulating bacteria in their matrix can be prepared by using extrusion or emulsion techniques.[4,5]

Herbal medicine has been commonly used over the years for treatment and prevention of diseases.[6,7] Psyllium is generally referred to seeds from some members of plants genus *Plantago* including but not limited to *Plantago ovata, Plantago psyllium, and Plantago indica*. It is native plant to Indian subcontinent and Iran, although psyllium is now commercially cultivated in many parts of the world.[8] Psyllium composed of a highly branched arabinoxylan forming gel mucilage. It is structurally consists of xylose units with arabinose and xylose in the side chains.[9] Psyllium seeds are primarily used in traditional herbal medicine to treat various disorders and some of its claimed health benefits have been scientifically approved now. There are several reports regarding the application of psyllium for treatment of constipation, diarrhea, irritable bowel syndrome, inflammatory bowel disease, ulcerative colitis, colon cancer, diabetes, and hypercholesterolemia.[8,10,11] Moreover, psyllium as a soluble fiber with the potential to stimulate bacterial growth in digestive system has been used as prebiotic.[12-14] Prebiotics are defined as "non-digestible food ingredients that beneficially affects the host by selectively stimulating the growth and/or activity of one or a limited number of bacteria in the colon, and thus improves host health".[15]

Considering the health benefits of psyllium in digestive system and its prebiotic activity, we have successfully incorporated psyllium (up to 0.5% w/v) in alginate beads containing probiotic bacteria *Lactobacillus acidophilus* in our previous work.[4] In the current study, we aimed to prepare alginate beads with maximum possible concentration of psyllium with a second layer of poly l lysine on top to improve the stability and protective capability. The physicochemical properties and viability of the bacteria in the prepared beads after exposing to acid, bile and freeze drying conditions were evaluated.

Materials and Methods
Materials
L. acidophilus was obtained from Pasteur institute (Iran), sodium alginate, poly l lysine, oxgall from Sigma-Aldrich (Germany), MRS broth and MRS agar, sodium hydrogen phosphate, calcium chloride, sodium hydroxide and hydrochloric acid from Merck (Germany), and psyllium seed husk was supplied from company Herbi Darou Tabriz-Iran.

Methods
Preparation of inoculum
L. acidophilus was cultured in MRS broth at 37°C for 18 h. Culture was harvested by centrifugation at 3000 rpm at 4°C for 7min and washed twice with saline and collected by centrifugation as above. The washed bacterial cells were resuspended in 7 mL saline, and the cell count was determined using pour plate technique in MRS agar in triplicate. The cell suspension was divided in some equal parts and consequently was used to prepare different formulations.[16]

Extraction of psyllium
Gel-forming fraction of the alkali-extractable polysaccharides of psyllium seed was extracted by a method described by[17] with some modifications which is depicted in Figure 1. First, 30 g of whole psyllium seed was grinded and then dispersed in 1000 mL water and placed it over night at 80°C water bath which led to swelling and gel formation. The gel phase was separated from solution and dissolved in 2 M NaOH solution at room temperature for 2 h; alkaline extract was separated from the residue by centrifugation (12000 rpm for 1h) and accordingly neutralized with 2 M HCl. During the neutralization, gel-like white precipitate was produced and separated by centrifugation (12000 rpm for 1 h) from the soluble fraction and washed three times with distilled water. The gel precipitate was evaporated for 3 h and then dried at 40°C oven for 48 h and after grinding

was used for beads preparation. The photographs of the extraction process are shown in Figures 1 and 2.

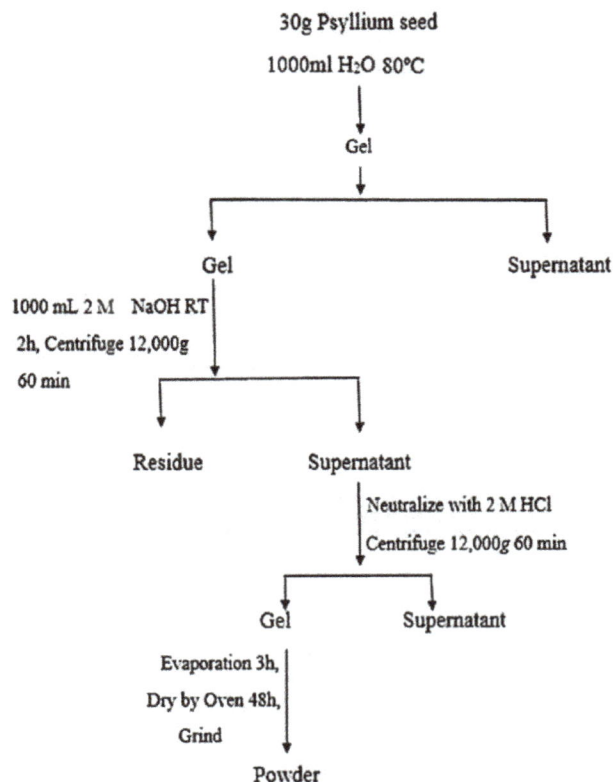

Figure1. Diagram of psyllium gel extraction process.

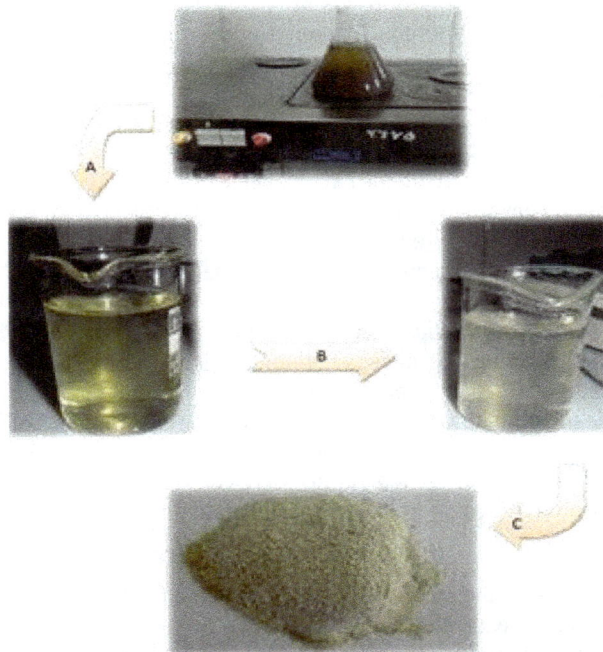

Figure 2. Procedure of psyllium gel extraction. A) psyllium gel and seed were separated from supernatant. NaOH was added to dissolve psyllium gel; alkaline solution was separated from the residue by centrifugation. B) Alkaline solution was neutralized by HCl 2M. C) White gel was harvested by centrifugation from supernatant; dried and grinded.

Preparation of beads

The extrusion technique was used to prepare alginate and alginate/psyllium beads (Lotfipour et al., 2012). Sodium alginate and psyllium were weighted, added to distilled water in different ratios and sterilized by steam at 121°C for15 min. The cooled alginate or alginate/psyllium gels (4.5 mL) were mixed with bacterial inoculum and gently stirred for 30 min to obtain a homogeneous suspension. The suspensions were extruded drop wise through a 27 gage nozzle into sterile hardening solution (CaCl₂) under shaking at 250 rpm for 15 min. The obtained beads were isolated, washed twice with sterile water, and kept in 0.5% w/v peptone solution at 4°C. Poly-l-lysine–(0.5% w/v) as the second coat was incorporated on the surface of the selective formulation, using immersion technique. The compositions of prepared formulations are shown in Table 1.

Table 1. Compositions of the studied formulation.

Formulation	Alginate/Psyllium (Total polymer 2.5% w/v)	CaCl2 (%w/v)
A1	3:0	2
A2	3:0	4
A3	3:0	6
A4	2:1	2
A5	2:1	4
A6	2:1	6
A7	1:2	2
A8	1:2	4
A9	1:2	6

Size and topographic analysis

The particle size of beads was assessed using optical microscopy (Dinolite, Taiwan) by scion image analyzer software. Data were collected from 50 beads in each sample, and mean particle size was reported. The topographical properties of prepared beads were investigated by scanning electron microscopy (SEM) (Philipse XL30, Holland) at an accelerating voltage of 20 KV. Prior to examination, samples were prepared on aluminum stubs and coated with gold under argon atmosphere by means of a sputter coater.

Encapsulation efficiency

To determine the encapsulation efficiency (EE), firstly prepared beads were mechanically disintegrated in phosphate buffer (pH = 6.8), then the number of entrapped cells after adequate dilution were measured by pour plate method, and counts were expressed as number of colony forming units (CFU), and calculated as:

$$EE= (Log_{10}N /Log_{10} N_0)$$

Where N is the number of viable entrapped cells released from the beads and N_0 is the number of free cells added to the biopolymer mixture immediately before the production procedure.

Viability of encapsulated and Free L. acidophilus at acid Condition

Acid conditions were produced using 50 mL of 14.91

g/L potassium chloride and 3.0 g/L of pepsin and pH adjusted to 2 with hydrochloric acid (Chávarri et al., 2010). 100 mg beads with entrapped bacteria or 1 mL of cell suspension were mixed in 10 mL of acid solution and incubated for 2 h at 37°C with constant agitation at 50 rpm. After incubation, beads were disintegrated in phosphate buffer (pH = 6.8), then 1.0 mL aliquot of the mixture removed and assayed using pour plate method. The survival (%) of the bacteria was calculated as follows:

%Survival= (log CFU/g beads after 2 h exposure to acidic condition/log CFU/g beads initial count) ×100

Viability of encapsulated and free L. acidophilus at bile salt condition

100 mg beads with entrapped bacteria or 1 mL of cell suspension were mixed in 10 mL of Bill condition containing 2% w/v oxgall for 2 h at 37°C with constant agitation at 50 rpm. After incubation, beads were disintegrated in phosphate buffer (pH = 6.8), samples were then taken, and bacterial growth was assayed using pour plate method.[18]

Incorporation poly l lysine as second coat

Selective formulation was washed by using sterile peptone. Poly l lysine (0.05% w/v) as a second coat was incorporated on the surface of alginate/psyllium beads using immersion technique. Hence, beads were dipped in poly l lysine (0.05% w/v) on stirrer at 250 rpm for 30 min.

Lyophilization of the prepared beads

Selective formulations were dipped in sucrose 10% and freezed for 24 h at -80°C. Accordingly, the samples were lyophilized using suction and second drying in a lyophilizer.

Statistical analyses

Statistical testing was carried out using SPSS19. All of the experiments were performed in triplicates. Data are presented as mean±SD. The One-Way ANOVA test was performed to assess the differences between beads and control groups and $P<0.05$ considered as a statistically significant difference.

Results
Characterization of prepared beads

Beads with different ratios of alginate: psyllium (3:0, 2:1, 1:2) and CaCl₂ as hardening solution (2, 4 and 6% w/v) were prepared. Table 2 shows the results for diameters and encapsulation efficiencies of the prepared beads. As can be seen, beads with narrow size distribution ranging from 1.85 ± 0.05 to 2.40 ± 0.18 mm were achieved. The initial *L. acidophilus* count in the inoculum and polymers mix used for bead preparation was 9 ± 0.01 log CFU/mL. The bacterial counts in the prepared beads showed more than 96% encapsulation efficiency of the method.

Table 2. Size, encapsulation efficiency, and % survival in acid condition of prepared formulation

Formulation	Diameter (mm)	Encapsulation efficiency (%)	Count (CFU/g) after acid exposure	Count (CFU/g) after bile exposure
A1	2.09±0.18	98.1 ±3.4	5.8 ± 0.4	8.6±0.3
A2	1.92±0.10	96.6± 5.7	5.6 ± 0.8	8.4±0.4
A3	1.96±0.15	98 ±3.5	5.5 ± 0.3	8.5±0.3
A4	2.03±0.09	97.4 ±2.6	5.4 ± 0.8	8.6±0.3
A5	1.85±0.05	99.5±0.8	5.5 ± 0.4	8.5±0.8
A6	1.92±0.12	98.5 ± 2.6	5.2 ± 0.1	8.5±0.5
A7	2.04±0.19	99.7 ± 0.5	5.9 ± 0.5	8.6±0.6
A8	2.23±0.15	99.8 ± 0.17	5.4 ± 0.2	8.9±0.1
A9	2.40±0.18	99.6 ± 1.1	5.5 ± 0.2	8.4±0.5
Untreated cells*	-	-	3.01 ± 0.068	8.4±0.1

* Initial count: 9 ± 0.01 Log CFU/mL

SEM images of the beads showed wrinkle beads (×90, Figure 3a), with rough and approximately porous surface characteristics (×2000, Figure 3c). On the other hand, it can be seen in Figures 3b and 3d that incorporation of psyllium resulted in more wrinkle appearance in lower resolutions (×90) (Figure 3b) and smoother and integrated beads (×2000) than their alginate counterparts (Figure 3d).

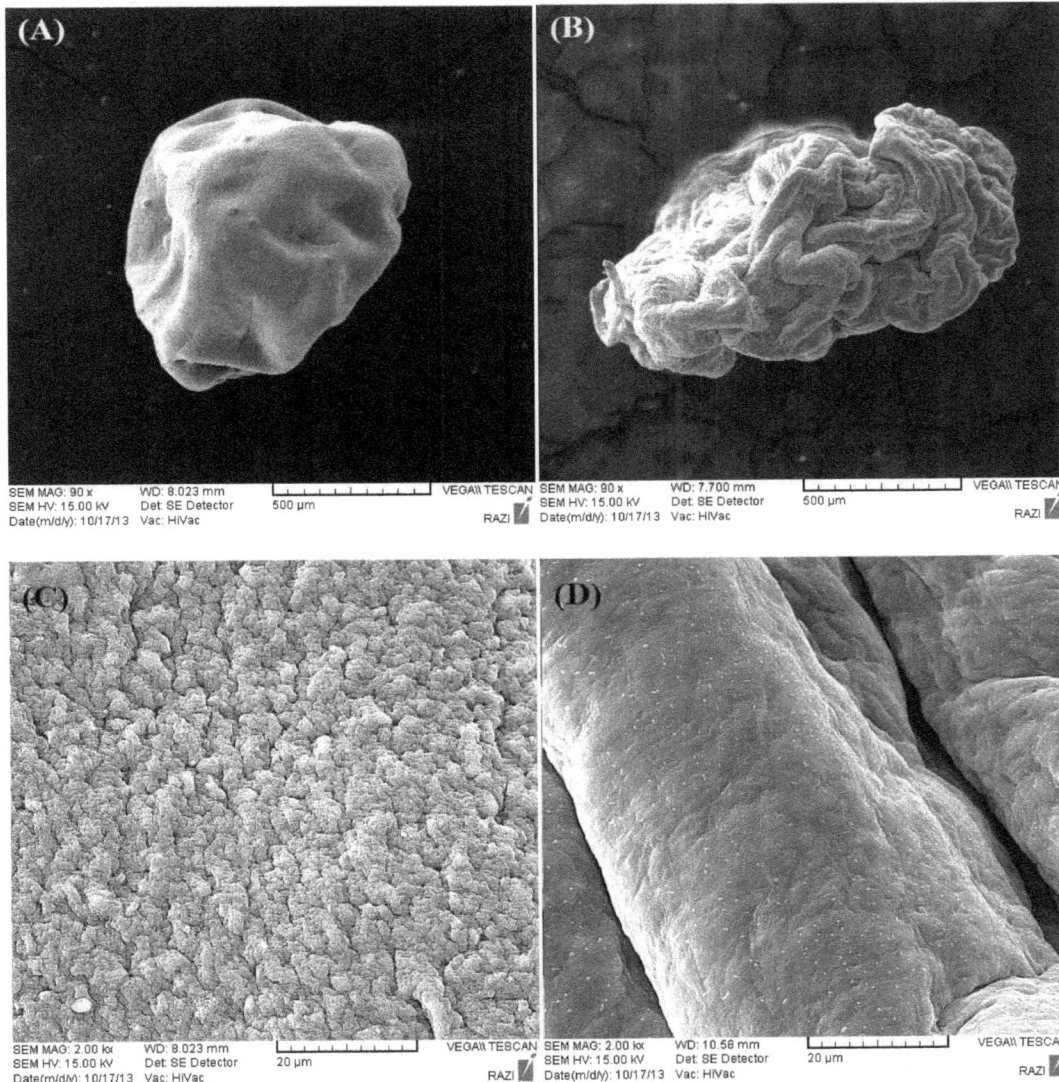

Figure 3. SEM pictures of A1(a) and A9(b) beads at a magnification of 90x , A1(c) and A4(d) at 2000x.

Viability of untreated and encapsulated bacteria in acid conditions

The protective effects of different coats of alginate and alginate/psyllium after 2 h exposure to acid conditions (pH=2) are compared to untreated bacteria, and results are expressed as log CFU/g in Table 2 and %survival in Figure 4.

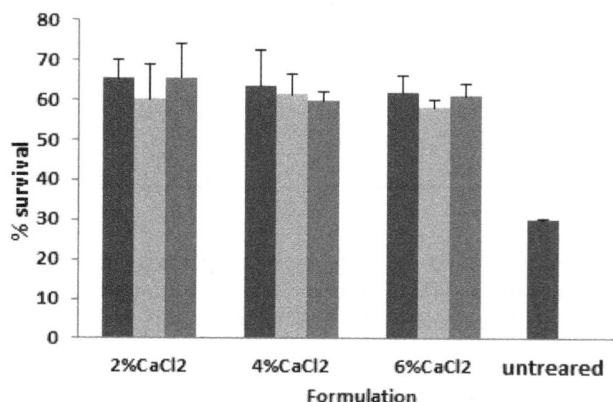

Figure 4. Percent of bacterial survival in the prepared beads after 2h acid exposure;
■: ALG; ■: ALG:PSL (2:1); ■: ALG:PSL (1:2)

As can be seen from Table 2, the initial inoculum count of untreated *L. acidophilus* was 9 ± 0.01 Log CFU/g which declined to 3.01 ± 0.068 Log CFU/g after acid exposure for 2 h (around 33% survival). On the other hand, in our prepared beads with the initial bacterial numbers of 9 ± 0.01 Log CFU/g, after 2 h acid exposure, the counts were 5.2 ± 0.15 to 5.9 ± 0.46 Log CFU/g indicating more than 58% survival in all the formulations.

Moreover, the effect of 2 h exposure to acid condition (pH=2) on the survival of *L. acidophilus* encapsulated in A8 with a second coat of poly l lysine (nominated as P8) are expressed as Log CFU/g and % survival in Table 3.

Table 3. % survival in acid condition of A8 and P8

Formulation	Count (CFU/g) after acid exposure	%Survival
A8	5.4±0.2	59.6±2.6
P8	7.5±0.3	83.3±1.2

Initial count: 9 ± 0.01 Log CFU/mL

Viability of untreated and Encapsulated Bacteria at High Bile Salt Concentration

The effect of 2 h exposure to 2% w/v oxgall on the survival of untreated *L. acidophilus* and in the prepared beads is demonstrated in Figure 5 and Table 2 as well. According to our results, viability of *L. acidophilus* after bile exposure was more than 90% in the case of untreated bacteria. Furthermore, the viability of the bacteria in all prepared beads was not significantly (*P*>0.05) different from those of untreated bacteria.

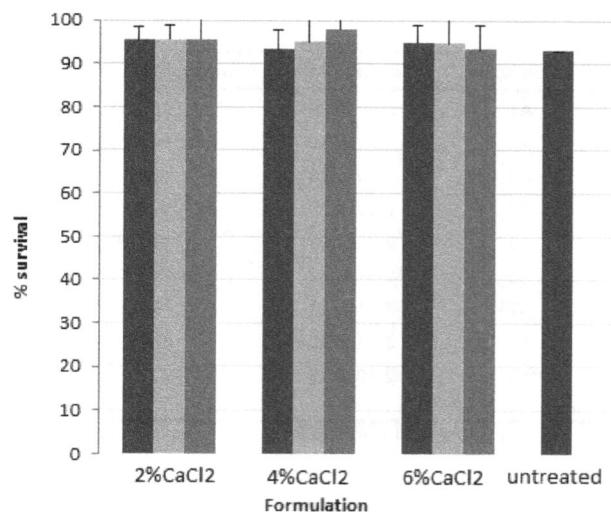

Figure 5. Percent of bacterial survival in the prepared beads after 2h bile exposure
■: ALG; ■: ALG:PSL (2:1); ■: ALG:PSL (1:2)

Effect of lyophilization in survival of L. acidophilus

A2, A5 and A8 beads with alginate/psyllium ratios of 3:0, 2:1 and 1:2 respectively and equal cross linker concentrations were subjected to lyophilization and the survival of the bacteria in the lyophilized beads were investigated. The results are expressed as log CFU/g and % survival in Table 4. According to the results, 2 log declines in bacterial count were observed. Our finding also concurs with the previous studies.[19]

Table 4. Viability of the bacteria before and after lyophilization

Formulation	Count (CFU/g) Before lyophilization	Count (CFU/g) After lyophilization	%survival
A2	10.0±0.1	8.0±0.1	80
A5	8.9±0.2	7.2±0.2	80.9
A8	8.8±0.3	7.3±0.1	82.9

Discussion

In the present study, we aimed to prepare alginate beads with maximum possible concentration of psyllium with a second layer of poly l lysine on top to protect the probiotic bacteria and to use the beneficial properties of psyllium as well.

According to ficsher et al. the extraction yield of alkali-extractable polysaccharides of psyllium was higher. Furthermore alkali-extractable polysaccharides of psyllium seem to have more potential for gel forming with Cacl2. Hence we used alkali-extractable polysaccharides of psyllium in this work.[9]

In the formulation experiments, total polymer concentration was selected to be 2.5% w/v according to our previous study.[4] Beads with narrow size distribution ranging from 1.85 ± 0.05 to 2.40 ± 0.18 mm were achieved. Inclusion of psyllium in different ratios or using of different concentrations of CaCl$_2$ as crosslinker, produced no constant trend in the sizes of obtained beads.

The results pertaining to EE indicated that more than

96% of cells were successfully entrapped in the beads. The obtained high EE indicated that there was no considerable loss of viability in the process of beads preparation, confirming the gentle propriety of the applied method.[20] Furthermore, there were no significant differences ($P>0.05$) regarding the EE between different formulations.

The rough and approximately porous surface characteristics of alginate beads shown in SEM pictures is in good agreement with the other studies which can be explained by the egg-box structure of calcium alginate beads.[21-24] Alginate is able to form gel by reaction with divalent cations such as Ca^{2+}. Gelation of alginate is mainly achieved by the exchange of Na^+ from the guluronic acids with Ca^{2+}, and stacking of these guluronic groups to form the characteristic egg-box structure. The Ca^{2+} binds to the α-L guluronic acid blocks in a highly cooperative manner and the size of the cooperative unit is more than 20 monomers. Each alginate chain dimerizes to form junctions with many other chains and accordingly gel networks are formed.[25,26]

According to our results, substitution of psyllium in the bead formulations (Figure 3d) gives a smoother surface to the beads. It can be assumable that psyllium gel as a cement like agent may fill the cracks and pores of the calcium alginate egg-box structure and can enhance the apparent integrity of the beads surface.

Based on the results shown in Table 2, it is clear that count of survived bacteria after acid exposure, in all prepared beads were significantly ($P<0.05$) higher than those of untreated bacteria. In fact, 6 log reductions in bacterial count in the case of untreated *L. acidophilus* decreased to 3 log reduction among bacteria encapsulated in the beads, and it can be concluded that coating of the bacteria as alginate or alginate/psyllium beads can improve the viability of *L. acidophilus* in acid conditions. This is in line with the previous studies for the probiotic encapsulation[27,28] Furthermore, replacement of alginate by psyllium, produced no significant changes in the bacterial viability ($P>0.05$) indicating an equal level of protection for the bacteria by using alginate/psyllium in comparison with alginate alone (Figure 4).

On the other hand, 2 h exposure to 2% w/v oxgall results in no significant difference in the case of untreated bacteria and bacteria encapsulated in the beads ($P>0.05$) indicating high resistance of our species against bile condition. The intrinsic resistance of *L. acidophilus* against bile condition has been reported previously.[29]

To evaluate the effect of second coat of poly l lysine, an optimum single coat formulation was selected. As the viability of the bacteria in acid and bile conditions were not significantly different between the formulations, the criteria for the selection of optimum formulation was based on the maximum replacement of alginate with psyllium (A7, A8 and A9). Among them A8 with 4% CaCl and maximum stability was chosen and subjected for incorporation of the second coat of poly l lysine by

immersion technique and nominated as P8. The results of 2 h exposure to acid condition showed a better survivability with P8, as around 2 log rise was observed in bacterial count among P8 beads in comparison with A8 beads. It can be concluded that coating of the bacteria as alginate/psyllium-poly l lysine beads can improve the viability of *L. acidophilus* in harsh conditions. Better protection of live bacteria in double and triple coated beads compared to single one has been shown by other studies. Thickening of the protection layer and lowering the porosity of the obtained beads resulted in production of more stable and integrated beads. Incorporation of poly l lysine on the alginate beads as the second layer and its effectiveness in the probiotics coating has also been studied.[30]

Conclusion

In the present study, replacement of alginate by psyllium in high ratio (alginate/psyllium 1:2) for encapsulation of *L. acidophilus* was carried out. Alginate/psyllium Beads with narrow size distribution and high encapsulation efficiency of the bacteria have been achieved. Presence of psyllium in the prepared beads produced a much smoother and integrated surface texture than alginate. Moreover, psyllium sufficiently protected the bacteria against acidic condition as much as alginate. Considering the pharmacological benefits of psyllium in gastrointestinal system and its prebiotic activity, it can be beneficially replaced in part for alginate in probiotic coating.

Conflict of Interest

The authors declare that there is no conflict of interests regarding the publication of this article.

References

1. Pineiro M, Stanton C. Probiotic bacteria: Legislative framework-- requirements to evidence basis. *J Nutr* 2007;137(3 Suppl 2):850S-3S.
2. Huq T, Khan A, Khan RA, Riedl B, Lacroix M. Encapsulation of probiotic bacteria in biopolymeric system. *Crit Rev Food Sci Nutr* 2013;53(9):909-16. doi: 10.1080/10408398.2011.573152
3. Kailasapathy K. Microencapsulation of probiotic bacteria: Technology and potential applications. *Curr Issues Intest Microbiol* 2002;3(2):39-48.
4. Lotfipour F, Mirzaeei S, Maghsoodi M. Preparation and characterization of alginate and psyllium beads containing lactobacillus acidophilus. *Sci World J* 2012;2012:680108. doi: 10.1100/2012/680108
5. Lotfipour F, Mirzaeei S, Maghsoodi M. Evaluation of the effect of cacl2 and alginate concentrations and hardening time on the characteristics of lactobacillus acidophilus loaded alginate beads using response surface analysis. *Adv Pharm Bull* 2012;2(1):71-8. doi: 10.5681/apb.2012.010

6. Nazemiyeh H, Lotfipoor F, Delazar A, Razavi SM, Asnaashari S, Kasebi N, et al. *Chemical composition, and antibacterial and free-radical- scavenging activities of the essential oils of a citronellol producing new chemotype of Thymus pubescens Boiss. & Kotschy ex Celak. Rec Nat Prod* 2011;5(3):184-92.

7. Khodaie L, Delazar A, Lotfipour F, Nazemiyeh H. Antioxidant and antimicrobial activity of pedicularis sibthorpii boiss. And pedicularis wilhelmsiana fisch ex. *Adv Pharm Bull* 2012;2(1):89-92. doi: 10.5681/apb.2012.012

8. Yu LL, Lutterodt H, Cheng Z. Beneficial health properties of psyllium and approaches to improve its functionalities. *Adv Food Nutr Res* 2009;55:193-220. doi: 10.1016/S1043-4526(08)00404-X

9. Fischer MH, Yu N, Gray GR, Ralph J, Anderson L, Marlett JA. The gel-forming polysaccharide of psyllium husk (plantago ovata forsk). *Carbohydr Res* 2004;339(11):2009-17. doi: 10.1016/j.carres.2004.05.023

10. Marlett JA, Fischer MH. The active fraction of psyllium seed husk. *Proc Nutr Soc* 2003;62(1):207-9.

11. Singh B. Psyllium as therapeutic and drug delivery agent. *Int J Pharm* 2007;334(1-2):1-14. doi: 10.1016/j.ijpharm.2007.01.028

12. Fujimori S, Tatsuguchi A, Gudis K, Kishida T, Mitsui K, Ehara A, et al. High dose probiotic and prebiotic cotherapy for remission induction of active crohn's disease. *J Gastroenterol Hepatol* 2007;22(8):1199-204. doi: 10.1111/j.1440-1746.2006.04535.x

13. Fujimori S, Gudis K, Mitsui K, Seo T, Yonezawa M, Tanaka S, et al. A randomized controlled trial on the efficacy of synbiotic versus probiotic or prebiotic treatment to improve the quality of life in patients with ulcerative colitis. *Nutrition* 2009;25(5):520-5. doi: 10.1016/j.nut.2008.11.017

14. Rishniw M, Wynn SG. Azodyl, a synbiotic, fails to alter azotemia in cats with chronic kidney disease when sprinkled onto food. *J Feline Med Surg* 2011;13(6):405-9. doi: 10.1016/j.jfms.2010.12.015

15. Gibson GR, Roberfroid MB. Dietary modulation of the human colonic microbiota: Introducing the concept of prebiotics. *J Nutr* 1995;125(6):1401-1

16. Farajnia S, Hassan M, Hallaj Nezhadi S, Mohammadnejad L, Milani M, Lotfipour F. Determination of indicator bacteria in pharmaceutical samples by multiplex PCR. *J Rapid Meth Aut Mic* 2009;17(3):328-38.

17. Guo Q, Cui SW, Wang Q, Young JC. Fractionation and physicochemical characterization of psyllium gum. *Carbohyd Polym* 2008;73(1):35-43. doi:10.1016/j.carbpol.2007.11.001

18. Ding WK, Shah NP. An improved method of microencapsulation of probiotic bacteria for their stability in acidic and bile conditions during storage. *J Food Sci* 2009;74(2):M53-61. doi: 10.1111/j.1750-3841.2008.01030.x

19. Bergenholtz AS, Wessman P, Wuttke A, Hakansson S. A case study on stress preconditioning of a lactobacillus strain prior to freeze-drying. *Cryobiology* 2012;64(3):152-9. doi: 10.1016/j.cryobiol.2012.01.002

20. Mokarram RR, Mortazavi SA, Habibi Najafi MB, Shahidi F. The influence of multi stage alginate coating on survivability of potential probiotic bacteria in simulated gastric and intestinal juice. *Food Res Int* 2009;42(8):1040-5. doi:10.1016/j.foodres.2009.04.023

21. Pluemsab W, Fukazawa Y, Furuike T, Nodasaka Y, Sakairi N. Cyclodextrin-linked alginate beads as supporting materials for sphingomonas cloacae, a nonylphenol degrading bacteria. *Bioresour Technol* 2007;98(11):2076-81. doi: 10.1016/j.biortech.2006.08.009

22. Jahan ST, Islam MS, Sadat SMA, Islam MK, Jalil RU, Chowdhury JA. Surface morphology and release behaviors of theophylline loaded sodium alginate gel beads. *Bangl Pharm J* 2010;13(2):41-6

23. Rasel MAT, Hasan M. Formulation and evaluation of floating alginate beads of diclofenac sodium. *Dhaka Univ J Pharm Sci* 2012;11(1):29-35. doi: 10.3329/dujps.v11i1.12484

24. Tzu TW, Tsuritani T, Sato K. Sorption of Pb (II), Cd (II), and Ni (II) toxic metal ions by alginate-bentonite. *J Environ Prot Ecol* 2013;4(1):51-5. doi: 10.4236/jep.2013.41B010

25. Singhal P, Kumar K, Pandey M, Saraf SA. Evaluation of acyclovir loaded oil entrapped calcium alginate beads prepared by ionotropic gelation method. *Int J Chem Tech Res* 2010;2(4):2076-85.

26. Verma A, Sharma M, Verma N, Pandit JK. Floating alginate beads: studies on formulation factors for improved drug entrapment efficiency and in vitro release. *Farmacia* 2013;61(1):143-61.

27. Pan LX, Fang XJ, Yu Z, Xin Y, Liu XY, Shi LE, et al. Encapsulation in alginate-skim milk microspheres improves viability of lactobacillus bulgaricus in stimulated gastrointestinal conditions. *Int J Food Sci Nutr* 2013;64(3):380-4. doi: 10.3109/09637486.2012.749841

28. Trabelsi I, Bejar W, Ayadi D, Chouayekh H, Kammoun R, Bejar S, et al. Encapsulation in alginate and alginate coated-chitosan improved the survival of newly probiotic in oxgall and gastric juice. *Int J Biol Macromol* 2013;61:36-42. doi: 10.1016/j.ijbiomac.2013.06.035

29. Ruiz L, Margolles A, Sanchez B. Bile resistance mechanisms in lactobacillus and bifidobacterium. *Front Microbiol* 2013;4:396. doi: 10.3389/fmicb.2013.00396

30. Chaikham P, Apichartsrangkoon A, George T, Jirarattanarangsri W. Efficacy of polymer coating of probiotic beads suspended in pressurized and pasteurized longan juices on the exposure to simulated gastrointestinal environment. *Int J Food Sci Nutr* 2013;64(7):862-9. doi: 10.3109/09637486.2013.799124

8

Melanogenesis Inhibitory and Antioxidant Effects of *Camellia oleifera* Seed Oil

Puxvadee Chaikul[1,2]*, Tawanun Sripisut[1,2], Setinee Chanpirom[1,2], Kanchanapa Sathirachawan[1], Naphatsorn Ditthawuthikul[1,2]

[1]*School of Cosmetic Science, Mae Fah Luang University, Chiang Rai 57100, Thailand.*
[2]*Phytocosmetics and Cosmeceuticals Research Group, Mae Fah Luang University, Chiang Rai 57100, Thailand.*

Article info

Keywords:
· Tea seed oil
· Cytotoxicity
· Melanogenesis
· Antioxidant
· Cosmetic

Abstract

Purpose: The study aimed to characterize the fatty acid profile of *Camellia oleifera* (tea) seed oil and evaluate for cytotoxicity and activities on melanogenesis and antioxidant activity assays in order to utilize as the functional oil.

Methods: The fatty acid profile of oil was analyzed by gas chromatography/mass spectrometry (GC/MS). The cytotoxicity was performed by sulforhodamine B (SRB) assay in B16-F10 melanoma cells and 3T3-L1 cells. The melanogenesis assay, including melanin content and activities of tyrosinase and tyrosinase-related protein-2 (TRP-2), and antioxidant activity were evaluated.

Results: Three major fatty acids of oil were oleic acid ($87.93\pm0.19\%$), stearic ($5.14\pm0.06\%$) and palmitic ($5.08\pm0.12\%$) acids. The non-cytotoxicity of 5% tea seed oil demonstrated the cell viabilities of $94.59\pm3.41\%$ in B16-F10 melanoma cells and $97.57\pm1.62\%$ in 3T3-L1 cells. Tea seed oil exhibited the inhibitory activity on melanogenesis assay via inhibition of tyrosinase and TRP-2 activities. The antioxidant activity of 3% tea seed oil appeared the cellular protection with cell viability of $90.38\pm7.77\%$.

Conclusion: The results of study have shown the potential utilization of tea seed oil as the functional oil in several products, including health, food and cosmetic products.

Introduction

Camellia spp., the native plants in Eastern Asia, have been cultivated worldwide and compose more than 200 species.[1] *Camellia oleifera*, a species of tea, is planted for oil-rich seeds. Tea seed oil has reported on several bioactive substances, including fatty acids, polyphenols and sesamin.[2] Due to the presence of variety of different compounds, tea seed oil has adopted to incorporate in health, food and cosmetic products. In the Chinese traditional medicine, tea seed oil has used in regimens for treatment of stomachache and burning injury.[3] The oil has employed as edible oil, because of acceptable taste and abundance of antioxidants. For cosmetics, the oil is the rich source of emollient for cosmetic preparation.[4] However, the study on biological activities of tea seed oil for utilization as the functional agent is limited.

The study aimed to characterize the fatty acid profile of *C. oleifera* seed oil and evaluate for cytotoxicity and activities on melanogenesis and antioxidant activity assays in order to utilize as the functional oil in health, food and cosmetic products.

Materials and Methods

Chemicals and reagents

C. oleifera seed oil was purchased from HallStar Company (Illinois, USA). The other reagents were of analytical grade.

Characterization of fatty acid profile

The fatty acid profile of oil was analyzed by GC/MS. The esterification of oil was prepared and analyzed as previously described.[5]

Cytotoxicity assay

Cytotoxicity assay was performed by SRB assay as previously described.[6]

Melanogenesis assay

Melanogenesis assay, including melanin content, tyrosinase and TRP-2 activities, was performed as previously described.[7]

Antioxidant activity assay

The antioxidant activity assay was performed as previous method.[7]

Statistical analysis

Data were expressed as mean $\pm$ S.E. One way analysis of variance (ANOVA) and LSD test were used to analyze the results at significant level of p-value <0.05.

Results and Discussion

Characterization of fatty acid profile

Table 1 is shown the fatty acid profile of tea seed oil. Three major fatty acids were oleic, stearic, and palmitic acids, respectively. Since triacylglycerols consisted of glycerol and three fatty acids are major components of plant oils, the content and types of fatty acids have been responsible for each plant oil characteristics.[8] The previous studies have been demonstrated the significant correlation of biological activities, including anti-inflammation, wound healing, and moisturizing effect,[9] and the proportion of unsaturated fatty acids in several functional oils.[10,11]

Table 1. Fatty acid profile of tea seed oil

Fatty acid	%
Myristic acid (C14:0)	0.04±0.00
Palmitic acid (C16:0)	5.08±0.12
Margaric acid (C17:0)	0.10±0.00
Stearic acid (C18:0)	5.14±0.06
Arachidic acid (C20:0)	0.34±0.01
Behenic acid (C22:0)	0.92±0.04
Lignoceric acid (C24:0)	0.25±0.01
Palmitoleic acid (C16:1)	0.19±0.02
Oleic acid (C18:1)	87.93±0.19
Linoleic acid (C18:2)	0.10±0.00

Cytotoxicity assay

The cytotoxicity assay of tea seed oil was performed in B16-F10 melanoma cells and 3T3-L1 cells. Figure 1 is shown the cytotoxicity assay of tea seed oil and oleic acid. The cytotoxicity of oil and oleic acid depended on treated concentrations. For B16-F10 melanoma cells, 1-5% tea seed oil and 0.0001-0.01 mg/mL oleic acid gave the greater cell viability than 90%, which indicated the non-cytotoxicity. However, the cell viabilities of 7% tea seed oil and 0.1-1 mg/mL oleic acid decreased to less than 80%, which indicated the cytotoxicity. The non-cytotoxic concentrations of oil and oleic acid were evaluated in 3T3-L1 cells in compared to vitamin C, a positive control in antioxidant activity assay (Figure 1). The cell viabilities of 3T3-L1 cells at non-cytotoxic concentrations of oil and oleic acid, and 0.0001-0.1 mg/mL vitamin C were greater than 85%, whereas 1 mg/mL vitamin C decreased cell viability to 69.38±1.99%.

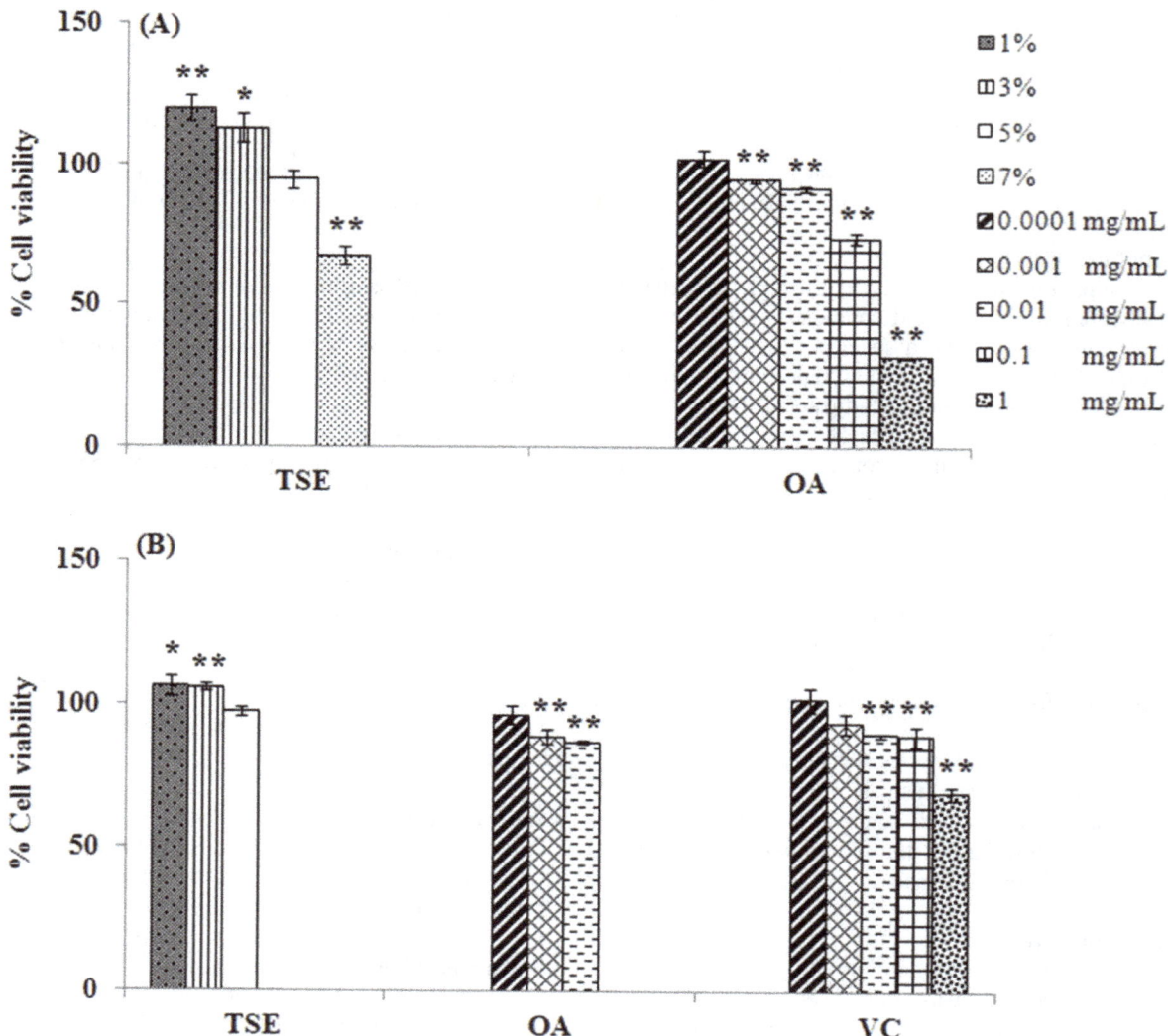

Figure 1. Cytotoxicity assay in B16-F10 melanoma cells (A) and 3T3-L1 cells (B) treated with tea seed oil (TSE), oleic acid (OA) and vitamin C (VC). * indicates significant difference from control (*$p<0.05$,**$p<0.01$).

The cytotoxicity of tea seed oil and oleic acid at high concentration may be due to the cell membrane damage. In fact, tea seed oil and oleic acid are lipophilic substances, they may pass through cell membrane and disturb the structure of membrane components.[12] The cytotoxicity of vitamin C may involve the acidic condition and lead to the inappropriate environment for cell proliferation.[12]

Melanogenesis assay

Tea seed oil and oleic acid were performed the melanogenesis assay in parallel with theophylline and kojic acid, which were used as positive and negative control, respectively.[7] The percentage of relative ratios of melanin content, tyrosinase activity, and TRP-2 activity are shown in Figure 2. Tea seed oil significantly decreased melanin content, whereas oleic acid gave the similar effect to control. The melanin contents of theophylline and kojic acid were of 167.09 ± 5.16 and $61.70 \pm 5.96\%$, respectively.

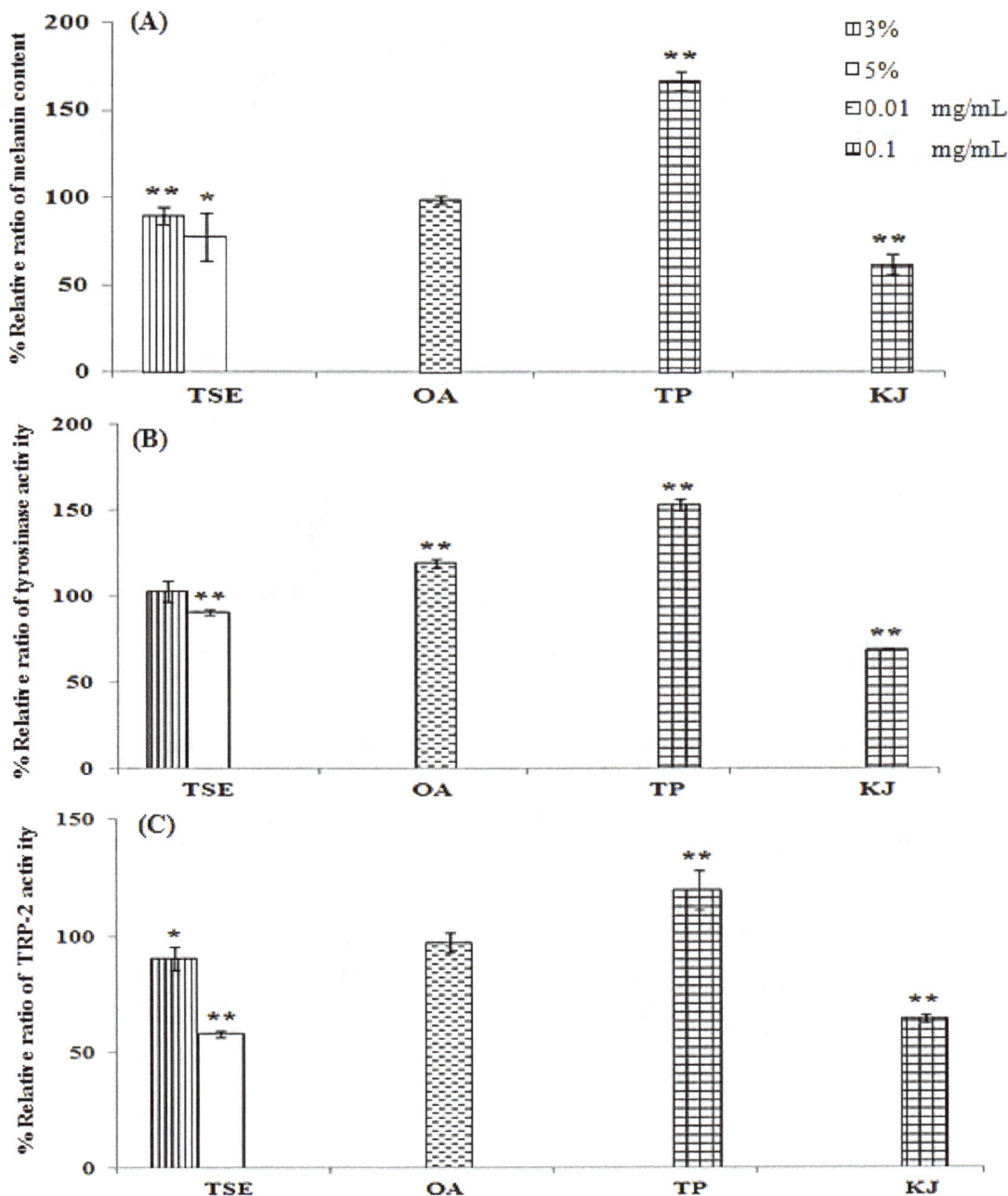

Figure 2. Percentage of relative ratio of melanin content (A), tyrosinase activity (B) and TRP-2 activity (C) in B16-F10 melanoma cells treated with tea seed oil (TSE), oleic acid (OA), theophylline (TP) and kojic acid (KJ). * indicates significant difference from control (*$p<0.05$, **$p<0.01$).

Tyrosinase and TRP-2 activities of tea seed oil were related to melanin content. 5% Tea seed oil significantly decreased the activities of tyrosinase and TRP-2 (p-value <0:001). However, tyrosinase activity of oleic acid was not in agreement with effect on melanin content and TRP-2 activity. Tyrosinase activity of oleic acid was significantly increased, whereas TRP-2 activity was similar to control. The tyrosinase and TRP-2 activities of theophylline and kojic acid were correlated with effects on melanin content.

Hyperpigmentation is one of skin problems in Asians that several researchers have investigated the compounds for treatment.[7,13] Tea seed oil appeared the pigment inhibition via inhibiting of melanogenic enzyme activities. Oleic acid exhibited no effect on melanin content and TRP-2 activity, except tyrosinase. The non-correlation between tyrosinase activity and the pigment regulatory agents have been demonstrated in previous study.[14] The different melanogenesis effect of oil and oleic acid may be due to the other bioactive compounds

of oil, in particularly to polyphenols.[3,15] The polyphenols of tea seed oil, such as epigallocatechin gallate and catechin gallate,[4] have shown the inhibitory activity on melanin synthesis and tyrosinase expression.[16] Theophylline is mediated the effect via cyclic adenosine monophosphate pathway,[17] whereas kojic acid is mediated via inhibition of tyrosinase in a non-classical manner.[18]

Antioxidant activity assay

Tea seed oil, oleic acid and vitamin C were evaluated for antioxidant activity in 3T3-L1 cells. The antioxidant activity demonstrated the cellular protection after hydrogen peroxide (H_2O_2) treatment. The cell viability after treatment with H_2O_2 was decreased to $76.50 \pm 1.08\%$. Tea seed oil, oleic acid and vitamin C exhibited the greater cell viability than H_2O_2 treatment (Figure 3). 3% Tea seed oil, 0.001 mg/mL oleic acid and 0.01 mg/mL vitamin C were shown the antioxidant characteristics.

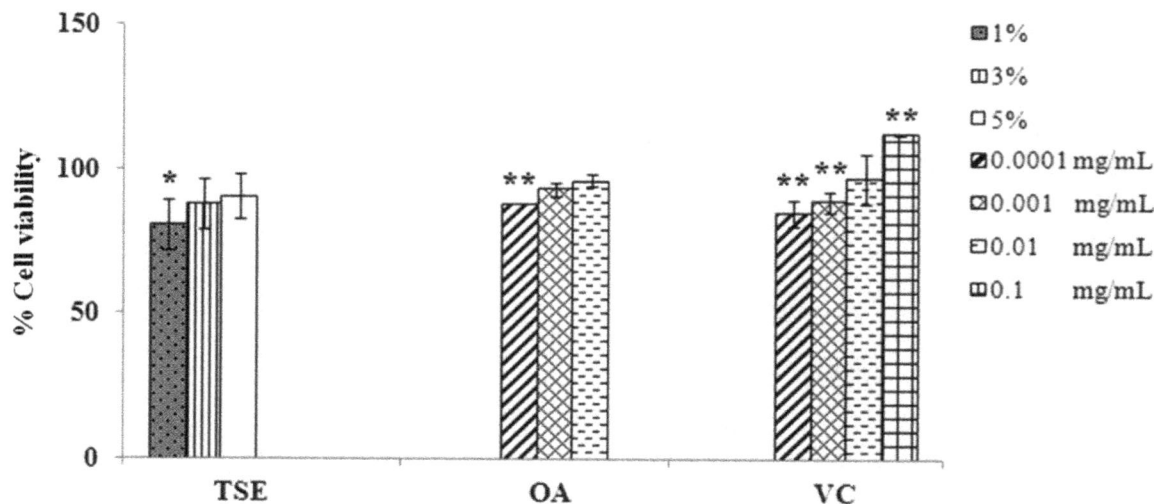

Figure 3. Antioxidant activity assay in 3T3-L1 cells treated with tea seed oil (TSE), oleic acid (OA), and vitamin C (VC). * indicates significant difference from control (*p<0.05,**p<0.01).

The free radicals have correlated with variety of human diseases, the antioxidant can relieve the oxidative stress damage. The antioxidant activity of tea seed oil and vitamin C was in agreement with previous studies.[3,11] Oleic acid also appeared the antioxidant activity similar to the previous study.[11] In addition, the other compounds of tea seed oil, including vitamin E, polyphenols, sesamin and compound B, may synergistically play the role in the antioxidant activity.[3] Vitamin C is mediated activity via reacting with aqueous peroxyl radicals and restoring the antioxidant properties of lipid-soluble vitamin E.[19]

Conclusion

Tea seed oil has exhibited the oleic acid as a major unsaturated fatty acid, the inhibitory activity on melanogenesis process via inhibition of tyrosinase and TRP-2 activities, and antioxidant activity. The results of

study have indicated the potential utilization of tea seed oil as the functional oil in several products, including health, food and cosmetic products.

Acknowledgments

The work was supported by Mae Fah Luang University [grant number. 58208050020, 2015].

Conflict of Interest

The authors declare no conflict of interests.

References

1. Ming TL, Bartholomew B. Theaceae. In: Wu ZY, Raven PH, Hong DY, editors. Flora of china. Missouri: Science Press; 2007.

2. Dimitrios B. Sources of natural phenolic antioxidants. *Trends Food Sci Tech* 2006;17(9):505-12. doi: 10.1016/j.tifs.2006.04.004

3. Lee CP, Yen GC. Antioxidant activity and bioactive compounds of tea seed (camellia oleifera abel.) oil. *J Agric Food Chem* 2006;54(3):779-84. doi: 10.1021/jf052325a

4. Sahari MA, Amooi M. Tea seed oil: Extraction, compositions, applications, functional and antioxidant properties. *Acad J Med Plants* 2013;1(4):068-79. doi: 10.15413/ajmp.2012.0113

5. Cert A, Moreda W, Perez-Camino MC. Methods of preparation of fatty acid methyl esters (FAME). Statistical assessment of the precision characteristics from a collaborative trial. *Grasas Aceites* 2000;51(6):447-56. doi: 10.3989/gya.2000.v51.i6.464

6. Papazisis KT, Geromichalos GD, Dimitriadis KA, Kortsaris AH. Optimization of the sulforhodamine b colorimetric assay. *J Immunol Methods* 1997;208(2):151-8.

7. Kanlayavattanakul M, Lourith N, Chaikul P. Jasmine rice panicle: A safe and efficient natural ingredient for skin aging treatments. *J Ethnopharmacol* 2016;193:607-16. doi: 10.1016/j.jep.2016.10.013

8. Montero de Espinosa L, Meier MAR. Plant oils: The perfect renewable resource for polymer science?! *Eur Polym J* 2011;47(5):837-52. doi: 10.1016/j.eurpolymj.2010.11.020

9. Sales-Campos H, Souza PR, Peghini BC, da Silva JS, Cardoso CR. An overview of the modulatory effects of oleic acid in health and disease. *Mini Rev Med Chem* 2013;13(2):201-10.

10. Aranda F, Gómez-Alonso S, Rivera del Álamo RM, Salvador MD, Fregapane G. Triglyceride, total and 2-position fatty acid composition of cornicabra virgin olive oil: Comparison with other spanish cultivars. *Food Chem* 2004;86(4):485-92. doi: 10.1016/j.foodchem.2003.09.021

11. Manosroi A, Ruksiriwanich W, Abe M, Sakai H, Manosroi W, Manosroi J. Biological activities of the rice bran extract and physical characteristics of its entrapment in niosomes by supercritical carbon dioxide fluid. *J Supercrit Fluid* 2010;54(2):137-44. doi: 10.1016/j.supflu.2010.05.002

12. Chaikul P, Manosroi J, Manosroi W, Manosroi A. Melanogenesis enhancement of saturated fatty acid methyl esters in B16F10 melanoma cell. *Adv Sci Lett* 2012;17(1):251-6. doi: 10.1166/asl.2012.4254

13. Ando H, Ryu A, Hashimoto A, Oka M, Ichihashi M. Linoleic acid and alpha-linolenic acid lightens ultraviolet-induced hyperpigmentation of the skin. *Arch Dermatol Res* 1998;290(7):375-81.

14. Ando H, Itoh A, Mishima Y, Ichihashi M. Correlation between the number of melanosomes, tyrosinase mrna levels, and tyrosinase activity in cultured murine melanoma cells in response to various melanogenesis regulatory agents. *J Cell Physiol* 1995;163(3):608-14. doi: 10.1002/jcp.1041630322

15. Kawabata T, Cui MY, Hasegawa T, Takano F, Ohta T. Anti-inflammatory and anti-melanogenic steroidal saponin glycosides from fenugreek (trigonella foenum-graecum l.) seeds. *Planta Med* 2011;77(7):705-10. doi: 10.1055/s-0030-1250477

16. Sato K, Toriyama M. Depigmenting effect of catechins. *Molecules* 2009;14(11):4425-32. doi: 10.3390/molecules14114425

17. Hu F. Theophylline and melanocyte-stimulating hormone effects on gamma-glutamyl transpeptidase and dopa reactions in cultured melanoma cells. *J Invest Dermatol* 1982;79(1):57-62.

18. Cabanes J, Chazarra S, Garcia-Carmona F. Kojic acid, a cosmetic skin whitening agent, is a slow-binding inhibitor of catecholase activity of tyrosinase. *J Pharm Pharmacol* 1994;46(12):982-5.

19. Bendich A, Machlin LJ, Scandurra O, Burton GW, Wayner DDM. The antioxidant role of vitamin C. *Adv Free Radical Bio Med* 1986;2(2):419-44. doi: 10.1016/S8755-9668(86)80021-7

9

Fisetin Protects DNA Against Oxidative Damage and Its Possible Mechanism

Tingting Wang, Huajuan Lin[†], Qian Tu[†], Jingjing Liu, Xican Li*

School of Chinese Herbal Medicine, Guangzhou University of Chinese Medicine, Waihuang East Road No.232, Guangzhou Higher Education Mega Center, 510006, Guangzhou, China.

Article info

Keywords:
· •OH-induced DNA damage
· Antioxidant mechanism
· Hydrogen atom transfer
· Single electron transfer mechanism
· 3',4'-dihydroxyl

Abstract

Purpose: The paper tries to assess the protective effect of fisetin against •OH-induced DNA damage, then to investigate the possible mechanism.

Methods: The protective effect was evaluated based on the content of malondialdehyde (MDA). The possible mechanism was analyzed using various antioxidant methods *in vitro*, including •OH scavenging (deoxyribose degradation), •O_2^- scavenging (pyrogallol autoxidation), DPPH• scavenging, ABTS•$^+$ scavenging, and Cu^{2+}-reducing power assays.

Results: Fisetin increased dose-dependently its protective percentages against •OH-induced DNA damage (IC_{50} value =1535.00±29.60 μM). It also increased its radical-scavenging percentages in a dose-dependent manner in various antioxidants assays. Its IC_{50} values in •OH scavenging, •O_2^- scavenging, DPPH• scavenging, ABTS•$^+$ scavenging, and Cu^{2+}-reducing power assays, were 47.41±4.50 μM, 34.05±0.87 μM, 9.69±0.53 μM, 2.43±0.14 μM, and 1.49±0.16 μM, respectively.

Conclusion: Fisetin can effectively protect DNA against •OH-induced oxidative damage possibly via reactive oxygen species (ROS) scavenging approach, which is assumed to be hydrogen atom (H•) and/or single electron (e) donation (HAT/SET) pathways. In the HAT pathway, the 3',4'-dihydroxyl moiety in B ring of fisetin is thought to play an important role, because it can be ultimately oxidized to a stable *ortho*-benzoquinone form.

Introduction

Reactive oxygen species (ROS), generated by normal cellular metabolism and exogenous agents (e.g. xenobiotics, ionising and nonionsing radiation), may lead to a condition of oxidative stress if its production overwhelms the antioxidant defences.[1,2] It has been considered as a significant promoter of cancer, cardiovascular malfunction, aging, and other diseases. Cellular DNA is a particularly sensitive target because of the potential to create cumulative mutations that can disrupt cellular homeostasis. However, the enzymatic repair in living organisms might be inadequate for protecting against permanent DNA mutations. Therefore, for the past few years, it has become a research focus to search for effective and safe antioxidants from natural sources.[3,4]

Most of natural antioxidants belong to the family of phenolic or polyphenolic compounds, which show their antioxidant activity via a hydrogen atom transfer (HAT) or single electron transfer (SET) mechanism.[5]

Fisetin (3,3',4',7-tetrahydroxyflavone, Figure 1) is a phenolic flavonoid in various food, such as strawberry, onion and persimmon.[6] It has a wide range of pharmacological effects, such as antitumor, antiinflammation,[7] anticoagulant and dissolving thrombus.[8] In recent years, its protective effect on the liver

in human body (especially patients with diabetes) attracted a wide spread attention. Researches showed that, the fisetin's liver protective effect and promoting glucose homeostasis effect were related to its antioxidant activity.[9] However, its antioxidant ability and mechanism remain unknown. Therefore, the present study used DNA protection model to investigate its antioxidant activity then further discuss the possible mechanisms.

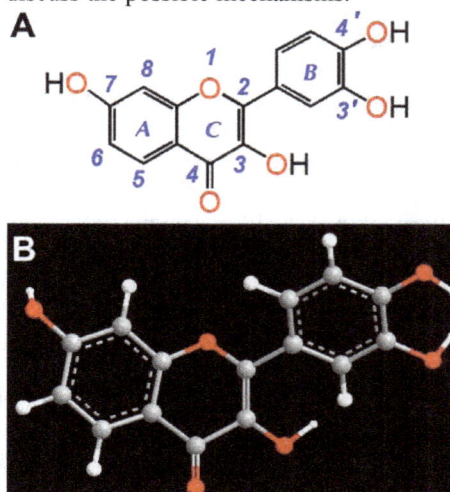

Figure 1. The structure of fisetin (A) and its ball-stick model (B)

*Corresponding author: Xican Li, Emails: lixican@126.com, lixc@gzucm.edu.cn
†: These authors contributed equally to this work.

Materials and Methods

Chemicals

Fisetin (98%, CAS 528-48-3) and DNA sodium salt (fish sperm) were obtained from Aladdin Co. (Shanghai, China). DPPH• (1,1-diphenyl-2-picryl-hydrazl), ABTS [2,2′-azino-bis(3-ethylbenzo- thiazoline-6-sulfonic acid diammonium salt)], neocuproine, BHA (butylated hydroxyanisole), Trolox [(±)-6-hydroxyl-2,5,7,8 - tetramethlychromane-2-carboxylic acid], pyrogallol and deoxyribise were purchased from Sigma Co. (Sigma-Aldrich Shanghai Trading Co., China). Other chemicals used in this study were of analytical grade and obtained from Guangzhou Chemical Reagent Factory (Guangzhou, China).

Methods

The protective effect of fisetin against •OH-induced DNA damage was determined by our method.[10] Mechanistic analysis experiments included •OH scavenging, •O_2^- scavenging, DPPH• scavenging, ABTS•$^+$ scavenging, and Cu^{2+}-reducing power assays. The •OH scavenging assay was based on the deoxyribose degradation, and improved by our laboratory;[11] in the improved deoxyribose degradation assay, all samples were pre-treated before determination. The •O_2^- scavenging assay was based on pyrogallol autoxidation reaction, and also improved by our laboratory; In the improved pyrogallol autoxidation assay, pH was modified as 7.4.[11] The other antioxidant assays were described in our previous paper.[10,11] In all these assays,

BHA and Trolox were used as the positive controls. The inhibition (or protecting DNA, reducing power) percentages were obtained according to the corresponding calculation formulas. The calculation formulas and experimental protocols were detailed in the Suppl. 1.

Results and Discussion

ROS can lead to the formation of single and double-strand breaks, as well as induce chemical and structural modifications to purine and pyrimidine bases, resulting in millions of lesions per cell each day.[4] Deoxythymineglycol (dTG), 8-hydroxy-deoxyguanine (8-OH-dG), malondialdehyde (MDA) and formamidopyrimidine (FAPy) constitute the important markers of DNA oxidative damage.[12,13] Among these fragments, MDA is usually used to reflect the DNA protective percentage, because MDA can be easily detected via combining with 2-thiobarbituric acid (TBA).[10]

As is seen in Figure 2A, the protective percentages of fisetin from •OH-induced DNA damage increased in a dose-dependent fashion. The IC_{50} values of fisetin, BHA and Trolox were respectively 1535.00±29.60 µM, 2469.00±96.69 µM and 1084.67±20.23 µM (Table 1). The results suggested that fisetin could protect DNA against •OH-induced damage. However, its protective effect is inferior to that of Trolox but stronger than that of BHA.

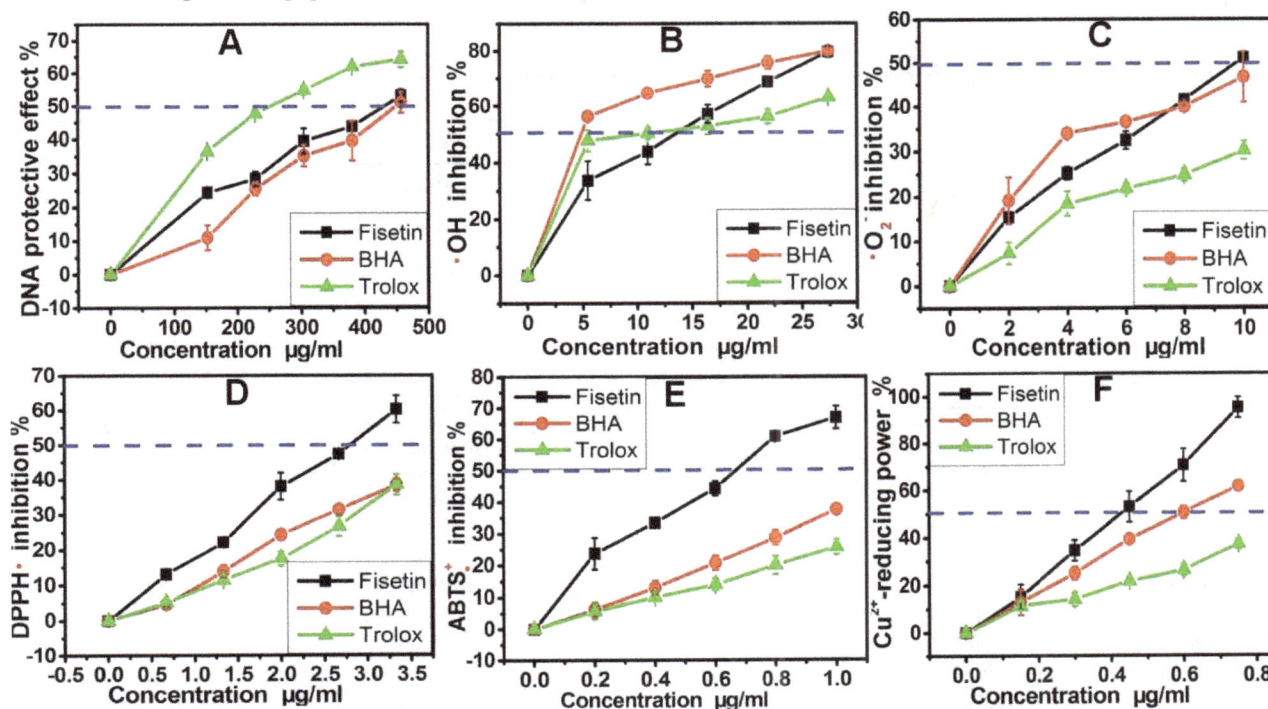

Figure 2. The dose response curves of fisetin in the assays: (A) protective effect against DNA damage; (B) hydroxyl (•OH) radical-scavenging; (C) superoxide anion (•O_2^-) radical-scavenging assay; (D) DPPH• radical-scavenging assay; (E) ABTS•$^+$ radical-scavenging assay; (F) Cu^{2+}-reducing power. Each value is expressed as the mean±SD (n=3). The concentration was the final concentration in the corresponding reaction system.

Some studies have shown that phenolic antioxidants protect DNA possibly through base-excision repair, which may arise from ROS (especially •OH and •O_2^-) scavenging at high reaction rates.[14-16] Therefore, the •OH and •O_2^- radical-scavenging capacities of fisetin were further measured in the study.

Our data in Figure 2B&C showed that fisetin could efficiently scavenge •OH and •O_2^- radicals dose-dependently. The IC_{50} values of fisetin, BHA and Trolox of •OH-scavenging were respectively 47.41±4.50 µM, 2.40±1.19 µM, and 41.84±9.55 µM. In the •O_2^- radical-scavenging assay, IC_{50} values of fisetin, BHA and Trolox were 34.05±0.87 µM, 76.02±5.22 µM and 66.75±2.25 µM, respectively (Table 1). This indicated that both •OH and •O_2^- radicals could be eliminated by fisetin at low concentration, and that ROS scavenging may be a possible approach for fisetin to protect DNA.

To confirm whether HAT and SET might happen in the ROS scavenging by fisetin, we further measured its radical-scavenging on DPPH•. The previous studies suggested that DPPH• may undergo HAT pathway to be scavenged to yield a stable DPPH-H molecule.[17] As illustrated in Figure 2D and Table 1, fisetin scavenged DPPH• radical with high efficiency. It clearly suggests a HAT pathway in the ROS scavenging by fisetin. The possible reaction of fisetin with DPPH• radical can be proposed as Figure 3.

In the process, since B ring is regarded as the active sites in the antioxidant process of flavonoids,[18] phenolic-OH in B ring of fisetin is thought to undergo homolysis prior to either the A or C ring, to produce H• and fisetin•

radical (I). Then DPPH-H molecule may be generated through H• combining with DPPH•. And the fisetin• radical might transform into a semi-quinone form (III), which could be further extracted H• by excess DPPH• to form the stable *ortho*-benzoquinone form. Now it is clear that, the 3',4'-dihydroxyl moiety in B ring of fisetin played an important role, because it could be ultimately oxidized to a stable *ortho*-benzoquinone form.

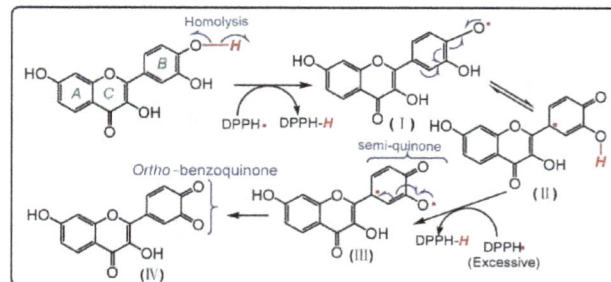

Figure 3. The proposed reaction of fisetin with DPPH• radical.

Since the formation of ABTS•$^+$ from ABTS was previously proven to be via one SET oxidation,[19] ABTS•$^+$ scavenging was also reported to be a SET mechanism.[20] The effective scavenging ABTS•$^+$ by fisetin indicate a SET possibility in its ROS scavenging reaction. The SET possibility was further supported by the Cu^{2+}-reducing power assay, in which fisetin efficiently reduced $Cu^{2+} \rightarrow Cu^+$ (Figure 2F and Table 1). Cu^{2+}-reducing however is well-known as an electron (e) transfer reaction.

Table 1. The IC_{50} values of fisetin and the positive controls (µM)

-	Fisetin	Positive controls	
		BHA	Trolox
DNA protective effect	1535.00±29.60[b]	2469.00±96.69[c]	1084.67±20.23[a]
•OH scavenging	47.41±4.50[c]	2.40±1.19[a]	41.84±9.55[b]
•O_2^- scavenging	34.05±0.87[a]	76.02±5.22[c]	66.75±2.25[b]
DPPH• scavenging	9.69±0.53[a]	22.84±0.34[c]	19.55±2.20[b]
ABTS$^+$• scavenging	2.43±0.14[a]	7.73±0.43[b]	7.54±0.57[b]
Cu^{2+}-reducing	1.49±0.16[a]	3.25±0.17[b]	4.31±0.21[c]

The IC_{50} value is defined as the concentration of 50% radical inhibition (or protection percentage, relative reducing percentage). These IC_{50} values were calculated by linear regression analysis based on the response curves in Figure 2 and converted from µg/mL to µM. Each value in this table is expressed as the *mean±SD* (*n*=3). Mean values with different superscripts (a, b, or c) in the same row are significantly different (*p* < 0.05), while those with same superscripts are not significantly different (*p* < 0.05).

Conclusion

Fisetin can effectively protect DNA against •OH-induced oxidative damage possibly via reactive ROS scavenging approach, which is assumed to be via HAT/SET pathways. In the HAT pathway, the 3',4'-dihydroxyl moiety in B ring of fisetin is thought to play an important role, because it can be ultimately oxidized to a stable *ortho*-benzoquinone form.

Conflict of Interest

Authors declare no conflict of interest in this study.

References

1. Dizdaroglu M, Jaruga P, Birincioglu M, Rodriguez H. Free radical-induced damage to DNA: Mechanisms and measurement. *Free Radic Biol Med* 2002;32(11):1102-15.

2. Cooke MS, Henderson PT, Evans MD. Sources of extracellular, oxidatively-modified DNA lesions: Implications for their measurement in urine. *J Clin Biochem Nutr* 2009;45(3):255-70. doi: 10.3164/jcbn.SR09-41

3. Cooke MS, Evans MD, Dizdaroglu M, Lunec J. Oxidative DNA damage: Mechanisms, mutation, and disease. *FASEB J* 2003;17(10):1195-214. doi: 10.1096/fj.02-0752rev

4. Silva JP, Gomes AC, Coutinho OP. Oxidative DNA damage protection and repair by polyphenolic compounds in pc12 cells. *Eur J Pharmacol* 2008;601(1-3):50-60. doi: 10.1016/j.ejphar.2008.10.046

5. Xue Y, Zheng Y, An L, Dou Y, Liu Y. Density functional theory study of the structure-antioxidant activity of polyphenolic deoxybenzoins. *Food Chem* 2014;151:198-206. doi: 10.1016/j.foodchem.2013.11.064

6. Sahu BD, Kumar JM, Sistla R. Fisetin, a dietary flavonoid, ameliorates experimental colitis in mice: Relevance of nf-kappab signaling. *J Nutr Biochem* 2016;28:171-82. doi: 10.1016/j.jnutbio.2015.10.004

7. Pal HC, Sharma S, Elmets CA, Athar M, Afaq F. Fisetin inhibits growth, induces g(2) /m arrest and apoptosis of human epidermoid carcinoma a431 cells: Role of mitochondrial membrane potential disruption and consequent caspases activation. *Exp Dermatol* 2013;22(7):470-5. doi: 10.1111/exd.12181

8. Perez-Vizcaino F, Duarte J. Flavonols and cardiovascular disease. *Mol Aspects Med* 2010;31(6):478-94. doi: 10.1016/j.mam.2010.09.002

9. Prasath GS, Pillai SI, Subramanian SP. Fisetin improves glucose homeostasis through the inhibition of gluconeogenic enzymes in hepatic tissues of streptozotocin induced diabetic rats. *Eur J Pharmacol* 2014;740:248-54. doi: 10.1016/j.ejphar.2014.06.065

10. Li X, Mai W, Wang L, Han W. A hydroxyl-scavenging assay based on DNA damage in vitro. *Anal Biochem* 2013;438(1):29-31. doi: 10.1016/j.ab.2013.03.014

11. Li X, Lin J, Gao Y, Han W, Chen D. Antioxidant activity and mechanism of rhizoma cimicifugae. *Chem Cent J* 2012;6(1):140. doi: 10.1186/1752-153X-6-140

12. Zheng RL, Huang ZY. Free-Radical Biology. 3rd ed. Beijing, China: Higher Education Press; 2007.

13. Sacheck JM, Milbury PE, Cannon JG, Roubenoff R, Blumberg JB. Effect of vitamin e and eccentric exercise on selected biomarkers of oxidative stress in young and elderly men. *Free Radic Biol Med* 2003;34(12):1575-88.

14. Alvarez-Idaboy JR, Galano A. On the chemical repair of DNA radicals by glutathione: Hydrogen vs electron transfer. *J Phys Chem B* 2012;116(31):9316-25. doi: 10.1021/jp303116n

15. Wallace SS. Enzymatic processing of radiation-induced free radical damage in DNA. *Radiat Res* 1998;150(5 Suppl):S60-79.

16. Zheng RL, Shi YM, Jia ZJ, Zhao CY, Zhang Q, Tan XR. Fast repair of DNA radicals. *Chem Soc Rev* 2010;39(8):2827-2834. doi: 10.1039/b924875g

17. Xie J, Schaich KM. Re-evaluation of the 2,2-diphenyl-1-picrylhydrazyl free radical (dpph) assay for antioxidant activity. *J Agric Food Chem* 2014;62(19):4251-60. doi: 10.1021/jf500180u

18. Tsimogiannis DI , Oreopoulou V. The contribution of flavonoid C-ring on the DPPH free radical scavenging efficiency: A kinetic approach for the 3'4'-hydroxy substituted members. *Innov Food Sci Emerg* 2006;7(4):140-6. doi: 10.1016/j.ifset.2005.09.001

19. Changha L, Jeyong Y. UV direct photolysis of 2,2'-azino-bis(3-ethylbenzothiazoline-6-sulfonate) (ABTS) in aqueous solution: Kinetics and mechanism. *J Photoch Photobio A* 2008;197(2-3):232-8. doi: 10.1016/j.jphotochem.2007.12.030

20. Villata LS, Berkovic AM, Gonzalez MC, Martire DO. One-electron oxidation of antioxidants: A kinetic-thermodynamic correlation. *Redox Rep* 2013;18(5):205-9. doi: 10.1179/1351000213Y.0000000063

10

Apoptosis Cell Death Effect of *Scrophularia Variegata* on Breast Cancer Cells via Mitochondrial Intrinsic Pathway

Abbas Azadmehr[1,2]**, Reza Hajiaghaee**[3]*****, Behzad Baradaran**[4]**, Hashem Haghdoost-Yazdi**[5]

[1] *Immunology Department, Qazvin University of Medical Sciences, Qazvin, Iran.*

[2] *Immunology Department, Babol University of Medical Sciences, Babol, Iran.*

[3] *Pharmacognosy and Pharmaceutics Department of Medicinal Plants Research Center, Institute of Medicinal Plants, ACECR, Karaj, Iran.*

[4] *Immunology Research Center, Tabriz University of Medical Sciences, Tabriz, Iran.*

[5] *Physiology Department, Qazvin University of Medical Sciences, Qazvin, Iran.*

Article info

Keywords:
· Scrophularia variegate
· Apoptosis
· Breast cancer cell line
· Caspase

Abstract

Purpose: Scrophularia variegata M. Beib. (Scrophulariaceae) is an Iranian medicinal plant which is used for various inflammatory disorders in traditional medicine. In this study we evaluated the anti-cancer and cytotoxic effects of the *Scrophularia variegata* (*S. variegata*) ethanolic extract on the human breast cancer cell line.

Methods: The cytotoxicity effect of the extract on MCF-7 cells was evaluated by MTT assay. In addition, Caspase activity, DNA ladder and Cell death were evaluated by ELISA, gel electrophoresis and Annexin V-FITC/PI staining, respectively.

Results: The *S. variegata* extract showed significant effect cytotoxicity on MCF-7 human breast cancer cell line. Treatment with the extract induced apoptosis on the breast cancer cells by cell cycle arrest in G2/M phase. The results indicated that cytotoxicity activity was associated with an increase of apoptosis as demonstrated by DNA fragmentation as well as an increase of the amount of caspase 3 and caspase 9. In addition, the phytochemical assay showed that the extract had antioxidant capacity and also flavonoids, phenolic compounds and phenyl propanoids were presented in the extract.

Conclusion: Our findings indicated that *S. variegata* extract induced apoptosis via mitochondrial intrinsic pathway on breast cancer by cell cycle arrest in G2/M phase and an increase of caspase 3 and caspase 9. However future studies are needed.

Introduction

Breast cancer is one of the leading causes of death among women in the world. At the present, using of natural compounds such as medicinal plants in cancer therapy has aroused general because of its minimal side effect, safety and efficiency.[1,2] *Scrophularia variegata* is an Iranian medicinal plant and which is used for various inflammatory disorders in traditional medicine. Our previous findings demonstrated that *Scrophularia* species had the anti-cancer activity by induction of apoptosis and inhibition of matrix metalloproteinases, anti-asthmatic, neuroprotective, inhibitory effect on the nitric oxide and pro-inflammatory cytokines production.[3-10] In the present study we investigated the cytotoxic effect and induction of apoptosis of *S. variegata* in the MCF-7 human breast cancer cell line.

Materials and Methods

Plant material and preparation

The plant was collected from Taleqan region (Alborz province) in May 2010, in Iran. A voucher specimen was deposited in the herbarium of the Institute of Medicinal Plants (IMP). Aerial parts of the plant were dried, powdered (100 g) and macerated with a 90% ethanol solution for 3 days with three changes of the solution. The resulting extract was filtered and evaporated under vacuum into a dried powder.

Phytochemical, anti-oxidant and total flavonoid assay

We analyzed the chemical components of extract by thin layer chromatocheraphy (TLC). In addition, the antioxidant capacity of the plant extract by the DPPH (2, 2-diphenylpicrylhydrazyl) test and also total flavonoid content were estimated by aluminum chloride colorimetric assay as described previously.[3]

Cell culture and cell viability assay with MTT test

The MCF-7 human breast cancer cell line and normal human fibroblast cells (L929) were prepared from the National Cell Bank of Iran (NCBI) and maintained by culturing in RPMI 1640 medium (Sigma, St Louis, USA) supplemented with 10% heat-inactivated fetal calf serum (Gibco, USA). The cell viability was assayed by MTT (3-(4, 5-dimethylthiazoyl)-2, 5- diphenyltetrazolium bromide) as previously described.[3]

*Corresponding author: Reza Hajiaghaee, Email: rhajiaghaee@yahoo.com

Cell apoptosis and cell cycle assay
Detection of apoptosis was evaluated with an Annexin V–FITC apoptosis Kit (Invitrogen, USA) according to the manufacturer's protocol. Moreover, the cell cycle distribution was measured by PI staining as previously described.[3]

DNA fragmentation analysis and measurement of caspase activity
To confirm breast cancer apoptosis, we evaluated the fragmented DNA from MCF-7 cells by gel electrophoresis as previously described.[3] In addition, caspase-3 and caspase-9 activity were assessed according to the manufacturer's instruction of the caspase colorimetric assay kit (R&D systems).

Statistical analysis
Data represented as mean±standard deviation. Statistical analyses were carried out by one-way analysis of variance (ANOVA) and a post–hoc Bonferroni's test to express the difference among the groups. All analyses performed using SPSS software16. Data considered statistically significant at $P<0.05$.

Results and Discussion
Antioxidant activity and total phenolic compounds
The results showed that the extract had the strong antioxidant and free radical scavenging capacities. These results are shown in Tables 1and 2.

Table 1. Antioxidant capacity and total phenolic compounds of *S. variegata* extract

Total flavonoids, (mg RE/1g de)	DPPH radical scavenging activity, IC50% (mg/l)	Ascorbic acid equivalent of the extract antioxidant capacity (mg/g)
51.93±4.43	299.22±0.03	31.5

Table 2. Phytochemical results of *Scrophularia variagata* extract

Compounds	Reagents	Standards	Results
Phenylpropanoids and Terpenoids	Vanillin sulfuric acid	Cinamic acid	+
Phenolic compounds	Ferric chloride	Nepitrin	+
Flavonoides	Natural product reagent	Quercetin	+

Cytotoxicity effect of S. variagata extract on MCF-7 tumor cell
In this study normal human fibroblast cells (L929) were used as normal cells compared with MCF-7 human breast cancer cell. In a preliminary experiment on L929, the results indicated that extract up to 200 μg/ ml did not any significant toxicity for 48 h (Data not shown). On the other hand, a successful antitumor drug should kill cancer cells without causing excessive side effects to normal cells that this ideal situation is achievable by apoptosis induction in cancer cells. As shown Figure 1, the extract significantly (p<0.05) inhibited MCF-7 cell

growth in dose and time dependent manner. So, the results indicate that the extract can induce a cytotoxicity effect in MCF-7 human breast cancer cell line.

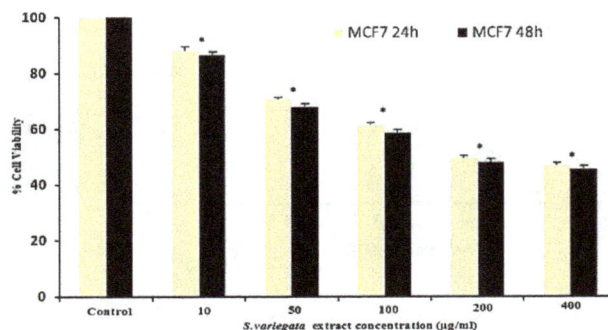

Figure 1. Cytotoxicity effect of *S. variegata* on MCF-7 tumor cell line.
The results showed that the extract significantly (*P<0.05) inhibited MCF-7 cell growth in dose and time dependent manner compared with non-treated (control group) after 48 h. The results shown are representative of three independent experiments.

Effect of S. variagata extract in MCF-7 apoptosis and cell cycle arrest
Apoptosis is a normal physiologic process that plays an important role in homeostasis and growth of the normal and cancer cells also dysregulation of apoptosis is usually considered as a major cancer property.[11,12]
In the present study, to determine whether the toxicity effect of *S. variagata* extract on MCF-7 cells was associated to apoptotic cell death, the apoptosis induction were measured by annexin V-FITC/PI staining. As shown in Figure 2, our findings indicated that the amount of apoptotic cells increased with increasing concentration of *S. variagata* extract. These results indicated that the cytotoxic effects of *S. variagata* extract could be mediated by the induction of apoptosis via mitochondrial intrinsic pathway in MCF-7 cells. Moreover, some studies showed that other genus of *scrophularia* such as *S. floribunda* and *S. striata* extract induced apoptosis in tumor cells through induction of cell cycle arrest.[3,13] Our findings demonstrated that *S. variagata* extract can induce a G2/M phase cell cycle arrest in MCF-7 cells in a dose-dependent manner.

Effects of S. variagata extract on caspases induction and DNA fragmentation
To confirm the effects of extract on the induction of apoptosis in the breast cancer cell line, the extract was examined for the appearance of DNA ladder and induction of caspases in treated cells. Our results demonstrated that increasing of the caspase-3 and caspase-9 activity and internucleosomal DNA fragmentation was dose dependently apparent in the cells indicating that the extract can cause apoptosis in the MCF-7 cells (Figure 3 A, B). Therefore, the findings in this study showed that the *Scrophularia variagata* could be as an anticancer agent against breast cancer by cell growth inhibition and apoptosis induction.

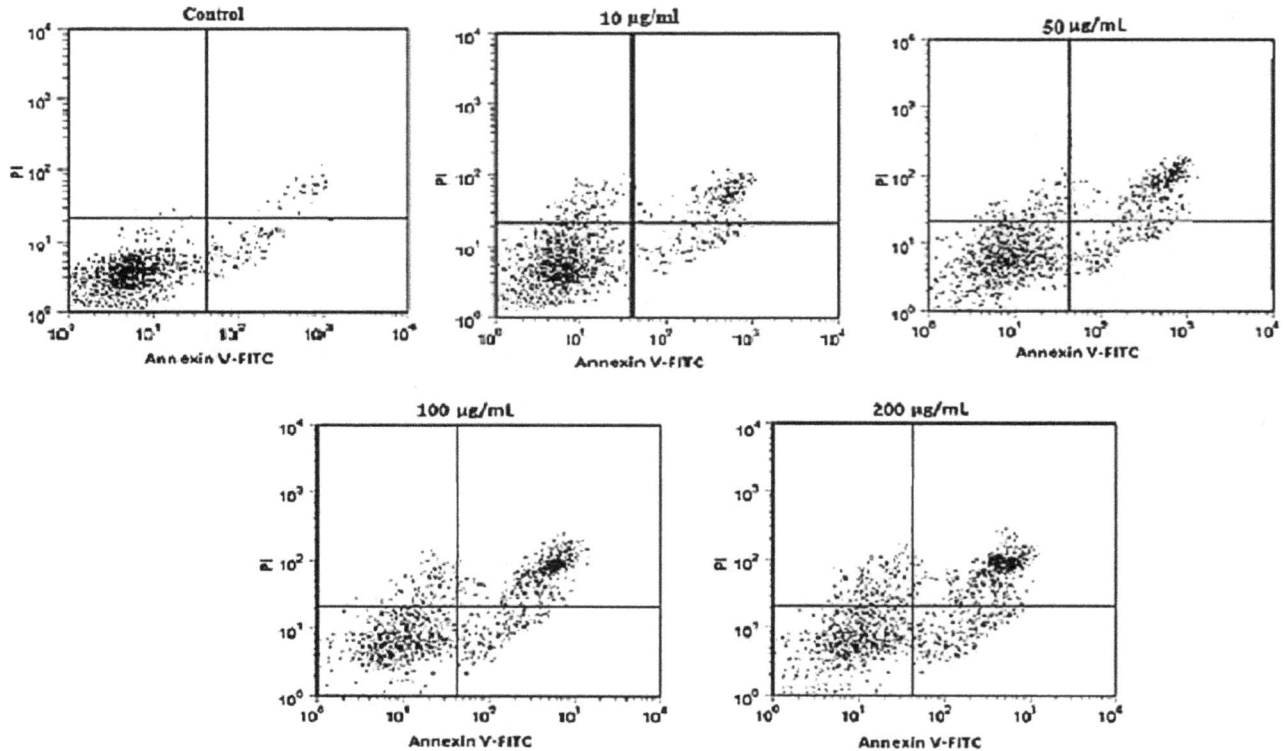

Figure 2. Effect of *S. variegata* extract on the inducing of apoptosis and cell cycle arrest.
Apoptosis inducing effect of *S. variegata* extract on MCF-7 human breast cancer cell line evaluated by Annexin V-FITC (AV)/PI method. The results shown are representative of three independent experiments.

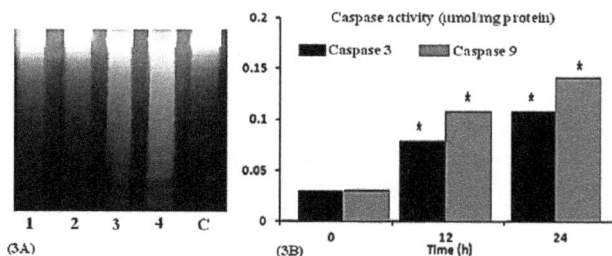

Figure 3. DNA fragmentation in MCF-7 tumor cell and caspases activation.
(A) DNA fragmentation in MCF-7 breast cancer cells after treatment with 0-200 µg/ml of the *S. variegata* extract 1; 10µg/ml, 2; 50µg/ml, 3; 100µg/ml, 4; 200µg/ml, C; negative control. DNA laddering typical for apoptotic cells is visible for cells treated with the *S. variegata* extract.
(B) The activity of caspase-3 and caspase-9 significantly (*$P<0.05$) is increased in time-dependent manner in MCF-7 cells after the treatment with extract.

Conclusion

Our in vitro study demonstrated that *S. variagata* has cytotoxic activity on MCF-7 breast cancer cell line. The ability of it medicinal plant to induce apoptosis through G2/M phase cell cycle arrest and an increase in caspases activity on human breast cancer cell line candidate it for further studies as a potential natural anti-cancer agent.

Acknowledgments

This study was supported by Iran National Science Foundation. We also thank of deputy for Research, Qazvin University of Medical Sciences, Qazvin, Iran and, Institute of Medicinal Plants (IMP), ACECR, Iran.

Conflict of Interest

The authors declare that there is no conflict of interests regarding the publication of this paper.

References

1. Ribereau-Gayon G, Jung ML, Frantz M, Anton R. Modulation of cytotoxicity and enhancement of cytokine release induced by viscum album l. Extracts or mistletoe lectins. *Anticancer Drugs* 1997;8 Suppl 1:S3-8.
2. Taixiang W, Munro AJ, Guanjian L. Chinese medical herbs for chemotherapy side effects in colorectal cancer patients. *Cochrane Database Syst Rev* 2005(1):CD004540. doi: 10.1002/14651858.CD004540.pub2
3. Azadmehr A, Hajiaghaee R, Mazandarani M. Induction of apoptosis and g2 /m cell cycle arrest by scrophularia striata in a human leukaemia cell line. *Cell Prolif* 2013;46(6):637-43. doi: 10.1111/cpr.12074
4. Azadmehr A, Oghyanous KA, Hajiaghaee R, Amirghofran Z, Azadbakht M. Antioxidant and neuroprotective effects of scrophularia striata extract against oxidative stress-induced neurotoxicity. *Cell Mol Neurobiol* 2013;33(8):1135-41. doi: 10.1007/s10571-013-9979-7
5. Azadmehr A, Hajiaghaee R, Zohal MA, Maliji G. Protective effects of scrophularia striata in ovalbumin-induced mice asthma model. *Daru* 2013;21(1):56. doi: 10.1186/2008-2231-21-56

6. Azadmehr A, Maliji G, Hajiaghaee R, Shahnazi M, Afaghi A. Inhibition of pro-inflammatory cytokines by ethyl acetate extract of *Scrophularia striata*. *Trop J Pharm Res* 2012;11(6):893-7.

7. Azadmehr A, Hajiaghaee R, Afshari A, Amirghofran Z, Refieian-Kopaei M, yousofi Darani H, et al. Evaluation of *in vivo* immune response activity and *in vitro* anti-cancer effect by *Scrophularia megalantha*. *J Med Plants Res* 2011;5:2365-8.

8. Amirghofran Z, Bahmani M, Azadmehr A, Ashouri E, Javidnia K. Antitumor activity and apoptosis induction in human cancer cell lines by dionysia termeana. *Cancer Invest* 2007;25(7):550-4. doi: 10.1080/07357900701518487

9. Azadmehr A, Afshari A, Baradaran B, Hajiaghaee R, Rezazadeh S, Monsef-Esfahani H. Suppression of nitric oxide production in activated murine peritoneal macrophages in vitro and ex vivo by scrophularia striata ethanolic extract. *J Ethnopharmacol* 2009;124(1):166-9. doi: 10.1016/j.jep.2009.03.042

10. Hajiaghaee R, Monsef-Esfahani HR, Khorramizadeh MR, Saadat F, Shahverdi AR, Attar F. Inhibitory effect of aerial parts of scrophularia striata on matrix metalloproteinases expression. *Phytother Res* 2007;21(12):1127-9. doi: 10.1002/ptr.2221

11. Asadi H, Orangi M, Shanehbandi D, Babaloo Z, Delazar A, Mohammadnejad L, et al. Methanolic fractions of ornithogalum cuspidatum induce apoptosis in pc-3 prostate cancer cell line and wehi-164 fibrosarcoma cancer cell line. *Adv Pharm Bull* 2014;4(Suppl 1):455-8. doi: 10.5681/apb.2014.067

12. Aghbali A, Moradi Abbasabadi F, Delazar A, Vosough Hosseini S, Zare Shahneh F, Baradaran B, et al. Induction of apoptosis and cytotoxic activities of iranian orthodox black tea extract (bte) using in vitro models. *Adv Pharm Bull* 2014;4(3):255-60. doi: 10.5681/apb.2014.037

13. Giessrigl B, Yazici G, Teichmann M, Kopf S, Ghassemi S, Atanasov AG, et al. Effects of scrophularia extracts on tumor cell proliferation, death and intravasation through lymphoendothelial cell barriers. *Int J Oncol* 2012;40(6):2063-74. doi: 10.3892/ijo.2012.1388

11

Preparation and Characterization of *Pistacia khinjuk* Gum Nanoparticles Using Response Surface Method: Evaluation of Its Anti-Bacterial Performance and Cytotoxicity

Ali Fattahi[1,2,3], Tahereh Sakvand[4], Marziyeh Hajialyani[3], Behzad Shahbazi[2], Mohammad Shakiba[5], Ahmad Tajehmiri[1], Ebrahim Shakiba[6]*

[1] *Medical Biology Research Center, Kermanshah University of Medical Sciences, Kermanshah, Iran.*
[2] *Nano Drug Delivery Research Center, Faculty of Pharmacy, Kermanshah University of Medical Sciences, Kermanshah, Iran.*
[3] *Pharmaceutical Sciences Research Center, Faculty of Pharmacy, Kermanshah University of Medical Sciences, Kermanshah, Iran.*
[4] *Department of Medicinal plants, Kermanshah Jahade-Daneshgahi, Institute of Higher Education, Kermanshah, Iran.*
[5] *Student Research Committee, Kermanshah University of Medical Sciences, Kermanshah, Iran.*
[6] *Department of Biochemistry, Medical School, Kermanshah University of Medical Sciences, Kermanshah, Iran.*

Article info

Keywords:
· Antibacterial activity
· Cytotoxicity
· Nanoparticle
· *Pistacia Khinjuk*
· Response Surface Model

Abstract

Purpose: This study aims to prepare a novel, natural nanoparticle (NP) as a drug carrier, which also has inherent therapeutic effects.

Methods: *Pistacia khinjuk* gum NPs were prepared and Response surface methodology (RSM) was used for statistical analysis of data and optimizing the size of NPs.

Results: NPs were in the range of 75.85–241.3 nm. The optimization study was carried out, and an optimized size (70.86nm) was obtained using DMSO as a solvent. The volume of the organic phase was 111.25µl, and the concentration of gum was 1% w/v. The cell viability assay was performed on the pure gum and NPs toward β-TC$_3$, MCF7, and HT29 cell lines. It was observed that NPs have higher cytotoxic activity in comparison with pure gum, and that the IC$_{50}$value was achieved at 1% of NPs in β-TC$_3$ cells. The obtained NPs demonstrated antibacterial activity against two bacterial strains (*Pseudomonas aeruginosa* and *Staphylococcus aureus).*

Conclusion: Altogether, according to the obtained results, these NPs with inherent cytotoxicity and antibacterial activity are an attractive carrier for drug delivery.

Introduction

Pistacia khinjuk is one of the major Pistacia species that grows in some of Mediterranean countries (they have especially been widely distributed in the *Zagrossian* region of Iran) and classified into the *Anacardiaceae* family. Different parts of the plant, including resin, leaf, bark, fruit, and aerial parts, can be used as traditional medicine.[1] They have been used for a long time as useful remedies for the treatment and prevention of different kinds of diseases such as asthma and stomach discomfort, throat infections, burns, nausea, eczema, vomiting, and toothaches;[2-5] specifically, the gum resin has exhibited wound healing activity that could be used for the treatment of brain and gastrointestinal disturbances.[2] Due to the literature reports, *p. khinjuk* has exhibited inherent anti-inflammatory, antileishmanial, antipyretic, antioxidant, antitumor, antiviral, antiasthmatic, and antimicrobial properties.[2,6,7] In addition to these common medical applications, *p.khinjuk* gum could be a candidate as a new natural biopolymer for drug delivery systems.

According to the literature review, the fabrication of p.khinjukgum NPs and using them as a novel delivery vehicle has not been previously investigated. Due to the numerous desirable characteristics and advantages of *p.khinjuk* gum in therapeutic objectives, the fabrication of *p.khinjuk* gum NPs as drug carriers was investigated in this study. The obtained data was statistically analyzed using RSM, which combines statistical and mathematical techniques to fit experimental data to the model for optimization processes.[8]

Materials and Methods

Materials

P.khinjuk gum was collected from the exudates of the trunk of *p.khinjuk* tree (from Oshtoran-Kooh Mountain, in Azna, Lorestan province, Iran) in July 2014. The organic solvents (acetone, ethanol and DMSO) were purchased from Merck (Germany). Trypsin-ethylenediamine tetra acetic acid (EDTA) was supplied from Ben Yakhte, Iran. DMEM (Dulbecco's Modified Eagle's Medium) and Roswell Park Memorial Institute

*Corresponding author: Ebrahim Shakiba, Email: eshakiba@kums.ac.ir

medium (RPMI) were procured from Gibco, Scotland. Thiazolyl blue (MTT) was purchased from Merck, Germany.All of the other compounds were of analytical grade from Merck.

Preparation of NPs

The organic solutions were prepared using three organic solvents (ethanol, acetone, and DMSO). *P.khinjuk* gum with three different amounts of 0.1, 0.55, and 1g, was dissolved in 100 ml of each organic solvent to prepare three different concentrations of *p.khinjuk* gum (0.1%, 0.55%, and 1%w/v).Then 100, 500, and 1000 µl of each stock solution was added dropwise to 10 ml of distilled water under stirring. The resulting solutions were stirred for 1 h at 2500 rpm and at room temperature.

Experimental design

In this study, optimization of the size of NPs was carried out according to the Central Composite Face-Centered Design (CCFD) and using Design-Expert software (Version 8.0.7.1, statEase, Inc., USA).

Characterization of NPs

The size of fabricated particles was assessed and analyzed by Zetasizer (Nano-ZS, Malvern, UK) using dynamic light scattering (DLS).
The morphology and structure of NPs were observed by a transmission election microscope (TEM, Zeiss-EM10C, 80 KV, Germany).

Cell viability assay

In this study, β-TC$_3$ (a mouse beta pancreatic cell line), was purchased from Iran genetic resources center. MCF7 (a human breast cancer cell line) and HT29 (a human colon adenocarcinoma cell line) were purchased from Pasteur Institute of Iran. The thiazolyl blue assay has been used in experiments for the assessment of cell viability. Briefly, cells were seeded at density of 5×10^4 cells/ml in 96-well tissue culture. After 24 h, cells were incubated with increasing concentrations of pure gum and NPs (1%, 0.5%, 0.25%, and 0.125% w/v) for 48 h separately. Then the MTT assay was performed to measure the cell viability according to previous study.[9]

Antibacterial test

Pseudomonas aeruginosa (ATCC27853), as a standard strain, and *Staphylococcus aureus*, as a clinicallyisolated strain, in the Microbiology Laboratory of Imam Khomeini Hospital (Kermanshah, Iran) were used in this study.
Serial dilutions (1.5%, 1.3%, 1.1%, 0.9%, and 0.7%) of the NPs were made in Mueller-Hinton Broth containing 5% DMSO for bacteria, in 96-well micro titer plates. 20 µl of fresh microbial suspensions was prepared from overnight grown cultures containing 1.5×10^8 organisms/ml and were added to each well. The final volume of culture was 200 µl per each well.
Ampicillin and water were used as positive and negative controls, respectively. The MTT assay was performed to

assess the (MIC) and MBC of the extract of NPs using MTT solution with concentration of 5.0 mg/ml.

Results and Discussion
Response Surface Model

Table 1 shows the actual form of factors and the experimental size of NPs, as the response. Based on the data, the range of responses was found from 75.85–241.3 nm. The response function was fitted by a quadratic polynomial model.

Table 1. Factors in actual form, and experimental size data

Organic phase volume (µl)	Concentration of gum (w/v%)	Solvent type	Size(nm)
1000	0.55	Ethanol	159
1000	0.55	Acetone	195.6
1000	0.55	DMSO	118.2
550	0.55	Acetone	189.66
550	0.55	DMSO	114.6
550	0.55	Acetone	183.3
550	0.55	Ethanol	117.1
550	0.55	Ethanol	116.5
550	0.55	Ethanol	113.5
550	0.55	Acetone	149.66
550	0.55	DMSO	105.9
550	0.55	Acetone	164.1
550	0.55	DMSO	100.9
550	0.55	DMSO	98.02
550	0.55	Ethanol	138
550	0.55	DMSO	107.3
550	0.55	Ethanol	134.1
550	0.55	Acetone	168.4
100	0.55	DMSO	78.86
100	0.55	Acetone	135.6
100	0.55	Ethanol	107.1
1000	1	DMSO	102
1000	1	Ethanol	186.6
1000	1	Acetone	241.3
550	1	DMSO	87.52
550	1	Acetone	202.3
550	1	Ethanol	164.5
100	1	Acetone	186.6
100	1	DMSO	97.2
100	0.1	Ethanol	144.8
1000	0.1	DMSO	155.2
1000	0.1	Acetone	140
1000	0.1	Ethanol	118
550	0.1	DMSO	114.5
550	0.1	Ethanol	82.96
550	0.1	Acetone	106.9
100	0.1	Acetone	96.32
100	0.1	DMSO	104.5
100	0.1	Ethanol	75.853

To find the best model correlating the response to process variables the analysis of variance (ANOVA) by calculating F-value was employed. It is important to note that the p-values< 0.05 indicate a better significance of model terms. The lack of fit F-value of 0.7007 revealed that the lack of fit is not significant in response, which indicates low error and accuracy of the model (Table 2). According to the experimental results and using RSM, the response function was fitted by a quadratic polynomial equation. This equation is given as follows in terms of coded factors:

$$Z \text{ average} = +50.85 + 0.05828A + 89.116B - 0.0145\ AB \text{ (ethanol)} \quad (1)$$

$$Z \text{ average} = +71.027 + 0.0666A + 114.2620B - 0.0145\ AB \text{ (acetone)} \quad (2)$$

$$Z \text{ average} = +100.63 + 0.0431A - 24.427B - 0.0145\ AB \text{ (DMSO)} \quad (3)$$

Where Z average is the average of size, A is the volume of the organic phase, and B is the percentage of gum in the solution.
The regression analysis shows that all the linear coefficients of the independent variables, and also the interaction of the volume of the organic phase and the percentage of gum in the solution, are significant (where $p<0.05$).
The coefficient of determination (R^2), adjusted R^2, and predicted R^2 of the model were found 0.93, 0.92, and 0.90, respectively.

Table 2. Analysis of Variance

Source	Sum of Squares	D_f	Mean Square	F-Value	p-value	Prob> F
Model	55183.41	6.00	9197.24	76.88	< 0.0001	Significant
A-Organic solvent volume	8409.62	1.00	8409.62	70.30	< 0.0001	
B-Concentration of gum	9734.17	1.00	9734.17	81.37	< 0.0001	
C-Type of solvent	23772.23	2.00	11886.12	99.36	< 0.0001	
BC	13267.39	2.00	6633.70	55.45	< 0.0001	
Residual	3827.95	32.00	119.62			
Lack of Fit	2143.51	20.00	107.18	0.76	0.7132	not significant
Pure Error	1684.44	12.00	140.37			
Cor Total	59011.36	38.00				

Figure 1 shows the distributed plot of the predicted amounts versus the actual amounts for the size of NPs. The closer the points are to the 45 degree line, the better the estimations of the RSM model. Based on this plot, the model could appropriately fit the data.

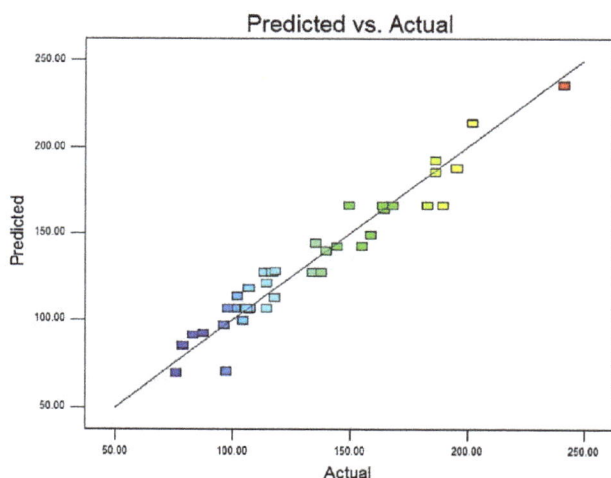

Figure 1. Predicted versus actual values of Zaverage for RSM mode

Figure 2 shows the response surface 3D plots exhibiting the effects of interactions between the volume of the organic phase and the concentration of gum in the organic phase.

Effect of process parameters on the size of NPs
The size of the fabricated NPs was measured and the results are tabulated in Table 1. In the presence of ethanol and acetone, increasing the gum concentration causes fabrication of larger NPs. But in the presence of DMSO, the results were the inverse, and increasing the concentration of gum resulted in the reduction in the size of NPs. As the concentration of gum in the organic phase increases, the size of fabricated NPs increases due to an increase in the viscosity of organic solution and the hindering of the diffusion of solvents to water. Diminution in viscosity leads to the facilitation of solvent diffusion to the outer aqueous solution and consequently, production of smaller particles.[10] This trend was conversely when DMSO was used as the organic solvent. This incongruity may arise from possible interactions between *p.khinjuk* gum and DMSO molecules.

B: The concentration of gum in organic phase (w/v%)   A: The volume of organic phase (µL)

B: The concentration of gum in organic phase (w/v%)   A: The volume of organic phase (µL)

B: The concentration of gum in organic phase (w/v%)   A: The volume of organic phase (µL)

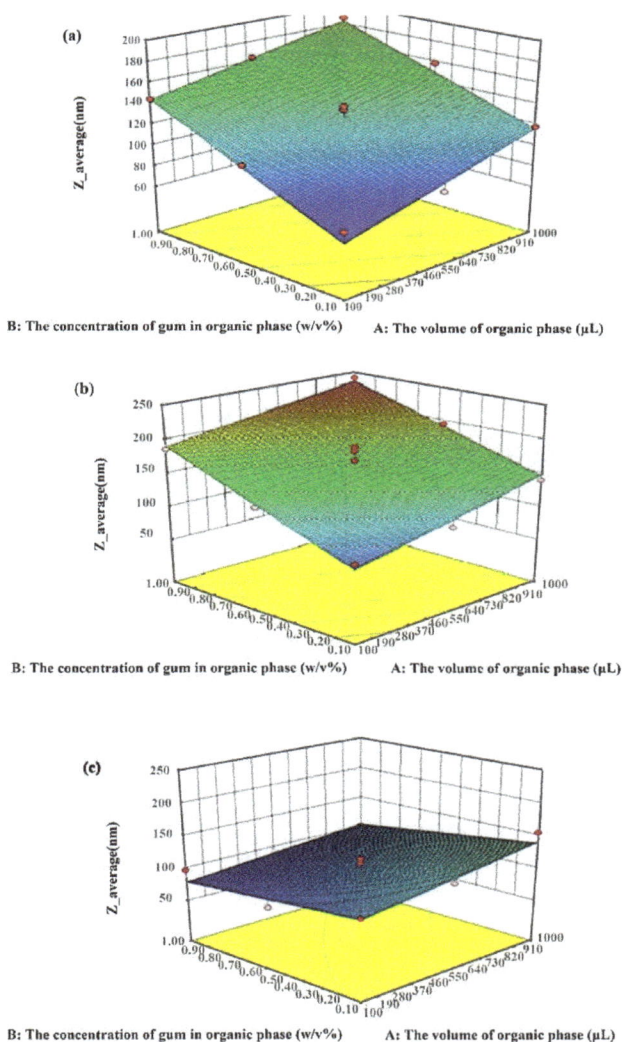

Figure 2. The effect of volume of organic phase and the concentration of gum in organic solution on Z average of NPs obtained by a) ethanol; b) acetone; and c) DMSO as organic solvent.

The results also revealed that, at constant volume of aqueous solution, increasing the volume of the organic phase (increasing the volume ratio of the organic to aqueous solutions) results in an increase in the size of fabricated NPs. Decreasing the ratio of organic to aqueous solutions can improve the diffusion of organic solvent, and it increases the distribution efficiency of the organic phase into the external phase, leading to formation of smaller NPs. This reason has been evoked in the similar studies.[11]

The size of NPs using different solvents is exhibited in Table 1. The comparison revealed that using DMSO as the solvent, results in smaller NPs at the highest concentration of gum. DMSO was chosen as the most suitable solvent due to the production of smaller particles. It is worthmentioning that the selection of organic solvent could be directly affected by individual key parameters, such as a solvent dielectric constant and the affinity of the solvent for water. The

miscibility of solvents in water is an important parameter that should be considered. The higher miscibility of the solvent in water causes the higher rate of diffusion into the aqueous phase, and consequently, the production of smaller NPs. The miscibility of solvents in water could be evaluated regarding the mutual solubility parameter ($\Delta\delta$), The smaller $\Delta\delta$ indicates the higher affinity.The $\Delta\delta$ has been evaluated 27, 28.7, and 34.4 MPa$^{1/2}$ for ethanol, DMSO, and acetone, respectively.[12]

Optimization and model validation

To determine the optimum condition for the lowest Z average, some solutions would be suggested by the software. Based on these results, the optimum size of NPs was obtained using DMSO as the organic solvent (using 111.25 µl of organic phase and 1% of gum). For model validation, experiments were performed by using the aforementioned optimum conditions. The experimental response for optimized NP size was 73.18 nm, and the prediction error was found 0.0327 (<0.05), which confirms the validity of model in optimizing the size of NPs.

Morphology of NPs

The TEM result of the suspension of NPs (at the concentration of 1% w/v using DMSO as organic phase) is visualized in Figure 3. The polydispersity index of these NPs was measured using Zetasizer. According to the TEM observation, particles were found to be relatively spherical, and the size of the obtained NPs was less than 100 nm. The obtained NPs were monodisperse, and the polydispersity of NPs was found 0.07, which confirms the narrow size distribution of NPs. The measured values resulted from TEM was comparable with the DLS results.

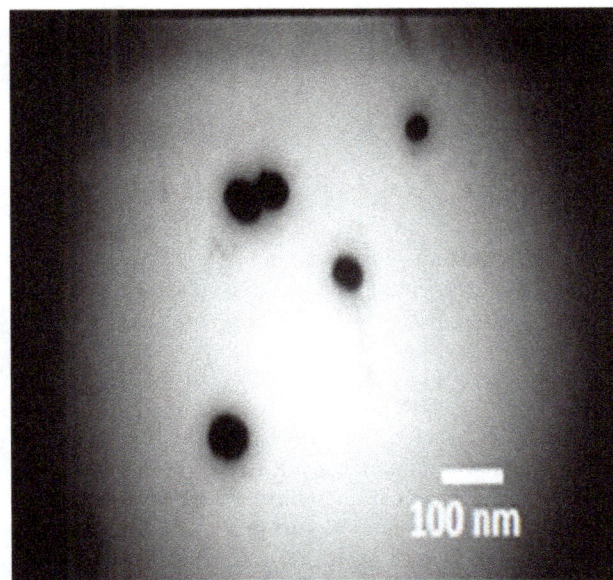

Figure 3. TEM of the suspension of NPs in DMSO with the concentration of 1% w/v.

The cytotoxicity test

The MTT results indicated that NPs have higher cytotoxic activity compare to pure gum in all three cell lines (β-TC$_3$, MCF7, and HT29), while NPs and gum exhibited the relatively highest cytotoxic activity towards β-TC$_3$ (Figure 4). The IC$_{50}$ value was achieved at 1% of NPs in β-TC$_3$. The results revealed that the cytotoxicity of pure gum and NPs does not reach IC$_{50}$ in HT29 and MCF7 cell line. The cytotoxic activity of NPs and pure gum can be attributed to the high content of terpenes in *p.khinjuk* gum structure.[13] The Hedgehog (Hh) signaling pathway is a critical element regulating cellular growth and organizing differentiation during embryonic development, which plays a significant role in different types of cancer.[14,15] Terpenes possess the ability to affect and target the Hh pathways and have been used for treating cancer. This pathway has been frequently discussed in the treatment of pancreatic cancer and has a significant effect on the treatment of this cancer, but it has no significant effect on HT29; the effect of this pathway on colon cancer is not clear. The Hh pathway also affects breast cancer, but there have some inconsistent reports on the effect of Hh on the MCF7 cell line. While this pathway has been found effective on the MCF7 cell line, its growth could not be inhibited by cyclopamine.[15,16] There is no clear report for the mechanism of Hh activation in breast cancer, and the mechanism of Hh effect on MCF7 is not clear yet.

The higher cytotoxic activity of NPs could be due to the small size of the particles and advantageous for nano-sized particles. Furthermore, it could be noted that pure gum is insoluble in water, while NPs could disperse homogenously in water and are able to transport more into cells, thus achieving lower cell viability and showing greater cytotoxicity compared to gum.

Measurement of antibacterial activity

Table 3 shows the results of antibacterial activity of NPs towards both performed bacterial strains.The inhibition activity of the samples can be attributed to the fact that the major constituent of gum is α-pinene. The antimicrobial activity of α-pinene has been reported in the literature.[17]

Conclusion

In the current study, *p.khinjuk* gum NPs, were prepared as novel drug carriers and the size of particles could be altered with different affecting parameters. The optimization was performed, and the optimum size was achieved using 111.25µl of DMSO, and 1% (w/v) of gum, with the NP size of 70.86 nm (obtained by model). The effect of experimental parameters on the size of NPs was obtained by fitting experimental data with a quadratic equation with a prediction error less than 0.05. The obtained NPs were found monodisperse and spherical, according to the DLS and TEM results. The obtained NPs had higher cytotoxic activity in comparison with pure gum and its IC$_{50}$ value was achieved at 1% of NPs in β-TC$_3$. These NPs also

possess inherent antibacterial activity and could be good candidates for treatment and as carriers in drug delivery systems.

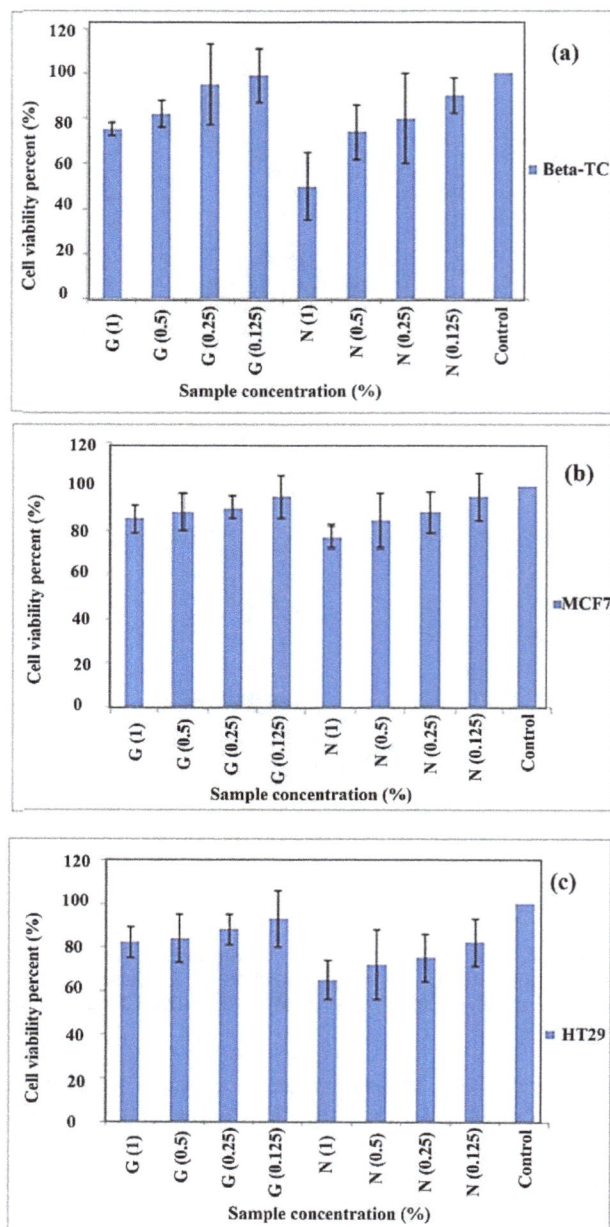

Figure 4. Cell viability of pure gum and NP on a) β-TC$_3$; b) MCF7; and c) HT29 cell lines (*G refers to Gum and N refers to NP).

Table 3. The antibacterial activity of NPs.

Bacterial Strains	Concentration				
	0.7%	0.9%	1.1%	1.3%	1.5%
Pseudomonas aeruginosa	+	+	MIC	+	MBC
staphylococcus aureus	+	+	MIC	MBC	–

Acknowledgments
The authors would like to acknowledge the Research Council of Kermanshah University of Medical Sciences for supporting this work (Research grant No.94219).

Conflict of Interest
The authors declare no conflict of interests.

References
1. Ezatpour B, Saedi Dezaki E, Mahmoudvand H, Azadpour M, Ezzatkhah F. In vitro and in vivo antileishmanial effects of Pistacia khinjuk against leishmania tropica and leishmania major. *Evid Based Complement Alternat Med* 2015;2015:149707. doi: 10.1155/2015/149707
2. Bozorgi M, Memariani Z, Mobli M, Salehi Surmaghi MH, Shams-Ardekani MR, Rahimi R. Five Pistacia species (P. vera, P. atlantica, P. terebinthus, P. khinjuk, and P. lentiscus): a review of their traditional uses, phytochemistry, and pharmacology. *Scientific World J* 2013;2013:219815. doi: 10.1155/2013/219815
3. Hacibekiroglu I, Yilmaz PK, Hasimi N, Kilinc E, Tolan V, Kolak U. In vitro biological activities and fatty acid profiles of Pistacia terebinthus fruits and Pistacia khinjuk seeds. *Nat Prod Res* 2015;29(5):444-6. doi: 10.1080/14786419.2014.947492
4. Ghasemi Pirbalouti A, Aghaee K. Chemical composition of essential oil of Pistacia khinjuk stocks grown in bakhtiari zagross mountains, iran. *Electron J Biol* 2011;7(4):67-9.
5. Tohidi M, Khayami M, Nejati V, Meftahizade H. Evaluation of antibacterial activity and wound healing of Pistacia atlantica and Pistacia khinjuk. *J Med Plant Res* 2011;5(17):4310-4.
6. Moussa AY, Labib RM, Ayoub NA. Isolation of chemical constituents and protective effect of Pistacia khinjuk against CCl4–induced damage on HepG2 cells. *Phytopharmacology* 2013;4(4):1-9.
7. Nazari H, Yavarmanesh M, Haddad Khodaparast MH. In vitro study to evaluate the antibacterial effect of Pistacia khinjuk stocks oil as compared with olive oil on food borne pathogenic bacteria (staphylococcus aureus, escherichia coli, listeria monocytogenes). *J Essent Oil Bear Plants* 2016;19(1):125-33. doi: 10.1080/0972060X.2014.971067
8. Bezerra MA, Santelli RE, Oliveira EP, Villar LS, Escaleira LA. Response surface methodology (RSM) as a tool for optimization in analytical chemistry. *Talanta* 2008;76(5):965-77. doi: 10.1016/j.talanta.2008.05.019
9. Shahbazi B, Taghipour M, Rahmani H, Sadrjavadi K, Fattahi A. Preparation and characterization of silk fibroin/oligochitosan nanoparticles for sirna delivery. *Colloids Surf B Biointerfaces* 2015;136:867-77. doi: 10.1016/j.colsurfb.2015.10.044
10. Chorny M, Fishbein I, Danenberg HD, Golomb G. Lipophilic drug loaded nanospheres prepared by nanoprecipitation: Effect of formulation variables on size, drug recovery and release kinetics. *J Control Release* 2002;83(3):389-400. doi: 10.1016/S0168-3659(02)00211-0
11. Budhian A, Siegel SJ, Winey KI. Haloperidol-loaded plga nanoparticles: Systematic study of particle size and drug content. *Int J Pharm* 2007;336(2):367-75. doi: 10.1016/j.ijpharm.2006.11.061
12. Galindo-Rodriguez S, Allemann E, Fessi H, Doelker E. Physicochemical parameters associated with nanoparticle formation in the salting-out, emulsification-diffusion, and nanoprecipitation methods. *Pharm Res* 2004;21(8):1428-39. doi: 10.1023/B:PHAM.0000036917.75634.be
13. Mirian M, Behrooeian M, Ghanadian M, Dana N, Sadeghi-Aliabadi H. Cytotoxicity and antiangiogenic effects of Rhus coriaria, Pistacia vera and Pistacia khinjuk oleoresin methanol extracts. *Res Pharm Sci* 2015;10(3):233-40.
14. Kubo M, Nakamura M, Tasaki A, Yamanaka N, Nakashima H, Nomura M, et al. Hedgehog signaling pathway is a new therapeutic target for patients with breast cancer. *Cancer Res* 2004;64(17):6071-4. doi: 10.1158/0008-5472.CAN-04-0416
15. Rifai Y, Arai MA, Koyano T, Kowithayakorn T, Ishibashi M. Terpenoids and a flavonoid glycoside from Acacia pennata leaves as hedgehog/GLI-mediated transcriptional inhibitors. *J Nat Prod* 2010;73(5):995-7. doi: 10.1021/np1000818
16. Zardawi SJ, O'Toole SA, Sutherland RL, Musgrove EA. Dysregulation of hedgehog, wnt and notch signalling pathways in breast cancer. *Histol Histopathol* 2009;24(3):385-98. doi: 10.14670/HH-24.385
17. Habibi Najafi MB, Hajimohamadi Farimani R, Tavakoli J, Madayeni S. GC-MS Analysis and Antimicrobial Activity of the Essential Oil of Trunk Exudates of Pistacia atlantica var. mutica. *Chem Nat Compd* 2014;50(2):376-8. doi: 10.1007/s10600-014-0959-z

12

Effects of Herbal Compound (IMOD) on Behavior and Expression of Alzheimer's Disease Related Genes in Streptozotocin-Rat Model of Sporadic Alzheimer's Disease

Niloofar Bazazzadegan[1], Marzieh Dehghan Shasaltaneh[2], Kioomars Saliminejad[3], Koorosh Kamali[3], Mehdi Banan[1], Hamid Reza Khorram Khorshid[1]*

[1] *Genetics Research Center, University of Social Welfare and Rehabilitation Sciences, Tehran, Iran.*
[2] *Laboratory of Neuro-organic Chemistry, Institute of Biochemistry and Biophysics (IBB), University of Tehran, Tehran, Iran.*
[3] *Reproductive Biotechnology Research Center, Avicenna Research Institute, ACECR, Tehran, Iran.*

Article info

Keywords:
· Alzheimer's disease
· Gene expression
· Herbal extract
· Rat model

Abstract

Purpose: Sporadic Alzheimer's disease (AD) accounts for over 95% of cases. Possible mechanisms of AD such as inflammation and oxidative stresses in the brain motivate researchers to follow many therapies which would be effective, especially in the early stages of the disease. IMOD, the herbal extract of *R. Canina*, *T. Vulgare* and *U. Dioica* plant species enriched with selenium, has anti-inflammatory, immunoregulatory and protective effects against oxidative stress.

Methods: In this study three AD-related genes, *DAXX*, *NFκβ* and *VEGF*, were chosen as candidate to investigate the neuroprotective effect of the extract by comparing their expression levels in the hippocampus of rat model of sporadic AD, using qPCR in the herbal-treated and control groups. The therapeutic effects on learning and memory levels were evaluated by Morris Water Maze (MWM) test.

Results: Gene expression results were indicative of significant up-regulation of *Vegf* in rat's hippocampus after treatment with the herbal extract comparing to model group (P-value= 0.001). The MWM results showed significant changes in path length and time for finding the hidden platform in all groups during test and the same change in the treated comparing to the control group in memory level.

Conclusion: It could be concluded that the herbal extract may have significant effect on gene expression but not on behavioral level.

Introduction

Sporadic Alzheimer's disease (AD) is a complex disorder which both genetic and environmental risk factors are involved.[1] An important event in pathogenesis of AD is aggregation of Aβ peptide in the brain. Most approaches to therapy in AD aimed at preventing aggregation of Aβ peptides.[2] Sporadic Alzheimer's disease (SAD) is an insulin-resistant brain state. It is proposed that direct injection of streptozotocin (STZ) into rat brain could be used as an AD model (type 3 diabetes).[3,4] STZ impairs brain glucose and energy metabolism and induces the impairment of learning and memory formation, and moreover lowering of choline acetyl transferase levels in the hippocampus.[3,5]

In AD it is essential to recognize the specific molecular pathways. The expression pattern of genes provides indirect information about function, drug target and cause of a disease. Among various genes related to pathology of SAD, *DAXX*, *NFκβ*, *VEGF* genes with the role in apoptosis, inflammation and angiogenesis represented significant differential expression in Alzheimer human brain.[6]

IMOD (Rose PharMed Co. (Iran)), the herbal extract of *Tanacetum vulgare*, *Rosa canina* and *Urtica dioica* plant species, which has been enriched with selenium, has anti-inflammatory, immunoregulatory and a protective effect against oxidative stress.[7-9] Several *in vitro* and *in vivo* studies in animal models and human have shown that *Urtica dioica* extracts decreases some inflammatory factors levels. Furthermore, its immunoregulatory properties in inflammatory bowel diseases, immunogenic type-1 diabetes in mouse, sepsis and HIV patients has been evaluated.[10-17] In this study according to the importance of molecular mechanisms of AD such as inflammation and oxidative stresses in the brain, the neuroprotective effect of this herbal extract was investigated by evaluating the expression levels of the three AD-related genes, *Daxx*, *Nfκβ* and *Vegf*, in the hippocampus of rat model of SAD using qPCR in treated and untreated groups. In addition, the therapeutic effects were checked on behavioral, learning and memory levels.

*Corresponding author: Hamid Reza Khorram Khorshid, Email: hrkk1@uswr.ac.ir

Materials and Methods

Thirty seven adult male *Wistar* rats with 250-300 g weight were used in this research. They were kept in cage with enough food and water, in a stable environment at 22°C and 12h light/dark cycle.[18] Animals were distributed into five groups each containing of six to eight rats. The control group (Eight rats) received no medication and had no surgery. The sham group (Eight rats) received bilateral intracerebroventricular (ICV) injection of aCSF as the vehicle of STZ, the Alzheimer group (Seven rats) with bilateral ICV infusion of STZ (3 mg/kg) five days after surgery as recovery. The ethanol-treated STZ group (Six rats) which received diluted ethanol 86% (10 fold dilution) as I.P. as the vehicle of herbal extract,[18] and the IMOD treated STZ group (Eight rats) received the compound as intrapritoneal (IP) at the dose of 20 mg/kg/day for 21 days after modeling.[19]

All groups of rats were examined for behavioral evaluation using Morris Water Maze (MWM) test.[20] They subsequently were sacrificed with stereotaxic surgery and all hippocampi were dissected and preserved in RNA protector solution at -20°C.[21] All procedures were carried out according to the National Institute of Health Guide for the care and use of laboratory animals.[22]

Total RNAs were extracted from all hippocampus tissues using UP100H ultrasonic processor (Germany) and RNeasy Plus Mini Kit (Qiagen, Hilden, Germany) according to the manufacturer's protocol. Purity and integrity of RNAs were specified using Nano-drop spectrophotometer and gel electrophoresis. cDNA synthesis was performed using RevertAid™ First Strand cDNA Synthesis Kit (Fermentas, Thermo Fisher Scientific) according to the manufacturer's protocol.

The relative expression levels of *Daxx, Nfkb* and *Vegf* in rat hippocampus of each group were assessed by SYBR green Real Time PCR (Takara SYBR Master Mix (Shiga, Japan) in an ABI 7500 Real-time PCR system (Applied Biosystem, Foster city, CA, USA). The normalization was done by *Actb* endogenous control.[23,24] Cycle threshold (Ct) values were used to calculate fold changes in gene expression between groups using REST 2009 software. P-values less than 0.01 for analysis by REST and in other analysis less than 0.05 were considered statistically significant. MWM test data were analyzed by GraphPad Prism 6 software; Kruskal Wallis (Dunn's multiple comparisons test) test was used for three recorded factors (path length, escape latency and swimming speed) in all treated and untreated groups separately during five days.

Results and Discussion

Behavioral Results

After assessing the learning and memory level changes by Morris Water Maze test, as it is obvious in Figure1, the results showed a significant reduction in swimming distance and time for finding the hidden platform during five days in all groups except alcohol group; however, no significant change was observed in the herbal-treated

comparing to the STZ-induced group in path length and escape latency during five days. Probe test indicated no significant change in the Herbal-treated comparing to the control group (Figure 2).

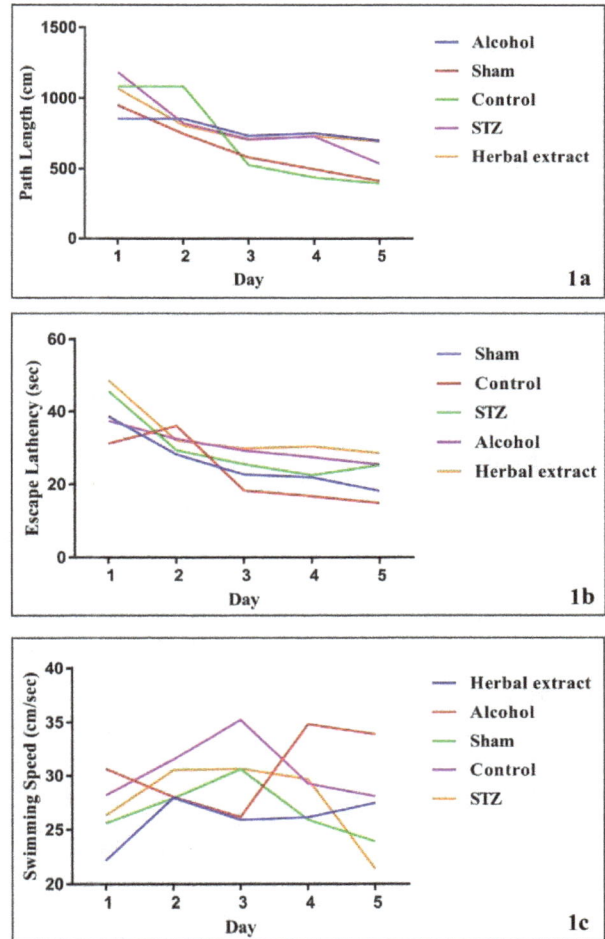

Figure 1. The mean of path length, time for finding hidden platform and swimming speed during five days in all treated and control groups were represented in 1A, 1B and 1C respectively

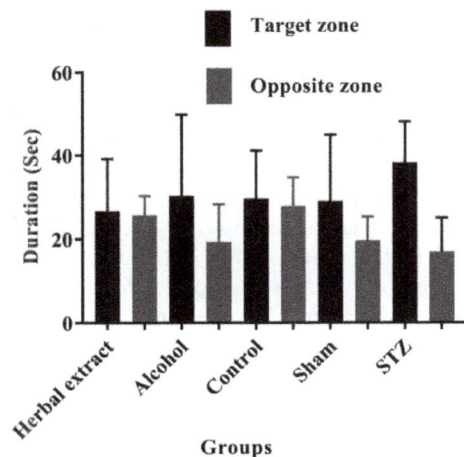

Figure 2. The median with interquartile range of duration time spending in target and opposite zone in the sixth day (four trials) of the test in all treated and control groups

Gene expression results

After evaluating the expression levels of three genes, only *Vegf* gene showed significant (p- value= 0.001) up-regulation in the herbal-treated versus the STZ-induced group (~2.5- fold). In addition, *Vegf* showed a significant down-regulation in the model compared to the control group (P- Value= 0) (Figure 3). Two other genes, *Daxx, Nfkb*, did not show any significant changes in expression level between the herbal-treated and the model group.

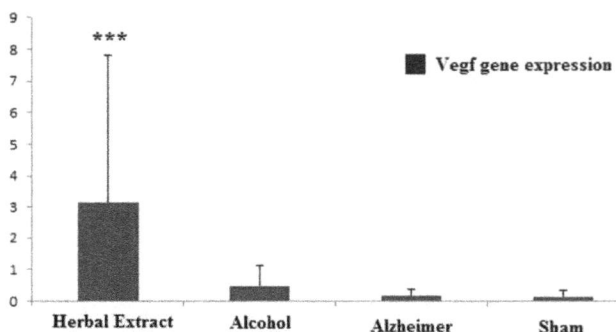

Figure 3. The expression level of *Vegf* gene in all treated and control groups were shown in this figure. * is representative of significant change of gene expression in herbal- treated comparing to Alzheimer group

In this study, we evaluated the expression of three candidate genes (*Daxx, Nfkb* and *Vegf*) for Alzheimr's disease in RNA level in rat models of AD. Our results showed that only *Vegf* gene was significantly up-regulated in the herbal-treated compared to the model group. According to the available data, it is postulated reduced *VEGF* expression in AD.[25] Furthermore, increased levels of VEGF has been reported in the hippocampal cortex of AD patients comparing to normal brain.[26] Therefore, VEGF levels are controversial in AD patient. In this study, *Vegf* expression showed significant down-regulation in model comparing to control group, but it showed inverse result in treated versus model group. Also, as it has been indicated, *Vegf* showed significant up-regulation in alcohol comparing to model group; whereas, no difference in the herbal comparing to its vehicle (alcohol) group was seen. Thus, alcohol may be an important factor which could be effective on expression level of *Vegf* gene in the herbal-treated group. In behavioral evaluation, as it has been shown in probe test graph (Figure 2), increasing of duration time spent in zone (target) where already the hidden platform has been located there, was observed in STZ group, whereas herbal-treated model showed decreased duration comparing to the model group but the same as control group. Regarding to the recent report by Daneshmand et al.[18] after evaluating rat treated with this herbal compound comparing to STZ-induced group in expression level and behavioral test, two other AD related genes, *Syp* and *Psen1* showed significant expression change in the herbal-treated group, and also significant increased memory was observed in this group comparing to the other groups.[18]

Conclusion

In summary, regarding to the both behavioral and gene expression analyses, it would be concluded that this extract may have significant effect on gene expression level related to angiogenesis but, not on clinical levels.

Acknowledgments

We would like to thank Rose PharMed Co. (Iran) for providing the herbal extract. The study was supported by the University of Social Welfare and Rehabilitation Sciences, Tehran, Iran.

Conflict of Interest

The authors declare no conflict of interest.

References

1. Blennow K, de Leon MJ, Zetterberg H. Alzheimer's disease. *Lancet* 2006;368(9533):387-403. doi: 10.1016/S0140-6736(06)69113-7
2. Liu R, Barkhordarian H, Emadi S, Park CB, Sierks MR. Trehalose differentially inhibits aggregation and neurotoxicity of beta-amyloid 40 and 42. *Neurobiol Dis* 2005;20(1):74-81. doi: 10.1016/j.nbd.2005.02.003
3. Lannert H, Hoyer S. Intracerebroventricular administration of streptozotocin causes long-term diminutions in learning and memory abilities and in cerebral energy metabolism in adult rats. *Behav Neurosci* 1998;112(5):1199-208. doi: 10.1037/0735-7044.112.5.1199
4. Lester-Coll N, Rivera EJ, Soscia SJ, Doiron K, Wands JR, de la Monte SM. Intracerebral streptozotocin model of type 3 diabetes: relevance to sporadic Alzheimer's disease. *J Alzheimers Dis* 2006;9(1):13-33. doi: 10.3233/jad-2006-9102
5. Hoyer S. Risk factors for Alzheimer's disease during aging. Impacts of glucose/energy metabolism. In: Gertz HJ, editor. Alzheimer's Disease. From Basic Research to Clinical Applications. Springer; 1998. PP. 187-94.
6. Lukiw WJ. Gene expression profiling in fetal, aged, and Alzheimer hippocampus: a continuum of stress-related signaling. *Neurochem Res* 2004;29(6):1287-97. doi: 10.1023/b:nere.0000023615.89699.63
7. Dügenci SK, Arda N, Candan A. Some medicinal plants as immunostimulant for fish. *J Ethnopharmacol* 2003;88(1):99-106. doi: 10.1016/s0378-8741(03)00182-x
8. Kanter M, Coskun O, Budancamanak M. Hepatoprotective effects of Nigella sativa L and Urtica dioica L on lipid peroxidation, antioxidant enzyme systems and liver enzymes in carbon tetrachloride-treated rats. *World J Gastroenterol* 2005;11(42):6684-8. doi: 10.3748/wjg.v11.i42.6684
9. Schinella GR, Giner RM, Recio MC, Mordujovich de Buschiazzo P, Rios JL, Manez S. Anti-inflammatory

Effects of South American Tanacetum vulgare. *J Pharm Pharmacol* 1998;50(9):1069-74. doi: 10.1111/j.2042-7158.1998.tb06924.x

10. Baghaei A, Esmaily H, Abdolghaffari AH, Baeeri M, Gharibdoost F, Abdollahi M. Efficacy of Setarud (IMOD®), a novel drug with potent anti-toxic stress potential in rat inflammatory bowel disease and comparison with dexamethasone and infliximab. *Indian J Biochem Biophys* 2010;47(4):219-26.

11. Khairandish P, Mohraz M, Farzamfar B, Abdollahi M, Shahhosseiny M, Madani H, et al. Preclinical and phase 1 clinical safety of Setarud (IMOD™), a novel immunomodulator. *DARU* 2009;17(3):148-56.

12. Khorram Khorshid HR, Novitsky YA, Abdollahi M, Shahhosseiny MH, Sadeghi B, Madani H, et al. Studies on potential mutagenic and genotoxic activity of Setarud. *DARU* 2008;16(4):223-8.

13. Look M, Rockstroh JK, Rao GS, Barton S, Lemoch H, Kaiser R, et al. Sodium selenite and N-acetylcysteine in antiretroviral-naive HIV-1-infected patients: a randomized, controlled pilot study. *Eur J Clin Invest* 1998;28(5):389-97. doi: 10.1046/j.1365-2362.1998.00301.x

14. Mahmoodpoor A, Eslami K, Mojtahedzadeh M, Najafi A, Ahmadi A, Dehnadi-Moghadam A, et al. Examination of Setarud (IMOD™) in the management of patients with severe sepsis. *DARU* 2010;18(1):23-8.

15. Mohseni-Salehi-Monfared SS, Habibollahzadeh E, Sadeghi H, Baeeri M, Abdollahi M. Efficacy of Setarud (IMOD™), a novel electromagnetically-treated multi-herbal compound, in mouse immunogenic type-1 diabetes. *Arch Med Sci* 2010;6(5):663-9. doi: 10.5114/aoms.2010.17078

16. Ogunro PS, Ogungbamigbe TO, Elemie PO, Egbewale BE, Adewole TA. Plasma selenium concentration and glutathione peroxidase activity in HIV-1/AIDS infected patients: a correlation with the disease progression. *Niger Postgrad Med J* 2006;13(1):1-5.

17. Paydary K, Emamzadeh-Fard S, Khorram Khorshid HR, Kamali K, SeyedAlinaghi S, Mohraz M. Safety and efficacy of Setarud (IMOD TM) among people living with HIV/AIDS: a review. *Recent Pat Antiinfect Drug Discov* 2012;7(1):66-72. doi: 10.2174/157489112799829756

18. Daneshmand P, Saliminejad K, Dehghan Shasaltaneh M, Kamali K, Riazi GH, Nazari R, et al. Neuroprotective Effects of Herbal Extract (Rosa canina, Tanacetum vulgare and Urtica dioica) on Rat Model of Sporadic Alzheimer's Disease. *Avicenna J Med Biotechnol* 2016;8(3):120-5.

19. Ghanbari S, Yonessi M, Mohammadirad A, Gholami M, Baeeri M, Khorram-Khorshid HR, et al. Effects of IMOD™ and Angipars™ on mouse D-galactose-induced model of aging. *DARU* 2012;20(1):68. doi: 10.1186/2008-2231-20-68

20. Morris RG. Morris water maze. *Scholarpedia* 2008;3(8):6315. doi: 10.4249/scholarpedia.6315

21. Paxinos G, Watson C. The Rat Nervous Coordinates: The New Coronal Set. New York: Elsevier; 2004.

22. National Research Council (US) Committee. Guide for the Care and Use of Laboratory Animals. 8th ed. Washington (DC): National Academies Press (US); 2011.

23. Moura AC, Lazzari VM, Agnes G, Almeida S, Giovenardi M, Veiga AB. Transcriptional expression study in the central nervous system of rats: what gene should be used as internal control? *Einstein (Sao Paulo)* 2014;12(3):336-41. doi: 10.1590/s1679-45082014ao3042

24. Silver N, Cotroneo E, Proctor G, Osailan S, Paterson KL, Carpenter GH. Selection of housekeeping genes for gene expression studies in the adult rat submandibular gland under normal, inflamed, atrophic and regenerative states. *BMC Mol Biol* 2008;9:64. doi: 10.1186/1471-2199-9-64

25. Mateo I, Llorca J, Infante J, Rodríguez-Rodríguez E, Fernández-Viadero C, Pena N, et al. Low serum VEGF levels are associated with Alzheimer's disease. *Acta Neurol Scand* 2007;116(1):56-8. doi: 10.1111/j.1600-0404.2006.00775.x

26. Tang H, Mao X, Xie L, Greenberg DA, Jin K. Expression level of vascular endothelial growth factor in hippocampus is associated with cognitive impairment in patients with Alzheimer's disease. *Neurobiol Aging* 2013;34(5):1412-5. doi: 10.1016/j.neurobiolaging.2012.10.029

13

Anti-Inflammatory and Antioxidant Activity of *Acalypha hispida* Leaf and Analysis of its Major Bioactive Polyphenols by HPLC

Md. Afjalus Siraj[1]*, Jamil A. Shilpi[2], Md. Golam Hossain[2], Shaikh Jamal Uddin[2], Md. Khirul Islam[3], Ismet Ara Jahan[4], Hemayet Hossain[4]

[1] *Department of Pharmaceutical Science, Daniel K. Inouye College of Pharmacy, University of Hawaii at Hilo, Hilo, HI 96720, USA.*
[2] *Faculty of Pharmacy Discipline, Life Science School, Khulna University, Khulna 9208, Bangladesh.*
[3] *Department of Biochemistry, Faculty of Mathematics and Natural Sciences, University of Turku, FI-20500, Finland.*
[4] *BCSIR Laboratories, Bangladesh Council of Scientific and Industrial Research (BCSIR), Dhaka 1205, Bangladesh.*

Article info

Keywords:
· Carrageenan
· Histamine
· Anti-inflammatory
· DPPH
· Ellagic acid

Abstract

Purpose: Inflammation and oxidative stress can lead to different chronic diseases including cancer and atherosclerosis. Many medicinal plants have the potential to show as anti-inflammatory activity. Present investigation was performed to investigate anti-inflammatory, antioxidant activity, and quantification of selected bioactive plant polyphenols of the ethanol (EAH) and aqueous (AAH) extracts of *Acalypha hispida* (Euphorbiaceae) leaves.

Methods: Anti-inflammatory activity was evaluated by carragenan and histamine induced rat paw edema models while antioxidant capacity was evaluated by DPPH free radical scavenging, Fe^{+2} chelating ability, reducing power, NO scavenging, total phenolic and total flavonoid content assay. Identification and quantification of bioactive polyphenols was done by HPLC.

Results: At the doses of 200 and 400 mg/kg, both EAH and AAH showed statistically significant inhibition of paw volume in the anti-inflammatory activity test. Both the extracts showed DPPH scavenging (IC_{50}: 14 and 17 µg/ml, respectively), Fe^{+2} ion chelating (IC_{50}: 40 and 46 µg/ml, respectively), NO scavenging activity (65.49 and 60.66% inhibition at 100 µg/ml), and concentration dependent reducing power ability. For EAH and AAH, flavonoid content was 126.30 and 149.72 mg QE/g dry extract, while phenolic content was 130.51 and 173.80 mg GAE/g dry extract, respectively. HPLC analysis of EAH and AAH indicated the presence of high content of ellagic acid along with other phenolic constituents.

Conclusion: High content of ellagic acid along with other phenolic constituents might have played an important role in the observed anti-inflammatory and antioxidant activity.

Introduction

Acalypha hispida Burm.f. (Euphorbiaceae) is an erect, sparsely branched shrub, locally known as sibjhul, sibjota or jotamangshi in Bangladesh. It grows in the coastal regions of Bangladesh. The plant is native to New Guinea, the Malay Archipelago and other islands in the East Indies.[1] It is commonly used as an ornamental plant in the garden and house. The leaves are laxative, diuretic and used in the treatment of leprosy and gonorrhea. Different part of the plant is also used in infectious diarrhoea, pulmonary problems, and as an expectorant in asthma.[2] The plant contains ellagitannins namely, acalyphidins M_1, M_2, and D_1, anthocyanins namely, cyanidin 3-*O*-(2″-galloyl-*β*-galactopyranoside), cyanidin 3-*O*-(2″-galloyl-β-galactopyranoside), and cyanidin 3-*O*-β-galactopyranoside.[3,4] Previous phytochemical screening of *A. hispida* leaves extract indicated the presence of reducing sugars, glycosides, steroids, flavonoids, and saponins.[3,4,5] The leaves of *A.*

hispida has been reported to possess cytotoxic, antibacterial,[5] antileprotic,[6] antimicrobial,[7] and antifungal[8] properties, while the flower extract was reported to have DPPH free radical scavenging and cytotoxic activity.[9] As a part of the continuation of our research on bioactivity screening of Bangladeshi medicinal plants,[10,11,12] here we report the anti-inflammatory, antioxidant activity and quantification of the major polyphenols of ethanol and water extracts of *A. hispida* leaves.

Materials and Methods

Plant collection and extraction

The leaves of *A. hispida* was collected from Khulna, Bangladesh during July, 2012 and identified by the experts at Bangladesh National Herbarium (voucher specimen no.: DACB 34471). Shade-dried leaves were ground into coarse powder with the help of a grinder.

---

*Corresponding author: Md. Afjalus Siraj, Email: masiraj@hawaii.edu , saeed_2567@yahoo.com

The powdered plant material was kept in an airtight container and preserved in a cool, dark and dry place until the extraction commenced. Powdered plant material (150 g) was soaked in 900 ml of ethanol and kept for 72 h with occasional shaking and stirring. The solvent was filtered through a cotton plug. The filtrate was evaporated to dryness using a rotary vacuum evaporator to get the ethanol extract (EAH). The plant material was dried from the residual solvent and macerated with MilliQ water. Upon filtration, the filtrate was freeze dried to get the aqueous extract (AAH).

Test animals

For the *in vivo* anti-inflammatory activity study, male rats of Wister strain weighing 179-205 g were used. The animals were housed at the Pharmacology Research Laboratory of Bangladesh Council of Scientific and Industrial Research (BCSIR), Chittagong under standard laboratory conditions maintained at 25±1°C and fed with rodent food and water *ad libitum*. Protocols approved by BCSIR Ethics Committee on research in animals were followed during all experimental procedures that involve animals.

Chemicals and drug

Indomethacin, carrageenan, histamine phosphate, (+)-catechin hydrate, gallic acid, vanillic acid, caffeic acid, *p*-coumaric acid, (-)-epicatechin, rutin hydrate, quercetin, ellagic acid, ascorbic acid, DPPH, and Folin-Ciocalteu's reagent were purchased from Sigma–Aldrich (St. Louis, MO, USA). Tween 80, chloroform (analytical grade), ethanol (analytical grade), acetonitrile (HPLC grade), methanol (HPLC grade), acetic acid (HPLC grade), trichloroacetic acid, phosphate buffer (pH 6.6), potassium ferricyanide, ferric chloride, sodium phosphate, EDTA, ammonium molybdate, and sodium carbonate were purchased from Merck (Darmstadt, Germany).

Tests for anti-inflammatory activity
Carrageenan-induced rat paw edema test
The rats were divided into control, positive control and test groups, consisting of five animals in each. Control and positive control groups were orally administered with 1% Tween-80 in normal saline (10 ml/kg), and indomethacin (10 mg/kg), respectively. Test groups received EAH and AAH orally at the doses of 200 and 400 mg/kg, respectively. Acute inflammation was induced in all the rats by injecting 0.1 ml of carrageenan (1% w/v in 1% Tween-80 in normal saline) in the right hind paw of the rats, 1 h post exposure of the treatments. The paw volume was determined with a micrometer screw gauge at 1, 2, 3, 4 and 5 h after carrageenan administration.[13]

Histamine-induced rat paw edema test
The rats were divided into groups, and treated in the same fashion as that of carrageenan-induced edema test. Acute inflammation was initiated in all test animals by injecting 0.1 ml of histamine (1% w/v in 1% Tween-80 in normal saline) in the right hind paw of the rats. The paw volume was measured with a micrometer screw gauge at 1, 2, 3, 4 and 5 h after histamine administration.[14]

Tests for antioxidant activity
DPPH free radical scavenging assay
Aliquots (1 ml) of EAH, AAH and ascorbic acid at different concentrations were added to 3 ml of a 0.004% w/v DPPH solution. The mixture was allowed to stand in the dark at 25°C for 30 min and the absorbance of the mixture was recorded against blank at 517 nm using a double beam UV/Visible spectrophotometer (Analykjena, Model 205, Jena, Germany). The IC_{50} was determined from the absorbance versus concentration plot.[15]

Fe^{2+} ion chelating assay
Aliquots of (5 ml) different concentrations (5-100 µg/ml) of EAH, AAH and standard (EDTA) were taken and 0.1 ml solution of 2 mM ferrous chloride was added to it, followed by the addition of 0.2 ml of 5 mM ferrozine. After an interval of 10 min to complete the reaction, the absorbance of the solution was measured at 562 nm.[16]

Reducing power assay
Different concentrations of EAH, AAH and standards (ascorbic acid and BHA) (5–100 µg/ml) in 1 ml of distilled water were mixed with phosphate buffer (2.5 ml, 0.2 M, pH 6.6) and potassium ferricyanide (2.5 ml, 1 %). The mixture was incubated at 50°C for 20 min. A 10 % solution of trichloroacetic acid (2.5 ml) was added to the mixture, which was then centrifuged at 3000 rpm for 10 min. The upper layer of the solution (2.5 ml) was mixed with distilled water (2.5 ml) and $FeCl_3$ (0.5 ml, 0.1 %) and the absorbance of the mixture was measured at 700 nm.[17]

Nitric oxide scavenging assay
Sodium nitroprusside in phosphate buffer was mixed with different concentrations of EAH and AAH (5-100 µg/ml), and incubated at 25°C for 30 min. The incubated solution (1.5 ml) was diluted with 1.5 ml of Griess reagent (1% sulphanilamide, 2% phosphoric acid, and 0.1% naphthylethylenediamine dihydrochloride). The absorbance of the resulting reaction mixture was measured at 546 nm.[18]

Total phenolic content assay
Aliquots (0.5 ml) of the extracts (1 mg/ml) and various concentrations of gallic acid solutions (500-15.62 mg/L) were mixed with 5 ml of Folin-Ciocaltu's reagent (1:10 v/v in distilled water) and 4 ml of sodium carbonate. The mixture was then vortexed for 15 sec and kept for 30 min at 40°C for the reaction to complete and the absorbance was measured at 765 nm. Total phenol content of the extracts were determined from the standard curve and

expressed as mg of gallic acid equivalent (GAE) per gram extract.[19]

Total flavonoid content assay
The extracts (5 ml, 1 mg/ml) were mixed with 2.5 ml of aluminium chloride reagent (133 mg of aluminium chloride and 400 mg of sodium acetate in 100 ml of de-ionised water) and kept for 30 min at room temperature. The absorbance of the reaction mixture was measured at 430 nm. Total flavonoids content was determined from the standard curve and expressed as mg of quercetin equivalent (QE) per gram extract.[20]

Quantification of polyphenolic compounds by HPLC
HPLC chromatographic analysis was done using a Thermo Scientific Dionex UltiMate 3000 Rapid Separation LC (RSLC) system (Thermo Fisher Scientific Inc., MA, USA), coupled to a quaternary rapid separation pump (LPG-3400RS), rapid separation diode array detector (DAD-3000RS) and ultimate 3000RS auto sampler (WPS-3000). Separation was accomplished on Acclaim® C18 (4.6 x 250 mm; 5μm) column (Dionex, USA), controlled at a constant temperature of 30°C. The separation was carried out using a gradient elution programme (0-10 min, 5%A/95%B; 10-20 min, 10%A/80%B/10%C; 20-30 min, 20%A/60%B/20%C; and 30 min, 100%A, where A is acetonitrile, B is acetic acid solution in water at pH 3.0, and C is methanol). The flow rate was maintained at 1 ml/min, and the injection volume was 20 μl. For the detection, UV detector was set to 280 nm and held for 18 min, changed to 320 nm and held for 6 min, finally to 380 nm and continued for the rest of the analysis while the diode array detector was set at an acquisition range of 200-700 nm. The standard solution was made by diluting the standard stock solutions in methanol to give a concentration of 20 μg/ml for each polyphenols, except for caffeic acid (8 μg/ml) and quercetin (6 μg/ml). Solution of the test extracts were prepared in ethanol having a concentration of 5 mg/ml. Spiking the sample solution with phenolic standards was done for further confirmation of individual polyphenols.[21]

Statistical analysis
Data were presented as mean ± standard deviation (SD). One-way ANOVA followed by Dunnett's test was performed and the results were considered statistically significant when $p < 0.05$.

Results
Anti-inflammatory activity test
Carrageenan-induced paw edema
At the doses of 200 and 400 mg/kg, both EAH and AAH significantly decreased the volume of carrageenan-induced rat paw edema. At the above dose levels, the maximum decrease in paw volume was 26 and 36%, respectively for EAH, in contrast to 29 and 40%, respectively for AAH as compared to control. Indomethacin showed statistically significant anti-inflammatory activity with the highest inhibition (64%) of paw edema at 5 h after carrageenan injection (Table 1).

Table 1. Effect of ethanol and aqueous extracts of *A. hispida* leaves on carrageenan-induced rat paw edema volume.

Treatment	Dose (mg/kg)	Right hind paw volume (% Inhibition)				
		1 h	2 h	3 h	4 h	5 h
Vehicle	10	0.95 ± 0.15	1.11 ± 0.21	1.28 ± 0.19	1.45 ± 0.27	1.51 ± 0.24
Indomethacin	10	0.51 ± 0.12 (46)*	0.53 ± 0.18 (52)*	0.55 ± 0.25 (57)*	0.59 ± 0.16 (59)**	0.60 ± 0.17 (60)**
Ethanol extract	200	0.82 ± 0.17 (14)*	0.95 ± 0.19 (14)*	1.04 ± 0.21 (19)*	1.13 ± 0.10 (22)*	1.12 ± 0.15 (26)**
	400	0.78 ± 0.17 (18)*	0.85 ± 0.19 (23)*	0.91 ± 0.13 (29)*	0.97 ± 0.20 (33)*	0.96 ± 0.14 (36)**
Aqueous extract	200	0.81 ± 0.18 (15)	0.92 ± 0.16 (17)*	1.01 ± 0.19 (21)	1.07 ± 0.21 (26)*	1.08 ± 0.14 (29)**
	400	0.73 ± 0.19 (23)	0.77 ± 0.16 (31)*	0.84 ± 0.15 (34)*	0.92 ± 0.17 (37)*	0.90 ± 0.13 (40)**

Value presented as the mean ± SE (*n*=5); *p<0.05, **p<0.01 versus control (Dunnett's test).

Histamine-induced paw edema
Rats pre-treated with EAH at 200 and 400 mg/kg, showed decrease in the histamine-induced paw edema volume with the maximum inhibition of 27 and 39%, respectively, while that of AAH was 31 and 45% inhibition, respectively as compared to control. Indomethacin showed a maximum inhibition of 64% at 5 h after histamine administration, and the results were statistically significant (Table 2).

Antioxidant activity test
DPPH free radical scavenging assay
In the quantitative DPPH free radical scavenging assay, EAH and AAH showed strong antioxidant activity with

IC_{50} values of 14 and 17 μg/ml, respectively, while that of ascorbic acid was 10 μg/ml.

Fe^{2+} ion chelating ability
Both EAH and AAH showed Fe^{2+} ion chelating ability with IC_{50} values of 40 and 46 μg/ml, respectively. The IC_{50} value of EDTA, used as the standard in this assay showed an IC_{50} of 17 μg/ml.

Reducing power assay
Concentration dependent reducing power was observed for both EAH and AAH with the maximum absorbance of 1.13 and 0.88, respectively at the highest concentration tested (100 ug/ml) (Figure 1).

Nitric oxide scavenging assay

Both the extracts EAH and AAH significantly scavenged NO radical. The IC_{50} value for EAH and AAH were found to be 43 and 50 μg/ml, respectively and were comparable to that of ascorbic acid (17 μg/ml) (Figure 2).

Total phenolic content assay

The total phenolic content of EAH and AAH were 130.5 and 173.8 mg GAE/g of dry extract, respectively (Figure 3).

Table 2. Effect of ethanol and aqueous extracts of *A. hispida* leaves on histamine-induced rat paw edema volume.

Treatment	Dose (mg/kg)	Right hind paw volume (% Inhibition)				
		1 h	2 h	3 h	4 h	5 h
Vehicle	10	1.10 ± 0.13	1.27 ± 0.11	1.36 ± 0.17	1.41 ± 0.22	1.48 ± 0.27
Indomethacin	10	0.54 ± 0.17 (51)*	0.58 ± 0.13 (54)*	0.59 ± 0.18 (57)*	0.56 ± 0.15 (60)**	0.53 ± 0.14 (64)**
Ethanol extract	200	0.92 ± 0.15 (16)*	1.01 ± 0.13 (20)*	1.04 ± 0.21 (24)	1.07 ± 0.12 (24)*	1.08 ± 0.16 (27)**
	400	0.82 ± 0.18 (26)	0.91 ± 0.15 (28)*	0.92 ± 0.19 (32)	0.89 ± 0.17 (37)*	0.90 ± 0.13 (39)**
Aqueous extract	200	0.87 ± 0.21 (21)	0.96 ± 0.13 (24)*	0.99 ± 0.20 (27)	1.01 ± 0.15 (28)*	1.02 ± 0.11 (31)**
	400	0.81 ± 0.19 (26)	0.88 ± 0.13 (31)*	0.89 ± 0.17 (35)*	0.84 ± 0.18 (40)*	0.82 ± 0.17 (45)**

Value presented as the mean ± SE (*n*=5); *p<0.05, **p<0.01 versus control (Dunnett's test).

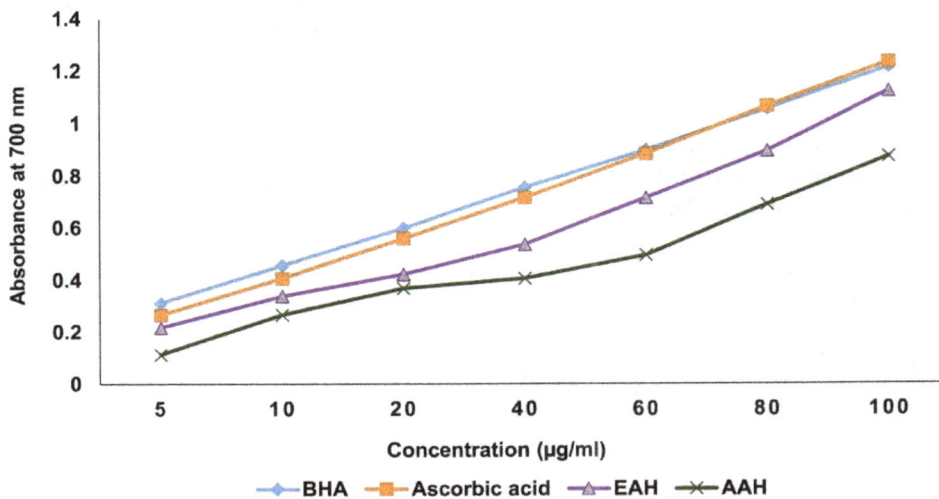

Figure 1. Reducing power of ethanol and aqueous extracts of *A. hispida* leaves.

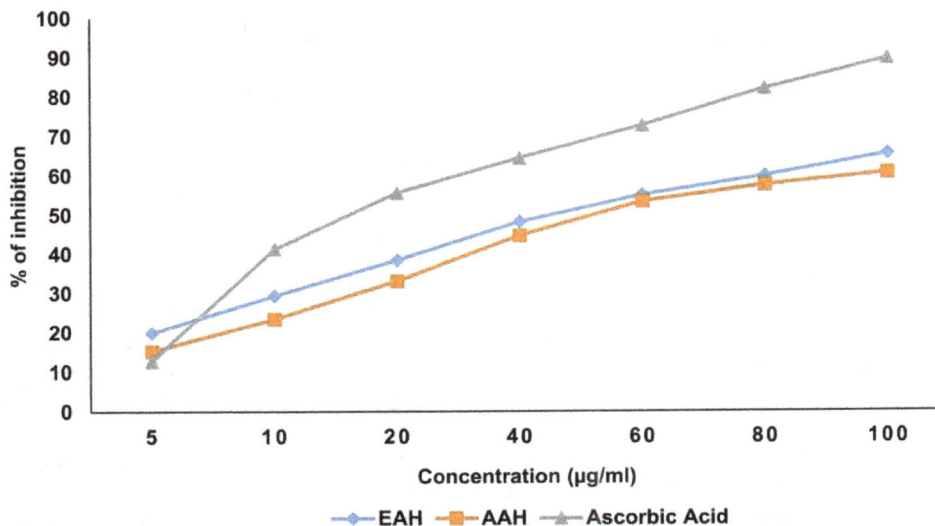

Figure 2. Nitric oxide (NO) scavenging activity of ethanol and aqueous extracts of *A. hispida* leaves.

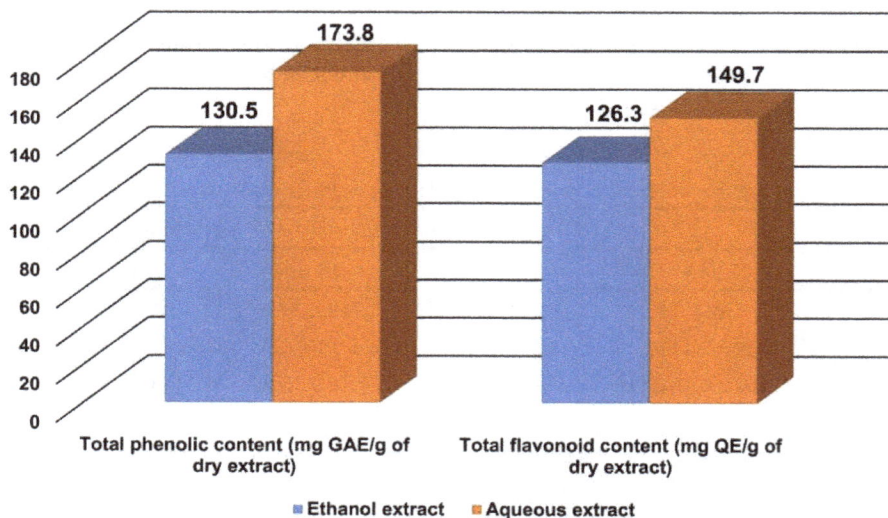

Figure 3. Total phenolic and flavonoid content of ethanol and aqueous extracts of *A. hispida* leaves.

Total flavonoid content assay

The total flavonoid content for EAH and AAH were 126.3 and 149.7 mg QE/g of dry extract, respectively (Figure 3).

Quantification of polyphenolic compounds by HPLC

The HPLC analysis indicated that both EAH and AAH are rich in ellagic acid content (119.40 and 540.90

mg/100 g dry extract). Gallic acid and quercetin were detected in both extracts but concentration was in lower amount (31.60 and 5.80 mg of gallic acid/100 g EAH extract, 0.50 and 0.60 mg of quercetin/100 g AAH extract, respectively). *p*-Coumaric acid and rutin were detected only in AAH (0.90 and 14.30 mg/100 g AAH, respectively) (Figure 4, Figure 5 and Figure 6).

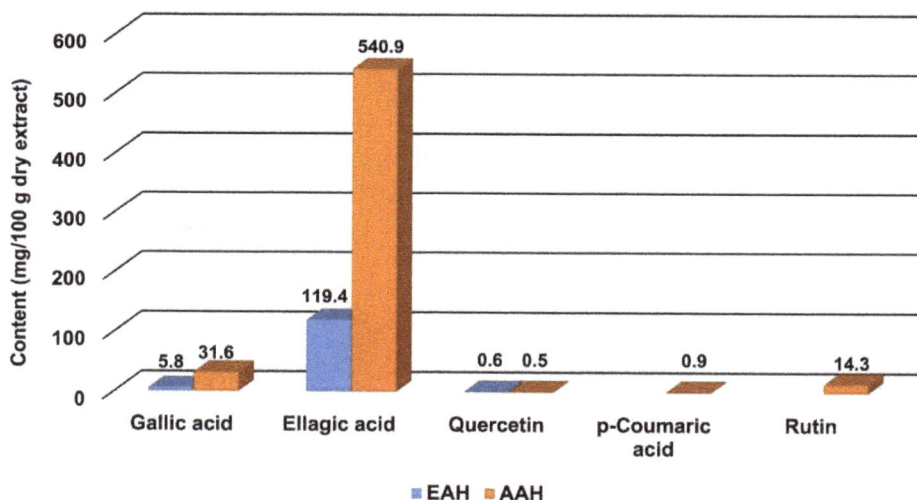

Figure 4. Polyphenolic contents of ethanol and aqueous extracts of *A. hispida* leaves.

Discussion

The inflammatory reaction induced by carrageenan in rats is recognised by a biphasic response. The key feature of marked edema formation is mediated by histamine, serotonin and bradykinins in the first phase, while the second phase is associated with the release of prostaglandins and nitric oxide, which is generated by cyclooxygenase-2 (COX-2), and inducible isoform of nitric oxide synthase (iNOS).[22,23] Histamine is an important mediator of inflammation, and act as a potent vasodilator, and vascular permeability

facilitator.[24] Administration of histamine in test animals results in an increase in the vascular penetrability of the host capillary venules at the site of injection. Agents that oppose the activity of histamine receptors reduce the swelling triggered by inflammation. In the present investigation, both the ethanol and aqueous extracts of *A. hispida* leaves significantly reduced the edema formation in carrageenan, as well as in histamine induced rat paw edema. Thus the anti-inflammatory activity of the extracts might involve antihistaminic activity. In addition, inhibition of other inflammatory pathway cannot be ruled out, since the extracts also inhibited

carrageenan induced inflammatory response, which involves several inflammatory pathways.

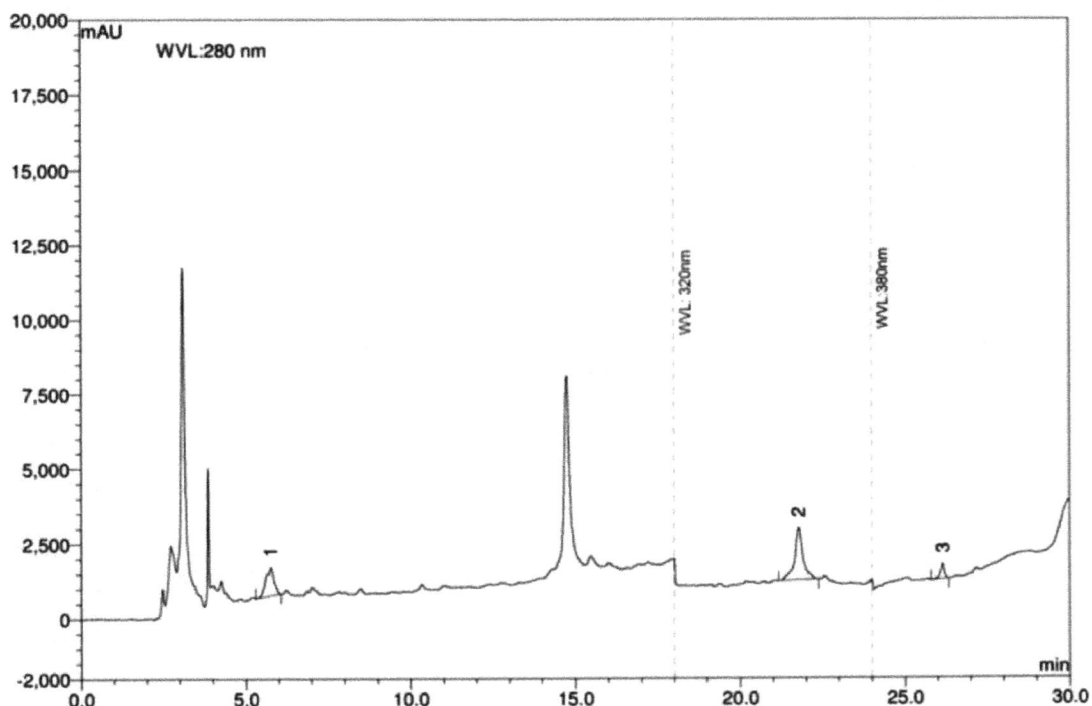

Figure 5. HPLC chromatogram of ethanol extract of *A. hispida* leaves. Peaks 1: gallic acid, 2: ellagic acid, 3: quercetin.

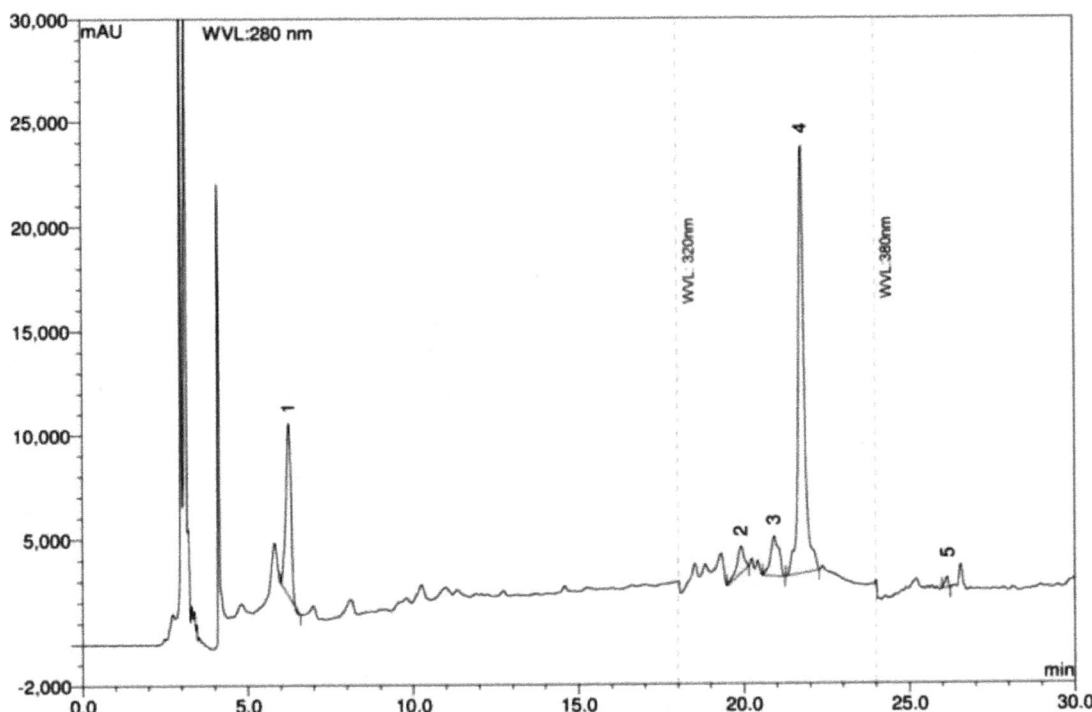

Figure 6. HPLC chromatogram of aqueous extract of *A. hispida* leaves. Peaks 1: gallic acid, 2: *p*-coumaric acid, 3: rutin, 4: ellagic acid, 5: quercetin.

Plant derived compounds with antioxidant activity often show anti-inflammatory activity.[25] The ability of antioxidants in protecting the cells from oxidative stress

can contribute towards the anti-inflammatory activity.[26] Commonly occurring plant phenolics and flavonoids are often associated with antioxidant activity.[27] Thus a number of assays were performed to investigate the antioxidant capacity of *A. hispida* leaves. In the DPPH radical scavenging assay, *A. hispida* leaves extracts showed a concentration dependent free radical scavenging activity. Saponins, flavonoids and tannins, which are also present in this plant, are known to show DPPH radical scavenging activity by donating proton to neutralise the free radicals.[28,29] Agents that form σ bond with a metal are active as secondary antioxidants, because they decrease the redox potential and steadying the oxidised form of the metal ion.[30] Results demonstrated that *A. hispida* leaf extracts have the capacity to reduce ferric ion, a further proof to the antioxidant potential of the extracts. Nitric oxide (NO) works as a neural modulator, which is involved in neurotransmitter release, neuronal excitability and other intellectual activities including learning and memory.[31] Though it has a role in physiologic processes, it also participates in pathogenic pathways underlying a large group of disorders including inflammation, inflammatory bowel disorder, primary headaches and stroke.[32] *A. hispida* leaf extracts showed NO scavenging activity suggesting the ability to ameliorate inflammatory response associated with NO.

With a view to justify the correlation between pharmacological activity and phenolic constituents of *A. hispida* leaf extracts, HPLC analysis was conducted to identify some of the biologically important antioxidant principles from plants. The HPLC analysis showed a high content of ellagic acid in both extracts. Previous studies revealed that ellagic acid possesses strong antioxidant and anti-inflammatory activities.[33,34] The anti-inflammatory activity of ellagic acid can be attributed due to its ability to inhibit one or more inflammatory pathways including inhibition of COX-2 and NO synthase expression.[35] Presence of phenolic hydroxyl group in the structure of ellagic acid enables the donation of proton to neutralise free radicals.[36] Trace amount of gallic acid, rutin and quercetin were also present in the leaf extracts. In addition to their antioxidant property, aforementioned compounds are also reported to have anti-inflammatory activity.[37-39]

The anti-inflammatory activity observed for the aqueous extract was higher than that of the ethanol extract. In the HPLC analysis, ellagic acid content, along with other phenolics were found higher for aqueous extract than the ethanol extract and it is also reflected by the total phenol and total flavonoid content assay. Therefore, stronger anti-inflammatory activity of the aqueous extract may be due its higher phenol and flavonoid content.

Conclusion
The ethanol and aqueous extracts of *A. hispida* leaf exhibited significant anti-inflammatory activity through the reduction of carrageenan and histamine induced edema formation in test rats. The extracts also showed potent antioxidant activity in a number of methods. The observed anti-inflammatory activity may be due to the presence of high concentration of ellagic acid in the plant extracts. In addition, other phenolic constituents present in the plant might have assisted towards the anti-inflammatory activity.

Acknowledgments
Authors are grateful to the Chemical Research Division of Bangladesh Council of Scientific and Industrial Research (BCSIR), Dhaka 1205, Bangladesh for allowing them to use their research facilities to perform these research works.

Conflict of Interest
The authors declare no conflict of interests.

References
1. Meyer S. Phytochemical methods A guide to modern techniques of plant analysis. USA: Champan and Hall; 1982.
2. Seebaluck R, Gurib-Fakim A, Mahomoodally F. Medicinal plants from the genus *Acalypha* (Euphorbiaceae)--a review of their ethnopharmacology and phytochemistry. *J Ethnopharmacol* 2015;159:137-57. doi: 10.1016/j.jep.2014.10.040
3. Amakura Y, Miyake M, Ito H, Murakaku S, Araki S, Itoh Y, et al. Acalyphidins M1, M2 and D1, ellagitannins from *Acalypha hispida*. *Phytochemistry* 1999;50(4):667-75. doi: 10.1016/s0031-9422(98)00579-2
4. Reiersen B, Kiremire BT, Byamukama R, Andersen MO. Anthocyanins acylated with gallic acid from chenille plant, *Acalypha hispida*. *Phytochemistry* 2003;64(4):867-71. doi: 10.1016/S0031-9422(03)00494-1
5. Bokshi B, Sayeed MAS, Ahmed MI, Karmakar UK, Sadhu SK. Assessment of antimicrobial and cytotoxic activities of ethanolic extract of leaves of *Acalypha hispida*. *IJPSR* 2012;3(6):1705-8.
6. McLaughlin JL, Rogers LL, Anderson JE. The use of biological assays to evaluate botanicals. *Drug Inf J* 1999;32:513-24.
7. Adesina SK, Idowu O, Ogundaini AO, Oladimeji H, Olugbade TA, Onawunmi GO, et al. Antimicrobial constituents of the leaves of *Acalypha wilkesiana* and *Aacalypha hispida*. *Phytother Res* 2000;14(5):371-4.
8. Ejechi BO, Souzey JA. Inhibition of biodeterioration of yam tuber *Dioscorea rotundata* Poir in storage with phenolic extract of *Acalypha hispida* Burm. f. leaves. *J Stored Prod Res* 1999;35(2):127-34. doi: 10.1016/s0022-474x(98)00038-1
9. Onocha PA, Oloyede GK, Afolabi QO. Chemical composition, cytotoxicity and antioxidant activity of essential oils of *Acalypha hispida* flowers. *Int J Pharmacol* 2011;7(1):144-8. doi: 10.3923/ijp.2011.144.148

10. Ahmed F, Selim MS, Shilpi JA. Antibacterial activity of *Ludwigia adscendens. Fitoterapia* 2005;76(5):473-5. doi: 10.1016/j.fitote.2005.04.007

11. Rouf R, Uddin SJ, Shilpi JA, Toufiq-Ur-Rahman M, Ferdous MM, Sarker SD. Anti-diarrhoeal properties of *Diospyros peregrina* in the castor oil-induced diarrhoea model in mice. *Ars Pharm* 2006;47:81-9.

12. Saha S, Shilpi JA, Mondal H, Gofur R, Billah M, Nahar L, et al. Bioactivity studies on *Musa seminifera* Lour. *Pharmacogn Mag* 2013;9(36):315-22. doi: 10.4103/0973-1296.117827

13. Sadeghi H, Mostafazadeh M, Sadeghi H, Naderian M, Barmak MJ, Talebianpoor MS, et al. *In vivo* anti-inflammatory properties of aerial parts of *Nasturtium officinale. Pharm Biol* 2014;52(2):169-74. doi: 10.3109/13880209.2013.821138

14. Perianayagam JB, Sharma SK, Pillai KK. Anti-inflammatory activity of *Trichodesma indicum* root extract in experimental animals. *J Ethnopharmacol* 2006;104(3):410-4. doi: 10.1016/j.jep.2005.08.077

15. Dehshiri MM, Aghamollaei H, Zarini M, Nabavi SM, Mirzaei M, Loizzo MR, et al. Antioxidant activity of different parts of *Tetrataenium lasiopetalum. Pharm Biol* 2013;51(8):1081-5. doi: 10.3109/13880209.2013.775594

16. Dinis TC, Maderia VM, Almeida LM. Action of phenolic derivatives (acetaminophen, salicylate, and 5-aminosalicylate) as inhibitors of membrane lipid peroxidation and as peroxyl radical scavengers. *Arch Biochem Biophys* 1994;315(1):161-9. doi: 10.1006/abbi.1994.1485

17. Dehpour AA, Ebrahimzadeh MA, Nabavi SF, Nabavi SM. Antioxidant activity of the methanol extract of *Ferula assafoetida* and its essential oil composition. *Grasas Aceites* 2009;60(4):405-12. doi: 10.3989/gya.010109

18. Govindarajan R, Rastogi S, Vijayakumar M, Shirwaikar A, Rawat AK, Mehrotra S, et al. Studies on the antioxidant activities of *Desmodium gangeticum. Biol Pharm Bull* 2003;26(10):1424-7. doi: 10.1248/bpb.26.1424

19. Wolfe K, Wu X, Liu RH. Antioxidant activity of apple peels. *J Agric Food Chem* 2003;51(3):609-14. doi: 10.1021/jf020782a

20. Hossain H, Karmakar UK, Biswas SK, Shahid-Ud-Daula AF, Jahan IA, Adnan T, et al. Antinociceptive and antioxidant potential of the crude ethanol extract of the leaves of *Ageratum conyzoides* grown in Bangladesh. *Pharm Biol* 2013;51(7):893-8. doi: 10.3109/13880209.2013.770535

21. Mondal H, Saha S, Awang K, Hossain H, Ablat A, Islam MK, et al. Central-stimulating and analgesic activity of the ethanolic extract of *Alternanthera sessilis* in mice. *BMC Complement Altern Med* 2014;14:398. doi: 10.1186/1472-6882-14-398

22. Seibert K, Zhang Y, Leahy K, Hauser S, Masferrer J, Perkins W, et al. Pharmacological and biochemical demonstration of the role of cyclooxygenase 2 in inflammation and pain. *Proc Natl Acad Sci U S A* 1994;91(25):12013-7. doi: 10.1073/pnas.91.25.12013

23. Sommer CV, Parth CM. Inflammation, tissue repair and fever. In: Porth C, editor. *Essential of Pathophysiology- Concepts of Altered Health Sciences.* 3rd ed. New York: Lippincott Williams and Wilkins; 2006. P. 495-514.

24. Cuman RKN, Bersani-Amadio CA, Fortes ZB. Influence of type 2 diabetes on the inflammatory response in rat. *Inflamm Res* 2001;50(9):460-5. doi: 10.1007/pl00000271

25. Tawaha K, Alali FQ, Gharaibeh M, Mohammad M, El-Elimat T. Antioxidant activity and total phenolic content of selected Jordanian species. *Food Chem* 2007;104(4):1372-8. doi: 10.1016/j.foodchem.2007.01.064

26. González R, Ballester I, López-Posadas R, Suárez MD, Zarzuelo A, Martinez-Augustin O, et al. Effects of flavonoids and other polyphenols on inflammation. *Crit Rev Food Sci Nutr* 2011;51(4):331-62. doi: 10.1080/10408390903584094

27. Ebrahimzadeh MA, Nabavi SM, Nabavi SF, Eslami B, Rahmani Z. Antioxidant and antihaemolytic activities of the leaves of Kefe cumin (*Laser trilobum* L) Umbelliferae. *Trop J Pharm Res* 2010;9(5):441-9. doi: 10.4314/tjpr.v9i5.61053

28. Ponou BK, Teponno RB, Ricciutelli M, Quassinti L, Bramucci M, Lupidi G, et al. Dimeric antioxidant and cytotoxic triterpenoid saponins from *Terminalia ivorensis* A. Chev. *Phytochemistry* 2010;71(17-18):2108-15. doi: 10.1016/j.phytochem.2010.08.020

29. Yokozawa T, Chen CP, Dong E, Tanaka T, Nonaka GI, Nishioka I. Study on the inhibitory effect of tannins and flavonoids against the 1,1-diphenyl-2-picrylhydrazyl radical. *Biochem Pharmacol* 1998;56(2):213-22. doi: 10.1016/S0006-2952(98)00128-2

30. Duh PD, Tu YY, Yen GC. Antioxidant activity of water extract of harng Jyur (*Chrysanthemum morifolium* Ramat). *LWT-Food Sci Technol* 1999;32(5):269-77. doi: 10.1006/fstl.1999.0548

31. Fossier P, Blanchard B, Ducrocq C, Leprince C, Tauc L, Baux G. Nitric oxide transforms serotonin into an inactive form and this affects neuromodulation. *Neuroscience* 1999;93(2):597-603. doi: 10.1016/S0306-4522(99)00165-7

32. Moncada S, Palmer RM, Higgs EA. Nitric oxide: physiology, pathophysiology, and pharmacology. *Pharmacol Rev* 1991;43(2):109-42.

33. Guruvayoorappan C, Kuttan G. (+)-Catechin inhibits tumour angiogenesis and regulates the production of nitric oxide and TNF-alpha in LPS-stimulated macrophages. *Innate Immun* 2008;14(3):160-74. doi: 10.1177/1753425908093295

34. Iñiguez-Franco F, Soto-Valdez H, Peralta E, Ayala-Zavala JF, Auras R, Gámez-Meza N. Antioxidant activity and diffusion of catechin and epicatechin from antioxidant active films made of poly(L-lactic

acid). *J Agric Food Chem* 2012;60(26):6515-23. doi: 10.1021/jf300668u

35. Gainok J, Daniels R, Golembiowski D, Kindred P, Post L, Strickland R, et al. Investigation of the anti-inflammatory, antinociceptive effect of ellagic acid as measured by digital paw pressure via the Randall-Selitto meter in male Sprague-Dawley rats. *AANA J* 2011;79(4 Suppl):S28-34.

36. Hatano T, Edamatsu R, Hiramatsu M, Mori A, Fujita Y, Yasuhara T, et al. Effects of the Interaction of Tannins with Co-existing Substances. VI. : Effects of Tannins and Related Polyphenols on Superoxide Anion Radical, and on 1, 1-Diphenyl-2-picrylhydrazyl Radical. *Chem Pharm Bull* 1989;37(8):2016-21. doi: 10.1248/cpb.37.2016

37. Kleemann R, Verschuren L, Morrison M, Zadelaar S, van Erk MJ, Wielinga PY, et al. Anti-inflammatory, anti-proliferative and anti-atherosclerotic effects of quercetin in human *in vitro* and *in vivo* models. *Atherosclerosis* 2011;218(1):44-52. doi: 10.1016/j.atherosclerosis.2011.04.023

38. Kroes BH, Van den Berg AJ, Quarles van Ufford HC, van Dijk H, Labadie RP. Anti-inflammatory activity of gallic acid. *Planta Med* 1992;58(6):499-504. doi: 10.1055/s-2006-961535

39. Selloum L, Bouriche H, Tigrine C, Boudoukha C. Anti-inflammatory effect of rutin on rat paw oedema, and on neutrophils chemotaxis and degranulation. *Exp Toxicol Pathol* 2003;54(4):313-8. doi: 10.1078/0940-2993-00260

14

Characterization of Terpenoids in the Essential Oil Extracted from the Aerial Parts of *Scrophularia Subaphylla* Growing in Iran

Parina Asgharian[1,2], Fariba Heshmati Afshar[1,3], Solmaz Asnaashari[1], Sedigheh Bamdad Moghaddam[1], Atefeh Ebrahimi[2], Abbas Delazar[1,2]*

[1] *Drug Applied Research Center, Tabriz University of Medical Sciences, Tabriz, Iran.*
[2] *Department of Pharmacognosy, Faculty of Pharmacy, Tabriz University of Medical Sciences, Tabriz, Iran.*
[3] *Faculty of Traditional Medicine, Tabriz University of Medical Sciences, Tabriz, Iran.*

Article info

Keywords:
· Scrophularia subaphylla
· Scrophulariaceae
· Essential oil composition
· GC-MS
· DPPH assay
· Antibacterial activity

Abstract

Purpose: The aim of this work was to investigate the volatiles released from aerial parts of *Scrophularia subaphylla* (*Scrophulariaceae*) which is a perennial herb growing in Azarbaijan province in Iran.

Methods: A combination of GC-MS and GC-FID were applied for analyzing the chemical compositions of the essential oil extracted by hydro-distillation from the aerial parts of *Scrophularia subaphylla* (*S. subaphylla*).

Results: Thirty six compounds, representing 97.32% of total oil were identified. High content of terpenoids (60.02%) were identified in the essential oil with Linalool (22.35%), phytol (15.74%) and geraniol (7.27%) as the most dominant compounds, while other main components were representatives of fatty acids (24.31%), indicated mainly by palmitinic acid (17.29%). DPPH assay was used for assessing the antioxidant properties of compounds. However, no remarkable free radical scavenging activity was observed. Furthermore, Disc diffusion method was applied for evaluating the antimicrobial activity of essential oil vs. gram positive and gram negative bacteria strains. The examined oil showed weak antibacterial effect.

Conclusion: Main constituents of *S. subaphylla* were terpenoids. In comparison with other genesis of *Scrophularia*, antioxidant and anti bacterial properties of *S. subaphylla* essential oil were not noticeable.

Introduction

The genus *Scrophularia* (commonly known as figworts) is one of the largest genera of the *Scrophulariaceae* family which is distributed widely in Asia, North America and central Europe, especially in the Mediterranean region.[1] This genus is represented in Iranian flora by 42 species, of which 19 are endemic.[1,2] *Scrophularia subaphylla* (*S. subaphylla*) is one of the endemic species growing in East Azarbaijan province of Iran. It is a multi- stemmed perennial herb with square stems, woody rhizomes, opposite leaves and open two-lipped flowers.[3] Several investigations on this genus have revealed various pharmacological activities such as wound healing, anti-inflammatory, antibacterial, cardiovascular, diuretic, protozoacidal, fungicidal, cytotoxic and anti-nociceptive.[4-10] Most of these mentioned characteristic were proven to attribute non-volatile components, which were known as secondary metabolites. Iridoids, phenylpropanoids, phenolic acids and flavonoids have been identified as main secondary metabolites.[4-10] Despite the high number of *Scrophularia* species, there are a few studies about the chemical composition of the essential oils of

these plants.[11-13] Moreover, to our knowledge, biological activities of the essential oils from *Scrophularia* genus, especially Iranian endemic taxa, have not yet been exhaustively investigated except two recent reports by Pasdaran et al which indicated antioxidant and antimicrobial properties of essential oils of *S. amplexicaulis* and, insecticidal effects of oil obtained from aerial parts of *S. oxycepala*.[11,12] Therefore, in this work we present for the first time the chemical composition of the essential oil from aerial parts of *S. subaphylla* occurring in East Azarbaijan province as well as its antioxidant and antimicrobial properties.

Material and Methods

Plant material

Flowering aerial parts of *S. subaphylla* was collected during July 2013 from Mishodagh Mountain near the Marand city (Yam) in East Azarbaijan province, Iran. Voucher specimen was identified and retained in the Herbarium of Faculty of Pharmacy, Tabriz University of Medical Sciences, Iran, under the accession code Tbz-fph 747.

---

*Corresponding author: Abbas Delazar, Email: delazara@tbzmed.ac.ir

Essential oil Isolation

The air-dried aerial parts of plant (100 g) were cut into small pieces and submitted to hydro-distillation for 3 h in a Clevenger-type apparatus using hexane (2 mL) as collector solvent. The pale yellow-colored essential oil was dried over anhydrous sodium sulphate, then the solvent was evaporated and the oil was stored in sealed vials at - 4° before analyses.

GC-MS analysis

GC-MS analysis was performed on a Shimadzu GCMS QP 5050A gas chromatograph-mass spectrometer fitted with a fused capillary column DB-1 (60 m, 0.25 mm id, film thickness 0.25 μm), with the following temperature program: 3 min at 50° C, then at 3 °C/min to 260°C, held for 5 min, for a total run of 80 min. Injector and transfer line temperatures were 240°C. Helium was utilized as the carrier gas, at a flow rate of 1.3 ml/min. Essential oil were diluted 1:100 in hexane, and the volume injected was 1μL; split ratio, 1:29; acquisition mass range, 30-600 m/z, ion source temperature 270 °C; quadrupole 100 °C; Solvent delay 2 min; scan speed 2000 amu/s and EV voltage 3000 volts. All mass spectra were acquired in electron-impact (EI) mode with an ionization voltage of 70 eV. Qualitative identification of essential oil constituents was based on direct comparison of the Kovats Indices (KI) and MS data with those for the standard compounds as well as using the spectrophotometer database like NIST NBS54K and Wily 229 library along with comparison of their retention indices (RT) and MS fragmentation pattern with the authentic reference compounds that were reported in the Adam'S literature.[14] Also flame ionization detector (FID) which was operated in ionization potential mode at 70 ev, was used for quantification purpose for calculating the relative area percentage (area %) without the use of correction factors.

Antimicrobial assay

Lyophilized form of two gram positive and gram negative bacteria, Staphylococcus aureus ATCC (6538) and Pseudomonas aeroginosa ATCC (9027) respectively, were purchased from institute of Pasture, Iran. They were used to evaluate the antibacterial activity of S. subaphylla essential oil. Activated bacteria were maintained in suitable agar media at 4°C as stock cultures for further uses. A single colony after transferring in to Muller Hinton Broth media incubated at 37°C for 24h then centrifuged. For providing an optical density equal to 10^8 CFU/ml of bacterial concentration, turbidity was corrected with adding a saline solution. After that, sterilized discs (6 mm diameter, Whatman paper) were impregnated with different concentration of test sample (which were dissolved in 10% aqueous DMSO previously) as well as positive reference (Amikacine). Negative control were prepared from the same solvent (DMSO) employed to dissolve the plant oil. Afterward, petridishes transferred in to the refrigerator to facilitate the diffusion of oil approximately for 30 min, thereafter, plates were incubated at 37 °C for starting the growth of bacteria. Finally, the diameter of the inhibition zones was considered as the antibacterial activity of the test sample.[15]

Antioxidant activity

The in vitro antioxidant property of the essential oil was evaluated through the modified DPPH assay. 2 ml of 0.08 gr/ml DPPH which was prepared in chloroform was added in to different dilutions of essential oil and negative control (chloroform). Afterwards, when the mixture was homogenous, was kept in room temperature for 30 min to any reaction to occur. The same procedure was repeated for positive control (quercetin). Finally, the absorbance of test specimens was recorded against negative control at 517 nm using UV/Visible Spectrophotometer 160A (USA). Percentage of DPPH reduction was calculated according to the following equation:

$$\% \text{ inhibition of DPPH} = \frac{\text{Abs control} - \text{Abs test}}{\text{Abs control}} \times 100$$

Also RC_{50} was extrapolated from dose-response curve. The experiment was performed in duplicate.[16]

Results and Discussion

The composition of the essential oil obtained from the aerial parts of S. subaphylla is compiled in Table 1, where the components are listed in order to their elution on the DB-1 column.

Hydro-distillation gave an odorous light yellow oil with a yield of 0.05 % W/W, based on the dry mass. The very low yield (0.05%) was consistent with those reported in the researches for other species of the genus Schrophularia.[11-13] so it seems that this genus contains oil-poor plants. A total of 36 volatiles were identified, accounting for 97.32% of the total volatiles. The components of essential oil were separated into two classes, which were terpenoids (60.02%) and non-terpenoid (37.30%) compounds. Terpenoids were represented mainly by oxygenated monoterpenes (39.42%), with Linalool (22.35%), geraniol (7.27%) and α-terpineol (5.25%) as the most abundant compounds, while the content of oxygenated sesquiterpenes was rather low (4.86%), represented mainly by nerolidol B (4.21%). Among oxygen containing components, alcohols were the most abundant. Moreover, as shown in Figure 1. The oil was characterized by high amount of diterpenes, notably phytol, which accounted for 15.74% of the oil. Among non-terpenoid compounds, fatty acids constituted the main fraction (20.53%) of this part, with palmitic acid (17.29%) as the major components. This finding previously was confirmed by Mitsuo Miyazawa et al in other species of Scrophularia.[13] Apart from the main compounds reported above, 1-Octen-3-ol (2.25%) and hexahydrofarnesyl acetone (3.75%) exceeded a content of 2% of the total oil composition, whilst the remaining compounds (n=27) were present in scant amount, most of them existing at contents lower than 1%.

Table1. Chemical constituent of the essential oil from aerial parts of *S. subaphylla*

Compounds[a]	K.I	Area %	Identification method
1-Octen-3-ol	963	2.25	GC-MS, I_s
n-Octan-3-ol	980	0.68	GC-MS, I_s
n-Nonanal	1083	0.85	GC-MS, I_s
L-Linalool	1086	**22.35**	GC-MS, I_s
α-Terpineol	1174	5.25	GC-MS, I_s
n-Decaldehyde	1185	0.52	GC-MS, I_s
4-α-dimethyl-3-Cyclohexene-1-acetaldehyde	1192	0.25	GC-MS, I_s
Z- geraniol	1211	1.94	GC-MS, I_s
Geraniol	1236	**7.27**	GC-MS, I_s
Z-2-Decenal	1238	0.49	GC-MS, I_s
Undecanal	1287	0.36	GC-MS, I_s
E,E-2,4-Decadienal	1290	0.27	GC-MS, I_s
Heptylidene acetone	1319	1.08	GC-MS, I_s
E-2-dodecenal	1341	0.2	GC-MS, I_s
β-Damascenone	1364	1.19	GC-MS, I_s
Palmitaldehyde	1389	0.5	GC-MS, I_s
Geranyl acetone	1430	0.56	GC-MS, I_s
β-Ionone	1466	1.22	GC-MS, I_s
Nerolidol B (E OR TZ)	1549	4.21	GC-MS, I_s
α-Bisabolol	1670	0.17	GC-MS, I_s
Tetradecanal	1696	0.24	GC-MS, I_s
Nerolidol	1702	0.48	GC-MS, I_s
Myristic acid	1743	1.02	GC-MS, I_s
n-Octadecane	1800	0.69	GC-MS, I_b
Hexahydrofarnesyl acetone	1831	3.75	GC-MS, I_s
Farnesyl acetone	1895	0.26	GC-MS, I_s
Methyl eicosanoate	1909	0.37	GC-MS, I_s
Palmitinic acid	1949	**17.29**	GC-MS, I_s
Palmitic acid ethyl ester	1978	0.49	GC-MS, I_s
Heneicosane	2100	0.62	GC-MS, I_b
Linoleic acid	2109	1.31	GC-MS, I_b
Oleic Acid	2116	0.91	GC-MS, I_b
Phytol	2124	**15.74**	GC-MS, I_b
Linolenic acid methyl ester	2125	1.68	GC-MS, I_b
Ethyl linoleate	2139	0.47	GC-MS, I_b
Hexadecanal diallyl acetal	-	0.39	GC-MS, I_b
Total identified	-	**97.32**	-
Non-terpenoid	-	**37.30**	-
Terpenoids	-	**60.02**	-

[a] Compounds listed in order of elution from a DB-1 column, [b] Identification Method (I_s = Kovats retention index according to authentic standard, I_b = Kovats retention index according to bibliography).

To the best of our knowledge, the current work represents the first study of the essential oil of *S. subaphylla* but there are some reports about chemical composition of other species of *Schrophularia*. The comparison of our results with previous researches illustrates considerable differences in terms of chemical composition of the oil. In our examined oil, linalool (22.35%), palmitic acid (17.29%) and phytol (15.74%) were identified as the main components whereas according to a report by Pasdaran et al, eugenol (53.8%), eugenol acetate (24.5%) and caryophyllen oxide (6.4%) were the main components of the essential oil of *S.*

amplexicaulis.[11] Moreover, the oil from the aerial parts of *S. oxy*cepala represented phytol (25.3%), methyl benzyl alcohol (9.3%) and dihydroeugenol (6.7%) as principle components.[12] It is notable that linalool was found at a relatively high level in our study whereas it was not detected in considerable amount in the oil of the other species.[11-13] Conversely, eugenol and its derivatives was absent in our examined oil compared with that of oil composition of other species.[11-13] It is noteworthy to mention that phytol as a diterpenoid compound present in all of the investigated *Scrophularia* species in variable value. [11-13] These findings showed that the genus *Schrophularia* had a remarkable variation in essential oil composition. Furthermore, in the current study was observed weak antibacterial activity of essential oil (Mean Inhibition Zone Diameter ± SD (MIZD 8 ± 0.3 mm) in comparison to Amikacin (MIZD 15 ± 0.1 mm). Our finding is in contrary to the previous study which were reported the significant antibacterial activity of *Scrophularia* genesis.[11] Also in the case of *S. subaphylla* was not found remarkable antioxidant activity (RC_{50} 5.2 $\times 10^{-2}$ mg/ml$^{)}$ in comparison to quercetine as a positive control and other species of *Scrophularia* like *S. amplexicaulis* oil.[11] Due to the fact that the phenolic compounds have been known the most likely constituents responsible for the free radical scavenging activity, lack of these sorts of constituents in our examined oil may be led to weak activity in this assay

Essential oil content

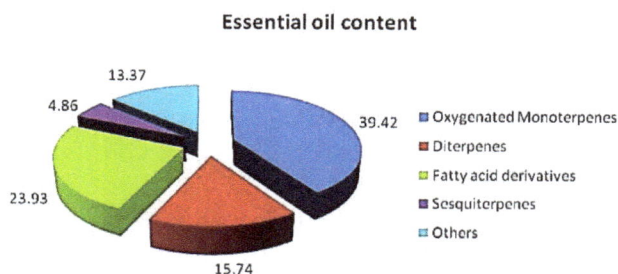

Figure 1. Identified chemical groups from the essential oil of *S. subaphylla*.

Conclusion
Main constituents of *S. subaphylla* were identified as terpenoides. In comparison with other species of *Scrophularia*, antioxidant and anti-bacterial properties of *S. subaphylla* essential oil were not remarkable.

Acknowledgments
This study was financially supported by grant no. 92/1114 from the Drug Applied Research Center of Tabriz University of Medical Sciences. This article was written based on data set of PhD thesis registered in Tabriz University of Medical Sciences (NO. 95).

Conflict of Interest
The authors report no conflicts of interest.

References
1. Ardeshiry Lajimi A, Rezaie-Tavirani M, Mortazavi SA, Barzegar M, Moghadamnia SH, Rezaee MB. Study of anti cancer property of scrophularia striata extract on the human astrocytoma cell line (1321). *Iran J Pharm Res* 2010;9(4):403-10.
2. Mozaffarian V. A dictionary of Iranian plant names, Latin, English, Persian. 4rd ed. Iran: Farhang Mo'aser; 1996.
3. Rechinger KH. Flora iranica 147. Austria: Graze: Akad. Druck. U. verlagsanstalt; 1981.
4. Akhmedov SG, Tkachenko DA, Kharchenko NS. pharmacology of flavonoid aglycones of scrophularia grossheimi. *Farmakol Toksikol* 1969;32(6):693-4.
5. Bermejo Benito P, Abad Martinez MJ, Silvan Sen AM, Sanz Gomez A, Fernandez Matellano L, Sanchez Contreras S, et al. In vivo and in vitro antiinflammatory activity of saikosaponins. *Life Sci* 1998;63(13):1147-56. doi: 10.1016/s0024-3205(98)00376-2
6. Emam AM, Diaz-Lanza AM, Matellano-Fernandez L, Faure R, Moussa AM, Balansard G. Biological activities of buddlejasaponin isolated from buddleja madagascariensis and scrophularia scorodonia. *Pharmazie* 1997;52(1):76-7.
7. Ghisalberti EL. Biological and pharmacological activity of naturally occurring iridoids and secoiridoids. *Phytomedicine* 1998;5(2):147-63. doi: 10.1016/S0944-7113(98)80012-3
8. Lacaille-Dubois M-A, Wagner H. Importance pharmacologique des dérivés polyphénoliques. *Acta botanica gallica* 1996;143(6):555-62. doi:10.1080/12538078.1996.10515353
9. Nishibe S. Bioactive phenolic compounds in traditional medicines. *Pure Appl Chem* 1994;66(10-11):2263-6. doi:10.1351/pac199466102263
10. Stevenson PC, Simmonds MS, Sampson J, Houghton PJ, Grice P. Wound healing activity of acylated iridoid glycosides from scrophularia nodosa. *Phytother Res* 2002;16(1):33-5. doi: 10.1002/ptr.798
11. Pasdaran A, Delazar A, Nazemiyeh H, Nahar L, Sarker SD. Chemical composition, and antibacterial (against staphylococcus aureus) and free-radical-scavenging activities of the essential oils of scrophularia amplexicaulis benth. *Rec Nat Prod* 2012;6:350-5.
12. Pasdaran A, Nahar L, Asnaashari S, Sarker SD, Delazar A. Gc-ms analysis, free-radical-scavenging and insecticidal activities of essential oil of scrophularia oxysepala boiss. *Pharm Sci* 2013;19(1):1-5.
13. Miyazawa M, Okuno Y. Volatile components from the roots of scrophularia ningpoensis hemsl. *Flavour Frag J* 2003;18(5):398-400. doi: 10.1002/ffj.1232
14. Adams R. Quadrupole mass spectra of compounds listed in order of their retention time on db-5. Identification of essential oils components by gas chromatography/quadrupole mass spectroscopy.

USA: Allured Publishing Corporation, Carol. Stream, IL; 2001.

15. Khodaie L, Delazar A, Lotfipour F, Nazemiyeh H. Antioxidant and antimicrobial activity of pedicularis sibthorpii boiss. And pedicularis wilhelmsiana fisch ex. *Adv Pharm Bull* 2012;2(1):89-92. doi: 10.5681/apb.2012.012

16. Takao T, Kitatani F, Watanabe N, Yagi A, Sakata K. A simple screening method for antioxidants and isolation of several antioxidants produced by marine bacteria from fish and shellfish. *Biosci Biotechnol Biochem* 1994;58(10):1780-3. doi:10.1271/bbb.58.1780

15

Cardioprotective Effect of Grape Seed Extract on Chronic Doxorubicin-Induced Cardiac Toxicity in Wistar Rats

Nasser Razmaraii[1,2], **Hossein Babaei**[1,3]*, **Alireza Mohajjel Nayebi**[3], **Gholamreza Assadnassab**[4], **Javad Ashrafi Helan**[5], **Yadollah Azarmi**[3]

[1] *Drug Applied Research Center, Tabriz University of Medical Sciences, Tabriz, 5165665811, Iran.*
[2] *Student Research Committee, Tabriz University of Medical Sciences, Tabriz, 5166614756, Iran.*
[3] *School of Pharmacy, Tabriz University of Medical Sciences, Tabriz, 5166414766, Iran.*
[4] *Department of Clinical Sciences, Tabriz Branch, Islamic Azad University, Tabriz, 5157944533, Iran.*
[5] *Department of Pathobiology, Faculty of Veterinary Medicine, University of Tabriz, Tabriz, 5166617564, Iran.*

Article info

Keywords:
· Grape Seed Extract
· Cardioprotective
· Doxorubicin
· Cardiotoxicity
· Cancer
· ECG

Abstract

Purpose: The aim of the present study was to determine the ability of grape seed extract (GSE) as a powerful antioxidant in preventing adverse effect of doxorubicin (DOX) on heart function.

Methods: Male rats were divided into three groups: control, DOX (2 mg/kg/48h, for 12 days) and GSE (100 mg/kg/24h, for 16 days) plus DOX. Left ventricular (LV) function and hemodynamic parameters were assessed using echocardiography, electrocardiography and a Millar pressure catheter. Histopathological analysis and *in vitro* antitumor activity were also evaluated.

Results: DOX induced heart damage in rats through decreasing the left ventricular systolic and diastolic pressures, rate of rise/decrease of LV pressure, ejection fraction, fractional shortening and contractility index as demonstrated by echocardiography, electrocardiography and hemodynamic parameters relative to control group. Our data demonstrated that GSE treatment markedly attenuated DOX-induced toxicity, structural changes in myocardium and improved ventricular function. Additionally, GSE did not intervene with the antitumor effect of DOX.

Conclusion: Collectively, the results suggest that GSE is potentially protective against DOX-induced toxicity in rat heart and maybe increase therapeutic index of DOX in human cancer treatment.

Introduction

Doxorubicin (DOX), an anthracycline antibiotic, is well-known as one of the most widely-used chemotherapeutic drugs which has been shown to be highly effective in the treatment of a broad spectrum of human cancers.[1] Despite its broad therapeutic effectiveness, clinical studies have reported that the major limiting factor of DOX chemotherapy is its significant cardiotoxic effects, which often results in irreversible degenerative cardiomyopathy and heart failure.[1,2] Although the exact mechanism by which DOX results in cardiotoxicity is not clearly understood, but most studies support the hypothesis that DOX induces oxidative stress through enhanced reactive oxygen species (ROS) production.[1-3] Considering that the heart is vulnerable to free radicals due to its less developed antioxidant defense mechanisms,[4] cellular injury can strongly be related to DOX-induced oxidative stress. Given that free radicals play a pivotal role in DOX-induced damage to the myocardium, antioxidants could protect the heart against DOX-toxicity.

One of the phytochemicals extensively investigated in recent years is grape seed extract (GSE). This extract, an excellent source of natural antioxidants, is used in the pharmaceutical, cosmetic and food industries.[5,6] Effects of GSE on improvement of liver function,[7] reducing infarct size and cardiac arrhythmias,[8] lipid profile[9] and lipid peroxidation[10] in patients with type II diabetes have been reported previously. Some studies have unequivocally demonstrated that GSE has substantial potential for scavenging free radicals in both *in vitro* and *in vivo* experimental models.[5,6,11] An excellent example comes from recent investigations where grape seed proanthocyanidins extract has been shown to be a superior scavenger against superoxide anion and hydroxyl radicals in comparison with vitamins C, E and β-carotene.[12]

In this context, a large number of preclinical and clinical studies have shown a broad spectrum of pharmacological and therapeutic benefits of GSE against oxidative stress,

---

*Corresponding author: Hossein Babaei, Email: babaeih@tbzmed.ac.ir, babaei42@yahoo.com

degenerative disease like cardiovascular dysfunctions and various types of cancers.[5,6,11-14]

Given that the protective effects of GSE on oxidative stress, cardiovascular diseases and neoplasm is dependent on its free radical scavenging capability and its antioxidant impacts and since the DOX-induced cardiotoxicity is mainly mediated through free radical production, natural antioxidants like GSE may offer an effective and safe means to counteract some of the problems and bolstering the antioxidant defense systems against cardiovascular diseases via neutralizing harmful free radicals. Therefore, the aim of the present study was to determine the ability of GSE to reduce the DOX-induced cardiotoxicity in a rat model.

Materials and Methods
Materials
The following materials were used in the experiments: DOX hydrochloride (Exir Nano Sina Company, Iran), Ketamine hydrochloride and Xylazxine (Alfasan, Netherlands), heparin (Hospira, USA), human breast adenocarcinoma MCF7 cell line (Pasteur Institute of Iran,), MTT (3-(4, 5-dimethylthiazol-2-yl)-2, 5-diphenyltetrazolium bromide), RPMI 1640, DPPH (1, 1-diphenyl-2-picrylhydrazyl; Sigma; Germany), fetal calf serum, DMSO (Dimethyl sulfoxide), penicillin, streptomycin, L-glutamine and sodium pyruvate (Gibco, USA).

Animals and ethics
Adult male Wistar rats (180–220 g, aged 8–10 weeks) were obtained from Pasteur institute of Iran. Animals were housed in a room with a 12:12-h light/dark cycle and had access to rodent chow and tap water ad libitum. All experiments were performed according to the protocols approved by the Committee on the Ethics of Animal Experiments of the Tabriz University of Medical Sciences. All efforts were made to minimize animal suffering.

Preparation of Grape Seed Extract
The GSE used in this study was prepared as described previously.[7,8] Briefly, grape seeds (Vitis vinifera) were washed with water and crushed, the crude extract was partitioned between H_2O and n-hexane for separating lipoid compounds, then GSE was prepared by using ethanol 95% and water (water/ethanol, 30/70) as solvents with mechanical agitation for 2 to 3 h, this process was repeated twice. Then the organic solvent was evaporated and dried extract residue was kept at 4 °C for treatments.

Drug Treatment and Experimental Groups
All experiments were conducted in a quiet room during the light period (between 8:00 a.m. and 1:00 p.m.). A summary of the experimental design is shown in Figure 1; eighteen rats were divided into three experimental groups (six animals in each group). Drug solutions were freshly prepared before administration. Group 1 received saline only intraperitoneally (IP) and served as control

(Ctrl), group 2 received DOX (2mg/kg/48h, IP for 12 days; DOX was dissolved in normal saline) and group 3 received GSE (100 mg/kg/day, IP for 16 days; GSE was administered in normal saline) and from day 4 received DOX (2 mg/kg/48h, IP for 12 days). The dose of GSE was chosen based on previous reports[15-18] and our pilot study.

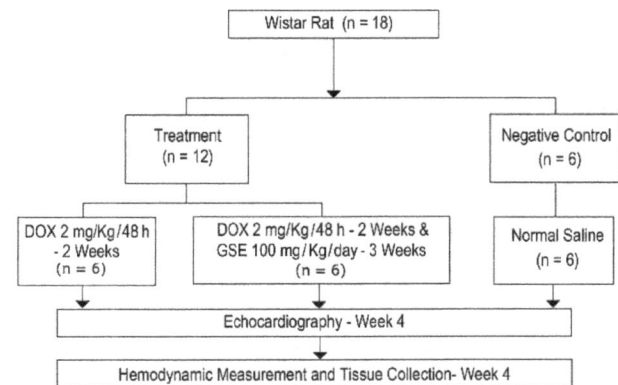

Figure 1. Experimental design, more details of the design are provided in section "Drug Treatment and Experimental Groups"

Echocardiography
Rats were sedated with ketamine (10-20 mg/kg IP) and transthoracic echocardiography was performed with a digital color Doppler ultrasound system (iVis 60 Expert Vet CHISON Medical Imaging, China) as described previously.[19] Briefly, animals were positioned in a chest closed supine form. The transducer was placed gently in the left parasternal position. The left ventricular end diastolic dimension (LVEDD) and left ventricular end systolic dimension (LVESD) were measured using M-mode tracing. The percentage of change in LV cavity dimension; fractional shortening (FS) and ejection fraction (EF) were measured as follows:[20]

Fractional shortening (%) = [(LVEDD - LVESD)/LVEDD] × 100;

Ejection fraction (%) = [(LVEDD^3 - LVESD^3)/LVEDD^3)] × 100.

Electrocardiography
Forty-eight hours after last DOX administration, rats were anesthetized with a combination of xylazine (10 mg/kg, IP) and ketamine (100 mg/kg, IP) and kept warm with a heating lamp. Electrocardiograms (ECG) were recorded using three stainless steel needle electrodes inserted subcutaneously into the left forepaw and hind paws of the rats.[19] They were connected to a bio-amplifier (Bio Amp ML136; ADInstruments; Australia) to record and analyze ECG data using Lab Chart7 software (ADInstruments; Australia).

Hemodynamic study
Animals were anesthetized with ketamine (100 mg/kg, IP) and xylazine (10 mg/kg, IP). In order to prevent blood coagulation, rats received a subcutaneous injection of heparin (2000 U/kg). After 10 min of ECG recording, the neck of the rat was opened longitudinally and the right

carotid artery was exposed and released, ligated distally and stay sutures were placed proximal to the carotid artery. A small opening was then made in the artery with mini-scissors and a 2F micromanometer-tipped pressure transducer catheter (SPR-407; Millar Instruments) was inserted to the artery for evaluation of arterial blood pressure (BP). A catheter was inserted gently into the LV to record data for hemodynamic analysis using Lab Chart 7 software (ADInstruments). The heart rate (HR), LV pressure at the ends of both systole and diastole (LVESP, LVEDP), maximum rate of rise of left ventricular pressure (max dP/dt), minimum rate of rise of left ventricular pressure (min dP/dt), end-diastolic pressure (EDP) and contractility index, a major determinant of cardiac output and an important factor in cardiac compensation, were calculated. The R-R interval, which is the interval from the peak of one QRS complex to the peak of the next and the QT interval on the surface electrocardiogram, an indirect measure of time between ventricular depolarization and repolarization, was also measured.

Body weight and heart/body weight ratio
We monitored body weight development at the beginning and end of the study in all groups. Heart weight (HW)/body weight (BW) ratio was calculated.[21]

Histopathological analysis
At the end of study, the animals were euthanized and the hearts were excised, weighted, then washed with normal saline and finally fixed in 10% neutral buffered formalin, as previously described.[21] After fixation, the tissues were processed using the standard histological method, embedded in paraffin and tissue sections were cut and stained with hematoxylin and eosin. The histopathologic slides were examined by a veterinary pathologist and compared under a light microscope. The hematoxylin-eosin (H&E) stained sections were used for the following purposes: 1) morphological analysis of the myocardium, 2) inflammation and tissue damage assessment. Inflammation and tissue damage were determined by counting the number of mononuclear inflammatory cells (Lymphocytes and Macrophages) in H&E stained sections by randomly counting 100 microscopic fields over a total area 1.5 mm^2 at 400 × magnifications.[22]

In vitro antitumor activity
In order to determine the effect of GSE on DOX-inhibited growth and proliferation of the malignant cell line MCF-7 (human breast cancer cells), cell viability was evaluated by MTT assay according to the manufacturer's instructions. Briefly, the cells were distributed (5000 cells/well) in 96-well plates and maintained in RPMI-1640 medium supplemented with 10% fetal-calf serum and antibiotics (Penicillin G 50,000 units/l. Streptomycin 38,850 units/l and Nystatin 9078 units/l), in an incubator at 37°C with a humidified atmosphere of 10% CO_2 and the cells were grown for 24 h. The cells were then exposed to a series of concentrations

of free DOX (0.1, 0.5, 1, 5 and 10 µg/ml) and/or GSE (250 and 500 µg/ml) and incubated for 24 h (the drugs were dissolved in 100 µl of DMSO and then diluted with RPMI 1640). At the end of incubation time, MTT (20 µl with the concentration of 5 mg/ml) was added to each well and the plates incubated for further 6 h. Then, the culture medium was removed, 200 µl of DMSO was added to each well and the plates were shaken for 10 min. Finally, the optical density was measured at 550 nm using a microplate reader (AD 340; Beckmann Coulter). All the experiments were performed in triplicate.[19,21]

Statistics
All data were analyzed using SPSS software (Version 13.0). Student's t-test or one-way analysis of variance (ANOVA) followed by a Tukey's HSD post hoc test were used to analyze the statistical significance of the differences between groups, as needed. All data are presented as the mean ± standard error of the mean (SEM) of at least 6 rats in each group. A p-value less than 0.05 was considered statistically significant.

Results
Echocardiographic analysis
To evaluate the influence of the GSE and DOX on LV remodeling and function, a series of echocardiography studies were conducted. As shown in Figure 2 and Table 1, statistical analysis revealed that DOX treatment significantly decreased the FS (p<0.01) and EF (p<0.01), as compared with the Ctrl group. In addition, data analysis indicated that GSE treatment significantly increased the FS (p<0.01) and EF (p<0.01) in comparison with DOX group. Increase of FS and EF in GSE group reached to normal values as in Ctrl group with no significant differences. Moreover, there was no significant change in LVDD and LVSD.

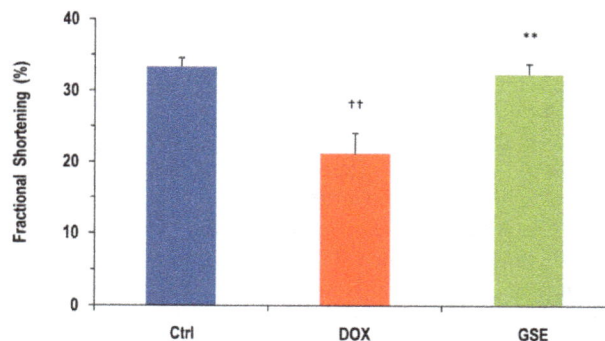

Figure 2. The effects of DOX (doxorubicin, 12 mg/kg) alone or in combination with GSE (grape seed extract, 100 mg/kg) on left ventricular fractional shortening in rats. Values are expressed as mean ± SEM. (n=6). ††: p<0.01 *vs*. Ctrl group; **: p<0.01 *vs*. DOX group.

Electrocardiographic recordings
Table 2 summarizes the significant changes in ECG recordings. ECG features in the Ctrl was normal. The data analysis revealed that DOX administration significantly changed the HR, RRI and QA parameters

(p<0.05) in comparison with Ctrl group. Moreover, statistical analysis demonstrated that GSE administration significantly improved the ECG parameters including HR and RRI, as compared to the DOX group (p<0.05).

Table 1. Echocardiographic analyses of left ventricular fractional shortening and ejection fraction in rat heart

Parameter	Group		
	Ctrl	DOX	GSE
LVDD (mm)	6.60±0.05	6.30±0.12	6.53±0.08
LVSD (mm)	4.40±0.07	4.97±0.217	4.41±0.07
FS (%)	33.31±1.24	21.16±2.88††	32.34±1.38**
EF (%)	70.19±1.71	50.03±5.10††	68.83±1.80**

Changes of left ventricular fractional shortening and ejection fraction in study groups, Ctrl=control, DOX=doxorubicin (12 mg/kg); GSE=grape seed extract (100 mg/kg), the values are expressed as mean ± SEM (n=6). ††: p<0.01 vs. Ctrl group and **: p<0.01 vs. DOX group.

Table 2. Electrocardiogram parameters

Parameter	Group		
	Ctrl	DOX	GSE
HR (BPM)	221.9±10.9	186.5±11.1†	233.9±9.100*
RRI (S)	0.274±.014	0.328±0.020†	0.270±0.010*
QA (µV)	1.171±3.18	14.07±5.760†	0.074±0.004
QTI (S)	0.072±0.005	0.076±0.004	0.074±0.004

Ctrl=control, DOX=doxorubicin, GSE=grape seed extract + DOX, RRI=RR interval, HR=heart rate, S=second, BPM=beats per minute. QA: Q amplitude, QTI: QT interval, the values are expressed as mean ± SEM (n=6). †: p<0.05 vs. Ctrl group,*: p< 0.05 vs. DOX group.

Blood pressure measuring

Table 3 shows that DOX treatment consistently and significantly decreased the systolic pressure (p<0.001), diastolic pressure (p<0.05) and mean pressure (p<0.01) in comparison with the Ctrl group. However, there was no significant change following GSE treatment, as compared to the DOX group.

Table 3. Arterial and left ventricular function parameters in study groups

Parameter		Group		
		Ctrl	DOX	GSE
Artery	Systolic pressure	88.06±1.85	71.74±1.84†††	81.08±1.85
	Diastolic pressure	68.25±2.28	53.32±4.66†	60.01±7.92
	Mean pressure (mmHg)	78.27±1.51	62.38±3.39††	70.46±7.42
Left Ventricle	Max Pressure (mmHg)	86.92±1.98	23.17±2.24†††	47.30±7.04**
	Min Pressure (mmHg)	1.03±0.86	5.01±0.95††	-2.44±1.25***
	Systolic Duration (s)	0.13±0.01	0.04±0.01†††	0.1±0.01***

Ctrl=control; DOX=doxorubicin (12 mg/kg); GSE=grape seed extract (100 mg/kg); the values are expressed as mean ± SEM (n=6). †: p<0.05, ††: p<0.01 and †††: p<0.001 vs. Ctrl group. *: p<0.05, **: p<0.01 and ***: p<0.001 vs. DOX group.

Left ventricular function analysis

DOX treatment markedly decreased the max pressure, (p<0.001, Table 3), contractility index (p<0.05, Figure 3) and the max dP/dt (p<0.05, Figure 4) and increased the EDP (p<0.001, Figure 5), min pressure (p<0.01, Table 3) and the min dP/dt (p<0.05, Figure 4) relative to the Ctrl group. In addition, GSE exposure significantly elevated the max pressure (Table 3), contractility index (Figure 3), min dP/dt (p<0.01, Figure 4), the min pressure (Table 3) and max dP/dt (p<0.001, Figure 4), while reduced the EDP (p<0.05, Figure 5), as compared to the DOX group.

Body weight development and heart/body weight ratio

As indicated in Table 4, the data analysis revealed that DOX treatment significantly resulted in decreased BW (p<0.001), HW (p<0.001) and HW/BW ratio (p<0.001) in comparison with the Ctrl group. Moreover, the results indicated that GSE treatment significantly increased BW (p<0.001), HW (p<0.001) and HW/BW ratio (p<0.01) relative to the DOX-treated group.

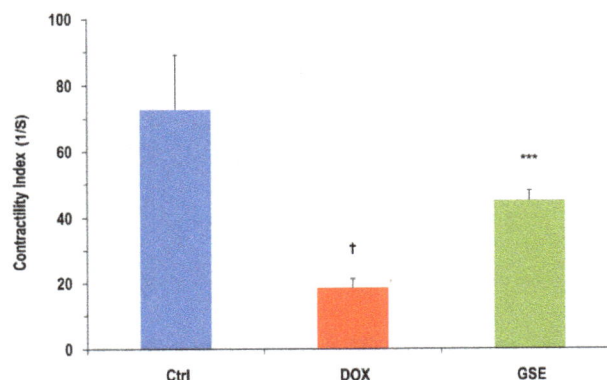

Figure 3. The effects of DOX (doxorubicin, 12 mg/kg) alone or in combination with GSE (grape seed extract, 100 mg/kg) on contractility index (1/S). Values are expressed as mean ± SEM. (n=6), †: p<0.05 vs. Ctrl group; ***: p<0.001 vs. DOX group.

Histopathological results of heart tissue

The histopathological changes in the rats' myocardium of all study groups are shown in Figure 6. The Ctrl group exhibited normal morphological findings. There were significant changes in DOX group including:

cytoplasmic vacuolization, interstitial edema, hyaline degeneration and Zenker's necrosis, as compared to the Ctrl group. Furthermore, DOX appeared to have significant adverse effects on rat cardiac tissue, i.e. focal to extensive hemorrhages, accumulation of acute inflammatory cells, injured vascular structures, necrotic changes in the nuclei of cardiomyocytes and mild cardiac fibrosis. In GSE group the myocardial damage was dramatically attenuated, as compared to the DOX group. There was also little evidence of pathological changes in the cardiomyocytes following GSE treatment. Therefore, it could be speculate that GSE leads to cell preservation and decreased necrosis, cytoplasmic vacuolization and maintained a normal morphology and structure for the cardiac muscle. The numbers of mononuclear inflammatory cells in study groups are illustrated in Figure 7. The numbers of inflammatory cells including lymphocytes and macrophages in DOX group were significantly higher than Ctrl group ($p < 0.001$) and GSE treatment significantly decreased the number of these cells in comparison with the DOX group ($p < 0.001$).

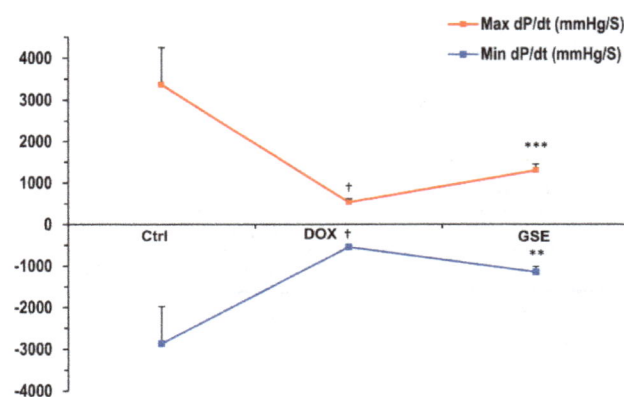

Figure 4. The effects of DOX (doxorubicin, 12 mg/kg) alone or in combination with GSE (grape seed extract, 100 mg/kg) on max dP/dt (mmHg/s) and min dP/dt (mmHg/s) alterations in rats. Values are expressed as mean ± SEM. (n=6). †: $p < 0.05$ vs. Ctrl group; **: $p < 0.01$ and ***: $p < 0.001$ vs. DOX group.

Table 4. Body weight and heart/weight ratio in study groups.

Group	IBW (gr)	FBW (gr)	HW (gr)	HW / BW
Ctrl	201.33±1.02	221.16±1.7000	0.90±0.0200	0.004±0.000100
DOX	210.00±0.89	181.17±1.61†††	0.54±0.02†††	0.003±0.0001†††
GSE	208.33±1.68	227.66±2.04***	0.78±0.02***	0.003±0.00001**

IBW=initial body weight; FBW=final body weight; HW=heart weight; BW=body weight.
Ctrl=control; DOX = doxorubicin (12 mg/kg); GSE = grape seed extract (100 mg/kg), the values are expressed as mean ± SEM (n=6).
†††: $p < 0.001$ vs. Ctrl group, **: $p < 0.01$ and ***: $p < 0.001$ vs. DOX group.

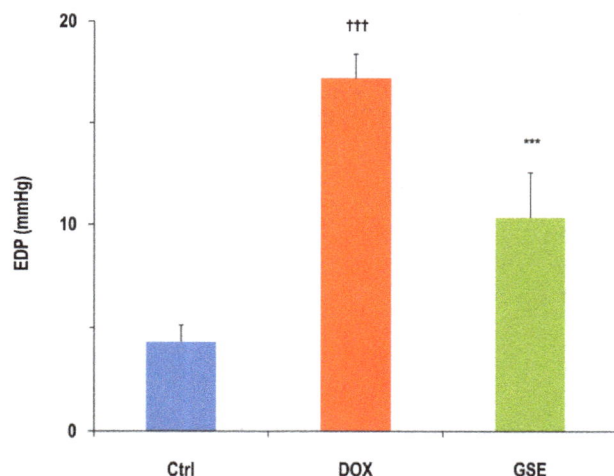

Figure 5. The effects of DOX (doxorubicin, 12 mg/kg) alone or in combination with GSE (grape seed extract, 100 mg/kg) on EDP (%). Values are expressed as mean ± SEM. (n=6). †††: $p < 0.001$ vs. Ctrl group and ***: $p < 0.001$ vs. DOX group.

Cytotoxicity assays
To evaluate the antitumor activities of GSE alone or in combination with DOX, MCF-7 cell line was used as tumor cells in MTT assay. As illustrated in Figure 8, the data analyses revealed that DOX produced cell toxicity dose-dependently. The results indicated that GSE alone, at dose 500 μg/ml, resulted in cell toxicity. However, co-

administration of GSE at this dose with DOX did not affect the cytotoxicity. Therefore, these findings demonstrate that GSE does not change the DOX-induced cell toxicity, *in vitro*, $p > 0.05$.

Discussion
DOX is widely used for the control and management of variety of human cancers, whereas, its consumption is limited by side effects. Cardiomyopathy is the most important toxic outcome in patients receiving DOX.[23,24] In the current study, it has been demonstrated that GSE has protective effect on DOX-induced cardiotoxicity in rat heart. The animal model used in this study was described previously[21] and characterized by injuries similar to what reported by others.[17,18,25-27] Alterations in physiological parameters are well known as one of the toxic effects of DOX, which is characterized by reduced body and heart weights.[28-30] Our findings here confirmed the literature reports that DOX treatment leads to decreased both body and heart weights in animals[31] and that GSE treatment increased body and heart weights, as compared to DOX group.
Our data supported previous findings in which DOX administration significantly resulted in increased left ventricular dysfunction and decreased the FS and EF in the echocardiographic assessment.[21,32] Treatment with GSE significantly reversed the effects of DOX on left

ventricular function, EF and FS, as compared to DOX group. In addition, in line with previous findings,[21,33-37] we found that DOX exposure resulted in reduced aortic, systolic, diastolic and mean pressure as well as decreased max pressure, min pressure, EDP, max dP/dt, min dP/dt and contractility. These adverse effects were reversed by GSE treatment.

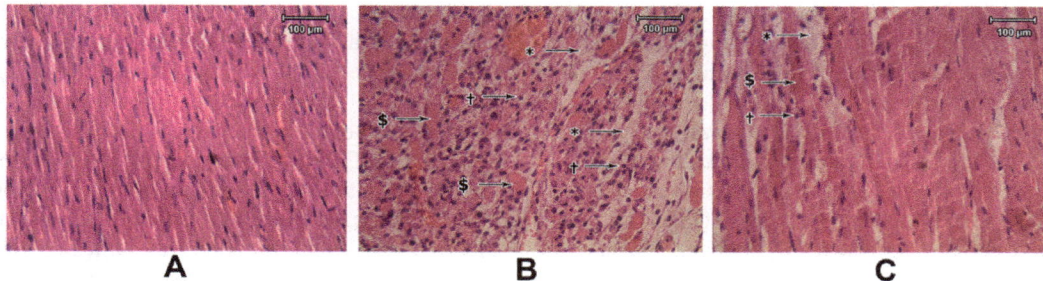

Figure 6. Effect of grape seed extract (GSE) on doxorubicin (DOX)-induced histopathological alterations in cardiac tissues (H&E, 400×). A: control group shows normal histological pattern. B: DOX group shows hyaline degeneration and Zenker's necrosis ($), infiltration of acute inflammatory cells (†) and inter cardiomyocytes edema (*): The lesions indicate severe pathological changes in the myocardium. C: GSE group shows hyaline degeneration and Zenker's necrosis ($), infiltration of acute inflammatory cells (†) and inter cardiomyocytes edema (*): These changes indicate slight histopathological injury in the cardiac tissue of GSE group.

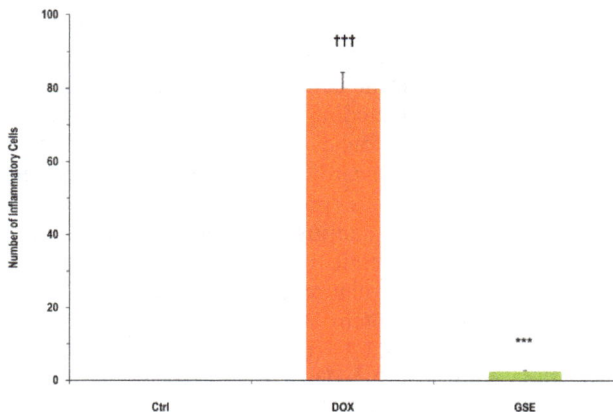

Figure 7. The numbers of mononuclear inflammatory cells (Lymphocytes and Macrophages) in study groups. DOX = doxorubicin (12 mg/kg) alone or in combination with GSE = grape seed extract (100 mg/kg). Values are expressed as mean ± SEM (n=6), †††: $p<0.001$ *vs.* Ctrl group and ***: $p<0.001$ *vs.* DOX group.

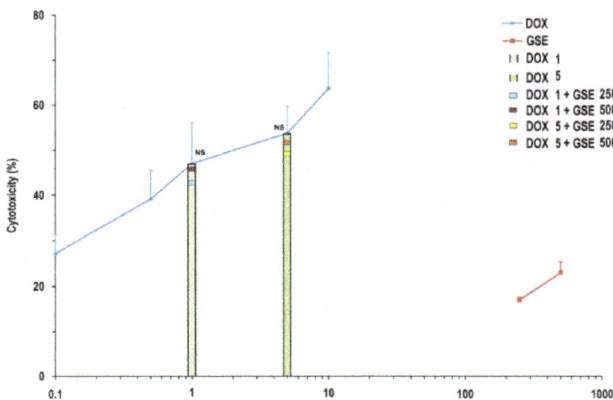

Figure 8. Cytotoxicity of DOX (doxorubicin; 1 and 5 µg/ml) alone or in combination with GSE (grape seed extract; 250 and 500 µg/ml) against MCF-7 cells. The results are mean values ± SEM of three independent experiments performed in triplicate. NS: There was no a significant difference between DOX alone or in combination with GSE, $p>0.05$.

A recent study provided interesting evidence indicating that GSE treatment has cardioprotective effect in high-fat diet-induced cardiac dysfunction and DOX-induced cardiotoxicity in animals. Treatment with GSE highly improved heart rate and pressure and this protection was associated with iron and calcium accumulation and ROS generation in the myocardium,[18,38] hence, they recommended GSE as an option for the prevention of DOX-induced cardiotoxicity. Further confirmation comes from another study showing that GSE treatment in combination with DOX in mice significantly protected the heart tissue by improving its antioxidant activity; leading to this conclusion that GSE acts as a potent antioxidant to prevent heart damage.[27,39]

In the line with this evidence, Karthikeyan et al have confirmed the efficacy of GSPE as a cardioprotective agent in alleviating isoproterenol-induced myocardial injury in rats.[40] They demonstrated that GSPE administration at doses of 100 and 150 mg/kg positively alters the levels of glutathione, ascorbic acid, a-tocopherol, ceruloplasmin, mitochondrial cytochrome, phospholipids and adenosine triphosphate and also restores normal mitochondrial function. This experimental evidence indicates that GSPE may serve as a potential therapeutic tool in promoting cardiovascular health.

We investigated ECG alterations because it was found that the severity of changes in ECG is directly related to the known DOX-induced cardiotoxicity in humans and animals.[41,42] Our results clearly indicate that DOX resulted in myocardial injury as indicated by the increase in the RR interval and QA and the decrease in HR of the ECG records. It has been documented that these ECG changes are associated with the prolongation of action potential duration and DOX could strongly affect the recovery phase of the transmembrane action potential, influencing preferentially Ca^{2+} movements across the cellular membrane.[26,43,44] In addition, it has been reported that DOX alters calcium homeostasis in the myocardium.[18] In fact, several previous studies demonstrated the role of Ca^{2+} disturbances in DOX-induced cardiotoxicity in vivo[45] and in vitro,[46] they also raise a major discrepancy as shown by lower levels of myocardial calcium following DOX administration compared to plethoric studies where higher levels of calcium after DOX treatment was observed. On the other hand, it was found that GSE affects the levels of calcium in the heart tissue,[18] it is possible that GSE normalized the DOX-induced ECG alterations in a positive way.[25] In the present study, GSE treatment was also able to prevent the development of ECG changes induced by DOX and to confirm that GSE has a cardioprotective effect against DOX-induced cardiac dysfunction.

In this study typical histopathological alterations such as noticeable interstitial edema, focal myocardial fibrosis, perinuclear vacuolation and myocardial necrosis was observed following DOX treatment as reported in different experimental animal models,[21,47-49] including noticeable interstitial edema, focal myocardial fibrosis, perinuclear vacuolation and myocardial necrosis. Treatment with GSE decreased the infiltration of inflammatory cells including lymphocytes and macrophages into the myocardium of rats significantly, in comparison to DOX group (Figure 7). Our data confirmed previous findings suggesting GSE attenuated the detrimental impacts of DOX on morphology and ultrastructure of heart tissues in histopathology studies.[27,31]

Furthermore, the results of the MTT assay indicated that DOX exerts a dose-dependent cytotoxic effect on MCF7 cells and that GSE treatment in combination with DOX had no significant effect on DOX-induced cell toxicity and GSE alone showed cytotoxicity effect on MCF7 cells.[50] In addition, it was reported that procyanidin, an antioxidant flavonoid of the GSE, exhibited antitumor activity on MCF7 cells. In this regard, other studies have demonstrated that procyanidins induce cytotoxicity on several tumor cells such as human adenocarcinoma cells A549,[31] human colorectal cancer HT29, LoVo cells,[51] A-427 human lung cancer cells, CRL-1739 human gastric adenocarcinoma cells and K562 chronic myelogenous leukemic cells.[52]

During the two past decades tremendous effort has been put into uncovering the molecular mechanisms and/or intracellular targets involved in the DOX-induced cardiotoxicity and different hypotheses have been developed to explain this phenomenon,[53-55] but no single one of these was able to fully explain it.[2] Rather, DOX cardiotoxicity appears to be a multifactorial process that results in cardiomyocytes death with typical apoptotic features and heart failure as the terminal downstream event.[53,56,57] It has long been established that DOX anticancer actions are closely associated with DNA intercalation, topoisomerase-II inhibition and apoptosis. The most important cardiotoxicity actions of DOX are related to oxidative

stress. It appears that such difference in mechanisms is not fully justified.[2,53] It seems there is some overlapping between the beneficial (anticancer/therapeutic) and detrimental (cardiotoxic) effects of DOX, in fact, they share common effectors such as oxidative stress and both involve apoptosis.[2] On the other side, it has been reported that antioxidants can be protective against DOX-induced cardiotoxicity through their free radical scavenging capability.[58,59] There are antioxidant flavonoids such as procyanidin B4, catechin and gallic acid in GSE which can protect DNA from oxidative damage in a dose-dependent manner.[60] For instance, GSPE treatment has been shown to significantly inhibit DOX-induced cardiotoxicity as indicated by decreased DNA damage and histopathological changes in the cardiac tissue of mice.[61] In addition, recent studies demonstrated the bioavailability of grape seed proanthocyanidins to the target organs exhibiting a superior protection against oxidative DNA damage and oxidative stress relative to vitamin C, E and β-carotene.[12] In support of our findings, it has been reported that various chemical compounds such as carvedilol,[62] rosmarinic acid,[63] dexrazoxane[64,65] as well as herbal agents including GSE,[18,39] saffron extract[66] and garlic extract[67] found to potentially be protective against DOX-induced cardiotoxicity. Based on reported studies GSE produces protective effect by several mechanisms including antioxidant effect,[68,69] decreasing the number of apoptotic cells,[70] prevention of DNA fragmentation,[15,71] regulation of the expression levels of the pro-apoptotic protein Bax-alpha,[72] increasing anti-apoptotic protein Bcl-2[73] and inhibition of apoptotic signaling pathways.[74,75] This study is a comprehensive descriptive study but did not aim to investigate the protection mechanism(s) of GSE on DOX-induced cardiomyopathy. Further mechanistically approach studies on GSE-induced cardioprotection and examining different doses of GSE will enrich the study.

Conclusion

In conclusion, hemodynamic, ECG, echocardiographic, histopathologic and MTT results in this study confirm the protective effects of GSE on DOX-induced cardiotoxicity, probably through antioxidant and anti-inflammatory mechanisms. Taken together, our results support the notion to introduce GSE as a potential drug candidate for co-administration with DOX in human chemotherapy in order to increase DOX therapeutic index. Further investigations by clinical trials to examine GSE cardioprotective effect in DOX users are necessary to confirm this claim.

Acknowledgments

The authors would like to acknowledge their funding support, provided by the Drug Applied Research Center (DARC) at Tabriz University of Medical Sciences (Grant No. 91.71). This study was part of a PhD thesis submitted by N. Razmaraii at DARC.

Conflict of Interest

The authors report no declaration of interest.

References

1. Octavia Y, Tocchetti CG, Gabrielson KL, Janssens S, Crijns HJ, Moens AL. Doxorubicin-induced cardiomyopathy: From molecular mechanisms to therapeutic strategies. *J Mol Cell Cardiol* 2012;52(6):1213-25. doi: 10.1016/j.yjmcc.2012.03.006

2. Tokarska-Schlattner M, Zaugg M, Zuppinger C, Wallimann T, Schlattner U. New insights into doxorubicin-induced cardiotoxicity: The critical role of cellular energetics. *J Mol Cell Cardiol* 2006;41(3):389-405. doi: 10.1016/j.yjmcc.2006.06.009

3. Gianni L, Herman EH, Lipshultz SE, Minotti G, Sarvazyan N, Sawyer DB. Anthracycline cardiotoxicity: From bench to bedside. *J Clin Oncol* 2008;26(22):3777-84. doi: 10.1200/JCO.2007.14.9401

4. Doroshow JH, Locker GY, Myers CE. Enzymatic defenses of the mouse heart against reactive oxygen metabolites: Alterations produced by doxorubicin. *J Clin Invest* 1980;65(1):128-35. doi: 10.1172/JCI109642

5. Baydar NG, Özkan G, Yaşar S. Evaluation of the antiradical and antioxidant potential of grape extracts. *Food Control* 2007;18(9):1131-6. doi: 10.1016/j.foodcont.2006.06.011

6. Leifert WR, Abeywardena MY. Cardioprotective actions of grape polyphenols. *Nutr Res* 2008;28(11):729-37. doi: 10.1016/j.nutres.2008.08.007

7. Khoshbaten M, Aliasgarzadeh A, Masnadi K, Farhang S, Tarzamani MK, Babaei H, et al. Grape seed extract to improve liver function in patients with nonalcoholic fatty liver change. *Saudi J Gastroenterol* 2010;16(3):194-7. doi: 10.4103/1319-3767.65197

8. Najafi M, Vaez H, Zahednezhad F, Samadzadeh M, Babaei H. Study the effects of hydroalcoholic extract of grape seed (vitis vinifera) on infarct size and cardiac arrhythmias in ischemic-reperfused isolated rat heart. *Pharm Sci* 2011;16(4):187- 94.

9. Abedini S, Pourghassem-Gargarri B, Babaei H, Aliasgarzadeh A, Pourabdollahi P. Effect of supplementation with grape seed extract (vitis vinifera) on serum lipid profiles in patient with type 2 diabetes. *Iran J Endocrinol Metab* 2013;15(1):59-66.

10. Pourghassem-Gargari B, Abedini S, Babaei H, Aliasgarzadeh A, Pourabdollahi P. Effect of supplementation with grape seed (vitis vinifera) extract on antioxidant status and lipid peroxidation in patient with type ıı diabetes. *J Med Plant Res* 2011;5(10):2029-34

11. Bagchi D, Swaroop A, Preuss HG, Bagchi M. Free radical scavenging, antioxidant and cancer chemoprevention by grape seed proanthocyanidin: An overview. *Mutat Res* 2014;768:69-73. doi: 10.1016/j.mrfmmm.2014.04.004

12. Bagchi D, Bagchi M, Stohs SJ, Das DK, Ray SD, Kuszynski CA, et al. Free radicals and grape seed proanthocyanidin extract: Importance in human health and disease prevention. *Toxicology* 2000;148(2-3):187-97. doi: 10.1016/S0300-483X(00)00210-9

13. Derry M, Raina K, Agarwal R, Agarwal C. Differential effects of grape seed extract against human colorectal cancer cell lines: The intricate role of death receptors and mitochondria. *Cancer Lett* 2013;334(1):69-78. doi: 10.1016/j.canlet.2012.12.015

14. Shrotriya S, Deep G, Gu M, Kaur M, Jain AK, Inturi S, et al. Generation of reactive oxygen species by grape seed extract causes irreparable DNA damage leading to g2/m arrest and apoptosis selectively in head and neck squamous cell carcinoma cells. *Carcinogenesis* 2012;33(4):848-58. doi: 10.1093/carcin/bgs019

15. Ray SD, Patel D, Wong V, Bagchi D. In vivo protection of dna damage associated apoptotic and necrotic cell deaths during acetaminophen-induced nephrotoxicity, amiodarone-induced lung toxicity and doxorubicin-induced cardiotoxicity by a novel ih636 grape seed proanthocyanidin extract. *Res Commun Mol Pathol Pharmacol* 2000;107(1-2):137-66.

16. Ganjali Z, Javadian F, Estakhr J, Heidari A. Anti-lipidimic and anti-hyperglycemic properties of methanolic extract of grape seed in diabetic rats. *Int J Anim Vet Adv* 2012;4(3):173-5.

17. Abd El Samad AA, Raafat MH. Comparative study on the effects of grape seed extract and telmisartan on doxorubicin-induced cardiotoxicity in adult male rats: Light and electron microscopic study. *Egypt J Histol* 2012;35(2):340-52. doi: 10.1097/01.ehx.0000414803.54664.e5

18. Mokni M, Hamlaoui-Guesmi S, Amri M, Marzouki L, Limam F, Aouani E. Grape seed and skin extract protects against acute chemotherapy toxicity induced by doxorubicin in rat heart. *Cardiovasc Toxicol* 2012;12(2):158-65. doi: 10.1007/s12012-012-9155-1

19. Razmaraii N, Babaei H, Mohajjel Nayebi A, Assadnassab G, Ashrafi Helan J, Azarmi Y. Crocin treatment prevents doxorubicin-induced cardiotoxicity in rats. *Life Sci* 2016;157:145-51. doi: 10.1016/j.lfs.2016.06.012

20. Bu'Lock FA, Gabriel HM, Oakhill A, Mott MG, Martin RP. Cardioprotection by icrf187 against high dose anthracycline toxicity in children with

malignant disease. *Br Heart J* 1993;70(2):185-8. doi: 10.1136/hrt.70.2.185

21. Razmaraii N, Babaei H, Mohajjel Nayebi A, Asadnasab G, Ashrafi Helan J, Azarmi Y. Cardioprotective effect of phenytoin on doxorubicin-induced cardiac toxicity in a rat model. *J Cardiovasc Pharmacol* 2016;67(3):237-45. doi: 10.1097/FJC.0000000000000339

22. Goncalves CC, Hernandes L, Bersani-Amado CA, Franco SL, Silva JF, Natali MR. Use of propolis hydroalcoholic extract to treat colitis experimentally induced in rats by 2,4,6-trinitrobenzenesulfonic acid. *Evid Based Complement Alternat Med* 2013;2013:853976. doi: 10.1155/2013/853976

23. Lefrak EA, Pitha J, Rosenheim S, Gottlieb JA. A clinicopathologic analysis of adriamycin cardiotoxicity. *Cancer* 1973;32(2):302-14.

24. Lenaz L, Page JA. Cardiotoxicity of adriamycin and related anthracyclines. *Cancer Treat Rev* 1976;3(3):111-20. doi: 10.1016/S0305-7372(76)80018-7

25. Ammar el SM, Said SA, El-Damarawy SL, Suddek GM. Cardioprotective effect of grape-seed proanthocyanidins on doxorubicin-induced cardiac toxicity in rats. *Pharm Biol* 2013;51(3):339-44. doi: 10.3109/13880209.2012.729065

26. Danesi R, Del Tacca M, Soldani G. Measurement of the $S\alpha T$ segment as the most reliable electrocardiogram parameter for the assessment of adriamycin-induced cardiotoxicity in the rat. *J Pharmacol Methods* 1986;16(3):251-9. doi: 10.1016/0160-5402(86)90046-X

27. Boghdady NA. Antioxidant and antiapoptotic effects of proanthocyanidin and ginkgo biloba extract against doxorubicin-induced cardiac injury in rats. *Cell Biochem Funct* 2013;31(4):344-51. doi: 10.1002/cbf.2907

28. Zhou S, Palmeira CM, Wallace KB. Doxorubicin-induced persistent oxidative stress to cardiac myocytes. *Toxicol Lett* 2001;121(3):151-7. doi: 10.1016/S0378-4274(01)00329-0

29. Kang J, Lee Y, No K, Jung E, Sung J, Kim Y, et al. Ginseng intestinal metabolite-I (GIM-I) reduces doxorubicin toxicity in the mouse testis. *Reprod Toxicol* 2002;16(3):291-8. doi: 10.1016/S0890-6238(02)00021-7

30. Herman EH, Zhang J, Chadwick DP, Ferrans VJ. Comparison of the protective effects of amifostine and dexrazoxane against the toxicity of doxorubicin in spontaneously hypertensive rats. *Cancer Chemother Pharmacol* 2000;45(4):329-34. doi: 10.1007/s002800050048

31. Li W, Xu B, Xu J, Wu XL. Procyanidins produce significant attenuation of doxorubicin-induced cardiotoxicity via suppression of oxidative stress. *Basic Clin Pharmacol Toxicol* 2009;104(3):192-7. doi: 10.1111/j.1742-7843.2008.00358.x

32. Pye MP, Black M, Cobbe SM. Comparison of in vivo and in vitro haemodynamic function in experimental heart failure: Use of echocardiography. *Cardiovasc Res* 1996;31(6):873-81. doi: 10.1016/S0008-6363(96)00051-X.

33. Platel D, Pouna P, Bonoron-Adèle S, Robert J. Comparative cardiotoxicity of idarubicin and doxorubicin using the isolated perfused rat heart model. *Anticancer Drugs* 1999;10(7):671-6. doi: 10.1097/00001813-199908000-00007

34. Sacco G, Bigioni M, Evangelista S, Goso C, Manzini S, Maggi CA. Cardioprotective effects of zofenopril, a new angiotensin-converting enzyme inhibitor, on doxorubicin-induced cardiotoxicity in the rat. *Eur J Pharmacol* 2001;414(1):71-8. doi: 10.1016/S0014-2999(01)00782-8

35. Thomas L, Bellmont S, Christen MO, La Roche B, Monassier L. Cardiovascular and survival effects of sympatho-inhibitors in adriamycin-induced cardiomyopathy in rats. *Fundam Clin Pharmacol* 2004;18(6):649-55. doi: 10.1111/j.1472-8206.2004.00282.x

36. Pacher P, Liaudet L, Bai P, Virag L, Mabley JG, Hasko G, et al. Activation of poly(ADP-ribose) polymerase contributes to development of doxorubicin-induced heart failure. *J Pharmacol Exp Ther* 2002;300(3):862-7. doi: 10.1124/jpet.300.3.862

37. Pacher P, Liaudet L, Mabley JG, Cziráki A, Haskó G, Szabó C. Beneficial effects of a novel ultrapotent poly(ADP-ribose) polymerase inhibitor in murine models of heart failure. *Int J Mol Med* 2006;17(2):369-75. doi: 10.3892/ijmm.17.2.369

38. Charradi K, Sebai H, Elkahoui S, Ben Hassine F, Limam F, Aouani E. Grape seed extract alleviates high-fat diet-induced obesity and heart dysfunction by preventing cardiac siderosis. *Cardiovasc Toxicol* 2011;11(1):28-37. doi: 10.1007/s12012-010-9101-z

39. Yalçin E, Oruç E, Çavuşoğlu K, Yapar K. Protective role of grape seed extract against doxorubicin-induced cardiotoxicity and genotoxicity in albino mice. *J Med Food* 2010;13(4):917-25. doi: 10.1089/jmf.2009.0162

40. Karthikeyan K, Bai BR, Devaraj SN. Efficacy of grape seed proanthocyanidins on cardioprotection during isoproterenol-induced myocardial injury in rats. *J Cardiovasc Pharmacol* 2009;53(2):109-15. doi: 10.1097/FJC.0b013e3181970c01

41. Larsen RL, Jakacki RI, Vetter VL, Meadows AT, Silber JH, Barber G. Electrocardiographic changes and arrhythmias after cancer therapy in children and young adults. *Am J Cardiol* 1992;70(1):73-7. doi: 10.1016/0002-9149(92)91393-I

42. Nousiainen T, Vanninen E, Rantala A, Jantunen E, Hartikainen J. QT dispersion and late potentials during doxorubicin therapy for non-hodgkin's lymphoma. *J Intern Med* 1999;245(4):359-64. doi: 10.1046/j.1365-2796.1999.00480.x

43. van Acker SA, Kramer K, Voest EE, Grimbergen JA, Zhang J, van der Vijgh WJ, et al. Doxorubicin-induced cardiotoxicity monitored by ECG in freely

moving mice. A new model to test potential protectors. *Cancer Chemother Pharmacol* 1996;38(1):95-101. doi: 10.1007/s002800050453

44. Villani F, Galimberti M, Monti E, Cova D, Lanza E, Rozza-Dionigi A, et al. Effect of ICRF-187 pretreatment against doxorubicin-induced delayed cardiotoxicity in the rat. *Toxicol Appl Pharmacol* 1990;102(2):292-9. doi: 10.1016/0041-008X(90)90028-S

45. Olson HM, Young DM, Prieur DJ, LeRoy AF, Reagan RL. Electrolyte and morphologic alterations of myocardium in adriamycin-treated rabbits. *Am J Pathol* 1974;77(3):439-54.

46. Yesair DW, Schwartzbach E, Shuck D, Denine EP, Asbell MA. Comparative pharmacokinetics of daunomycin and adriamycin in several animal species. *Cancer Res* 1972;32(6):1177-83.

47. Dogan I, Sonmez B, Turker O, Yenilmez E, Uçar U, Zengin A, et al. Decreased myocardial Tl-201 uptake in rats: Early sign of doxorubicin induced myocardial damage and the relation to inflammation. *Eur J Gen Med* 2010;7(1):43-9.

48. Klimtová I, Šimůnek T, Mazurová Y, Hrdina R, Gerš V, Adamcová M. Comparative study of chronic toxic effects of daunorubicin and doxorubicin in rabbits. *Hum Exp Toxicol* 2002;21(12):649-57. doi: 10.1191/0960327102ht311oa

49. Yilmaz S, Atessahin A, Sahna E, Karahan I, Ozer S. Protective effect of lycopene on adriamycin-induced cardiotoxicity and nephrotoxicity. *Toxicology* 2006;218(2-3):164-71. doi: 10.1016/j.tox.2005.10.015

50. Sharma G, Tyagi AK, Singh RP, Chan DC, Agarwal R. Synergistic anti-cancer effects of grape seed extract and conventional cytotoxic agent doxorubicin against human breast carcinoma cells. *Breast Cancer Res Treat* 2004;85(1):1-12. doi: 10.1023/B:BREA.0000020991.55659.59

51. Kaur M, Singh RP, Gu M, Agarwal R, Agarwal C. Grape seed extract inhibits in vitro and in vivo growth of human colorectal carcinoma cells. *Clin Cancer Res* 2006;12(20 Pt 1):6194-202. doi: 10.1158/1078-0432.CCR-06-1465

52. Ye X, Krohn RL, Liu W, Joshi SS, Kuszynski CA, McGinn TR, et al. The cytotoxic effects of a novel ih636 grape seed proanthocyanidin extract on cultured human cancer cells. *Mol Cell Biochem* 1999;196(1-2):99-108. doi: 10.1023/A:1006926414683

53. Minotti G, Menna P, Salvatorelli E, Cairo G, Gianni L. Anthracyclines: Molecular advances and pharmacologic developments in antitumor activity and cardiotoxicity. *Pharmacol Rev* 2004;56(2):185-229. doi: 10.1124/pr.56.2.6

54. Olson RD, Mushlin PS. Doxorubicin cardiotoxicity: Analysis of prevailing hypotheses. *FASEB J* 1990;4(13):3076-86.

55. Singal PK, Iliskovic N, Li T, Kumar D. Adriamycin cardiomyopathy: Pathophysiology and prevention. *FASEB J* 1997;11(12):931-6.

56. Kalyanaraman B, Joseph J, Kalivendi S, Wang S, Konorev E, Kotamraju S. Doxorubicin-induced apoptosis: Implications in cardiotoxicity. In: Vallyathan V, Castranova V, Shi X, editors. Oxygen/nitrogen radicals: Cell injury and disease. USA: Springer; 2002. P. 119-24.

57. Fukazawa R, Miller TA, Kuramochi Y, Frantz S, Kim YD, Marchionni MA, et al. Neuregulin-1 protects ventricular myocytes from anthracycline-induced apoptosis via erbb4-dependent activation of PI3-kinase/Akt. *J Mol Cell Cardiol* 2003;35(12):1473-9. doi: 10.1016/j.yjmcc.2003.09.012

58. Horenstein MS, Vander Heide RS, L'Ecuyer TJ. Molecular basis of anthracycline-induced cardiotoxicity and its prevention. *Mol Genet Metab* 2000;71(1-2):436-44. doi: 10.1006/mgme.2000.3043

59. Ferreira AL, Matsubara LS, Matsubara BB. Anthracycline-induced cardiotoxicity. *Cardiovasc Hematol Agents Med Chem* 2008;6(4):278-81. doi: 10.2174/187152508785909474

60. Fan P, Lou H. Effects of polyphenols from grape seeds on oxidative damage to cellular DNA. *Mol Cell Biochem* 2004;267(1-2):67-74. doi: 10.1023/B:MCBI.0000049366.75461.00

61. Bagchi D, Sen CK, Ray SD, Das DK, Bagchi M, Preuss HG, et al. Molecular mechanisms of cardioprotection by a novel grape seed proanthocyanidin extract. *Mutat Res* 2003;523-524:87-97. doi: 10.1016/S0027-5107(02)00324-X

62. Spallarossa P, Garibaldi S, Altieri P, Fabbi P, Manca V, Nasti S, et al. Carvedilol prevents doxorubicin-induced free radical release and apoptosis in cardiomyocytes in vitro. *J Mol Cell Cardiol* 2004;37(4):837-46. doi: 10.1016/j.yjmcc.2004.05.024

63. Kim DS, Kim HR, Woo ER, Hong ST, Chae HJ, Chae SW. Inhibitory effects of rosmarinic acid on adriamycin-induced apoptosis in H9c2 cardiac muscle cells by inhibiting reactive oxygen species and the activations of c-Jun N-terminal kinase and extracellular signal-regulated kinase. *Biochem Pharmacol* 2005;70(7):1066-78. doi: 10.1016/j.bcp.2005.06.026

64. Ducroq J, Moha ou Maati H, Guilbot S, Dilly S, Laemmel E, Pons-Himbert C, et al. Dexrazoxane protects the heart from acute doxorubicin-induced QT prolongation: A key role for I(ks). *Br J Pharmacol* 2010;159(1):93-101. doi: 10.1111/j.1476-5381.2009.00371.x

65. Sawyer DB, Fukazawa R, Arstall MA, Kelly RA. Daunorubicin-induced apoptosis in rat cardiac myocytes is inhibited by dexrazoxane. *Circ Res* 1999;84(3):257-65. doi: 10.1161/01.RES.84.3.257

66. Chahine N, Hanna J, Makhlouf H, Duca L, Martiny L, Chahine R. Protective effect of saffron extract against doxorubicin cardiotoxicity in isolated rabbit heart. *Pharm Biol* 2013;51(12):1564-71. doi: 10.3109/13880209.2013.802812

67. Alkreathy H, Damanhouri ZA, Ahmed N, Slevin M, Ali SS, Osman AM. Aged garlic extract protects against doxorubicin-induced cardiotoxicity in rats. *Food Chem Toxicol* 2010;48(3):951-6. doi: 10.1016/j.fct.2010.01.005

68. Cetin A, Kaynar L, Kocyigit I, Hacioglu SK, Saraymen R, Ozturk A, et al. Role of grape seed extract on methotrexate induced oxidative stress in rat liver. *Am J Chin Med* 2008;36(5):861-72. doi: 10.1142/S0192415X08006302

69. Da Silva JMR, Darmon N, Fernandez Y, Mitjavila S. Oxygen free radical scavenger capacity in aqueous models of different procyanidins from grape seeds. *J Agric Food Chem* 1991;39(9):1549-52. doi: 10.1021/jf00009a002

70. Sato M, Bagchi D, Tosaki A, Das DK. Grape seed proanthocyanidin reduces cardiomyocyte apoptosis by inhibiting ischemia/reperfusion-induced activation of JNK-1 and C-JUN. *Free Radic Biol Med* 2001;31(6):729-37. doi: 10.1016/S0891-5849(01)00626-8

71. Bagchi D, Garg A, Krohn RL, Bagchi M, Bagchi DJ, Balmoori J, et al. Protective effects of grape seed proanthocyanidins and selected antioxidants against TPA-induced hepatic and brain lipid peroxidation and DNA fragmentation, and peritoneal macrophage activation in mice. *Gen Pharmacol* 1998;30(5):771-6. doi: 10.1016/S0306-3623(97)00332-7

72. Decean H, Fischer-Fodor E, Tatomir C, Perde-Schrepler M, Somfelean L, Burz C, et al. Vitis vinifera seeds extract for the modulation of cytosolic factors bax-alpha and nf-kb involved in uvb-induced oxidative stress and apoptosis of human skin cells. *Clujul Med* 2016;89(1):72-81. doi: 10.15386/cjmed-508

73. Baiomy AA. Protective role of grape seeds extract against cadmium toxicity in the lung of male wistar rats. *J Cytol Histol* 2016;S5:004. doi: 10.4172/2157-7099.S5-004

74. Joshi SS, Kuszynski CA, Bagchi D. The cellular and molecular basis of health benefits of grape seed proanthocyanidin extract. *Curr Pharm Biotechnol* 2001;2(2):187-200. doi: 10.2174/1389201013378725

75. Filip GA, Postescu ID, Bolfa P, Catoi C, Muresan A, Clichici S. Inhibition of uvb-induced skin phototoxicity by a grape seed extract as modulator of nitrosative stress, erk/nf-kb signaling pathway and apoptosis, in skh-1 mice. *Food Chem Toxicol* 2013;57:296-306. doi: 10.1016/j.fct.2013.03.031

16

Determination of Four Major Saponins in Skin and Endosperm of Seeds of Horse Chestnut (*Aesculus Hippocastanum* L.) Using High Performance Liquid Chromatography with Positive Confirmation by Thin Layer Chromatography

Zead Helmi Mahmoud Abudayeh[1]*****, **Khaldun Mohammad Al Azzam**[2]*****, **Ahmad Naddaf**[1], **Uliana Vladimirovna Karpiuk**[3], **Viktoria Sergeevna Kislichenko**[4]

[1]*Faculty of Pharmacy, Isra University, 11622 Amman, Jordan.*
[2]*Department of Pharmaceutical Chemistry, Pharmacy Program, Batterjee Medical College for Sciences and Technology (BMC), 21442 Jeddah, Kingdom of Saudi Arabia.*
[3]*Department of pharmacognosy and botany, National Medical University is the name of O.O.Bogomolets, Ukraine.*
[4]*National University of Pharmacy, Kharkiv, Ukraine.*

Article info

Keywords:
· Horse chestnut
· *Aesculus hippocastanum* L.
· Saponins
· HPLC
· TLC
· Ultrasonic extraction

Abstract

Purpose: To separate and quantify four major saponins in the extracts of the skin and the endosperm of seeds of horse chestnut (*Aesculus hippocastanum* L.) using ultrasonic solvent extraction followed by a high performance liquid chromatography-diode array detector (HPLC-DAD) with positive confirmation by thin layer chromatography (TLC).

Methods: The saponins: escin Ia, escin Ib, isoescin Ia and isoescin Ib were extracted using ultrasonic extraction method. The optimized extraction conditions were: 70% methanol as extraction solvent, 80 °C as extraction temperature, and the extraction time was achieved in 4 hours. The HPLC conditions used: Zorbax SB-ODS-(150 mm × 2.1 mm, 3 µm) column, acetonitrile and 0.10% phosphoric acid solution (39:61 v/v) as mobile phase, flow rate was 0.5 mL min^{-1} at 210 nm and 230 nm detection. The injection volume was 10 µL, and the separation was carried out isothermally at 30 °C in a heated chamber.

Results: The results indicated that the developed HPLC method is simple, sensitive and reliable. Moreover, the content of escins in seeds decreased by more than 30% in endosperm and by more than 40% in skin upon storage for two years.

Conclusion: This assay can be readily utilized as a quality control method for horse chestnut and other related medicinal plants.

Introduction

The use of medicinal plants to heal diseases has been a common practice worldwide.[1] Its popularity is still maintained due to the cultural and historical reasons, and to the primary health care needs added by modern medicine.[1,2] For instance, beneficial effects including antimutagenicity,[3] chemoprotection, and antioxidant activity have been reported.[4]

Aesculus hippocastanum L., commonly known as "horse chestnut", is a native, stable and important elements of urban and rural landscapes, which is widely distributed all over the world.[1,5] It is used for a variety medical conditions, including malary, fever, bladder and gastrointestinal disorders. Moreover, the seeds extract have been prescribed traditionally for the treatment of several chronic venous insufficiency, to reduce its associated symptoms, including leg swelling and heaviness as well as vascular problems.[1,6] This extract consists mainly of escins and a mixture of triterpenoid saponins (α- and β-escin).

Saponins consist of four substances make up 60% of the total mixture, namely: escin Ia 24%, escin Ib 17%, escin IIa 13% and escin IIb 6%.[7] Thus, due to the different pharmacological properties and their wide use in the pharmaceutical, β-escin (which all are dependent on its concentration) has significant role making its analysis in herbal medicines important and deemed necessary.

Literature survey reveals that saponins in *Aesculus hippocastanum* L., plant have been widely studied, and about 30 individual compounds of saponins have been isolated and identified. Only escin Ia among the four escins is assigned as the marker species for Semen Aesculi as prescribed by the official Chinese

*****Corresponding authors:** Khaldun Mohammad Al Azzam, Email: azzamkha@yahoo.com,
Zead Helmi Mahmoud Abudayeh, Email: zead09@meta.ua, These two authors contributed equally to this work.

Pharmacopoeia of 2005 edition.[8] The structures of the four compounds are illustrated in Figure 1.

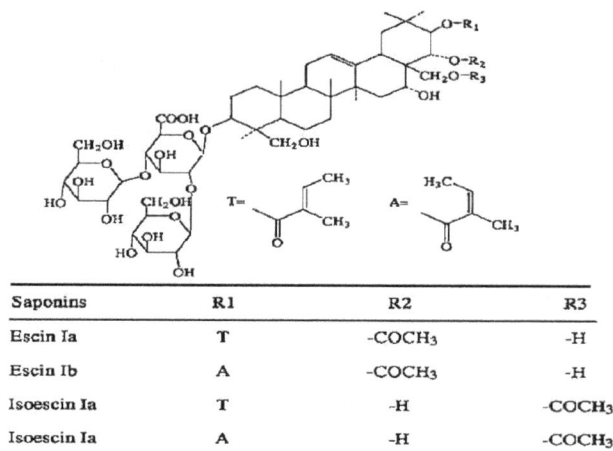

Saponins	R1	R2	R3
Escin Ia	T	-COCH₃	-H
Escin Ib	A	-COCH₃	-H
Isoescin Ia	T	-H	-COCH₃
Isoescin Ia	A	-H	-COCH₃

Figure 1. Chemical structures of four escins: escin Ia, escin Ib, isoescin Ia and isoescin Ib.

Several analytical methods for the analysis of *Aesculus hippocastanum* L., have been reported whether for the determination of the phenolic compounds, organic acids, and sugars in the dry extracts from the leaves using high performance liquid chromatography (HPLC) coupled with UV detector at 190 nm,[9] or at 340 nm for the analysis of esculin and fraxin in bark,[10] or at 210 nm for the analysis of β-escin extract.[11] Ultra performance liquid chromatography (UPLC) coupled with UV detector at 365 nm for coumarins analysis in *Aesculus hippocastanum* L. flowers has also been reported.[12] Ultraviolet (UV) method at 265 nm for the estimation of *Aesculus hippocastanum* L. extract has also been developed.[13] Capillary electrophoresis (CE) coupled with UV detector at 226 nm in dry, hydroalcoholic and hydroglycolic extracts of *Aesculus hippocastanum* L. have been reported.[14] Additionally, liquid chromatography coupled with mass spectrometry (LC-MSQT) for the determination of the content of phenolic compounds in leaf tissues of white and red *Aesculus hippocastanum* L. with leaf miner larvae before and after cameraria ohridella attack has been conducted.[15] Recently, the application of ultrasound sonication has showed up promising results in plant extraction area. Moreover, ultrasound-assisted extraction, as an innovative technology, could enhance mass and heat transfer by disrupting the matrix cell walls mechanically, through creation shear forces, to promote the release of bioactive components from natural products.[16,17] It has been reported that a variety of nutritional materials such as saponins, phenolics, polysaccharides, essential oils, and carotenoids have been extracted successively with the aid of ultrasound methods.[18,19] Once compared to conventional solvent extraction, ultrasound sonication is considered a useful, inexpensive method in addition it can increase extraction yield and extraction efficiency, thus a noticeable reduction in solvent consumption

resulting in saving extraction time and energy input with high reproducibility.[17] Additionally, the advantages of ultrasound sonication, compared with supercritical fluid (CO₂) extraction, are that ultrasound sonication can accelerate mass transfer by mechanical effects and simplify manipulation with cheaper equipment.[20]
In the present paper, HPLC method has been developed for the quantitative determination of four major saponins: escin Ia, escin Ib, isoescin Ia and isoescin Ib in the skin and the endosperm of seeds of *Aesculus hippocastanum* L. extract. TLC has also been conducted herein for the identification of individual escins.

Materials and Methods
Chemicals and reagents
Standards of escin Ia, escin Ib, isoescin Ia and isoescin Ib were obtained from National Institute for the Control of Pharmaceutical and Biological Products of China. HPLC-grade methanol (≥99.96%), acetonitrile (≥99.96%), ethyl acetate, and isopropanol were purchased from Merck (Merck, Darmstadt, Germany). Ortho-phosphoric acid (85%) was purchased from Sigma-Aldrich (St Louis, MO, USA). Phosphotungstic acid ($H_3PW_{12}O_{40}$, HPW) was purchased from Sinopham Chemical Reagent Co., Ltd. Ultrapure water (resistivity, 18.2 $M\Omega cm^{-1}$) was produced by a Milli-Q system (Millipore, USA) and was used throughout for the preparation of solutions. Centrifuge (model 2100) was purchased from Kubota (Tokyo, Japan).

Sample preparation
Seeds of *Aesculus hippocastanum* L. growing in Ukraine were collected from healthy trees that were harvested in September, 2012 and 2014. The dried seeds were divided into two parts; skin and endosperm. The two parts were air-dried, ground, sifted through 0.30 mm mesh screen before extraction to obtain a uniform particle size. After collected, the samples were immediately submitted to the ultrasonic extraction step.

Ultrasonic extraction
Ultrasonic extraction was conducted by mixing 2 g of the powdered sample and 150 mL of 70% methanol in a flask. It was then placed in an ultrasonic bath for 4 hours at 80 °C. The extraction was repeated three additional times in order to enhance the extraction yield and the extracts were then combined. The combined extracts was centrifuged (2580 rcf) for 10 min. The obtained supernatant was evaporated to dryness using a rotary evaporator at 50 °C. Finally, the residue was dissolved in 50 mL of 70% methanol and then filtered through a 0.2 μm nylon membrane filter prior HPLC analysis.

Standard solutions preparation
Standard stock solutions containing 1 mg mL^{-1} were prepared by dissolving approximately 10 mg of each pure compound in 10 mL methanol. The calculations were carried out using the following equation:

$$x = \frac{Cx \times Vs \times 1000}{k \times M} \left[\frac{g}{kg}\right]$$

C_x – concentration of escin in the test sample
V_s – volume of extract
M – mass of prepared sample
k - coefficient of concentration of the extract
x – content of escin (g) per 1 kg of plant material

HPLC conditions

HPLC analysis was carried out using Agilent instrument (Agilent1200, USA) equipped with a quaternary solvent delivery system, autosampler, column oven and diode array UV/Vis detector. Zorbax SB-ODS-150 mm×2.1 mm, 3 µm column, (Agilent Technologies, USA) was used isocratically with a binary mixture of acetonitrile and 0.10% orthophosphoric acid solution (39:61 v/v) at a flow rate of 0.5 mL min^{-1}. Detection was achieved at 210 and 230 nm. The injection volume was 10 µL, and separation was carried out isothermally at 30 ˚C in a heated chamber. Identification was conducted by comparing the retention times of the components of the sample and standards of escins. The quantitative determination was conducted by external calibration method.

Identification by TLC

Standards of escins (100 µg mL^{-1} each) and the extract obtained were spotted on RP-18 Silica coated TLC plate (Merck, 20 × 20 cm) with a 10 mm space between each spot. The spots were then air dried before solvent development. The plate was developed in a mixture of ethyl acetate, isopropanol, and water at a ratio of (40:40:30 v/v) for approximately 60 min in a developing chamber. After the plate was air dried, a 25% alcoholic solution of phosphotungstic acid reagent was used to develop escin spots. The identification of escins was confirmed based on comparison with the R_f values with the escin standards and the quantitative concentrations were obtained from the HPLC analysis.

Results and Discussion

The HPLC chromatographic conditions were developed and optimized using saponin standards and real *Aesculus hippocastanum* L. sample to get the best separation in a reasonable separation time. Reversed phase HPLC was applied according to the previous work reported by Chen *et al.*, 2007 by varying the ratios of water and acetonitrile in the mobile phase which provided a better improvement in separation and significant enhancement in peak shape.[13]
Figure 2 (A and B) shows the chromatograms of the *Aesculus hippocastanum* L. samples (endosperm & skin) harvested in 2014 under the same HPLC conditions. All the saponin peaks are well resolved from each other.

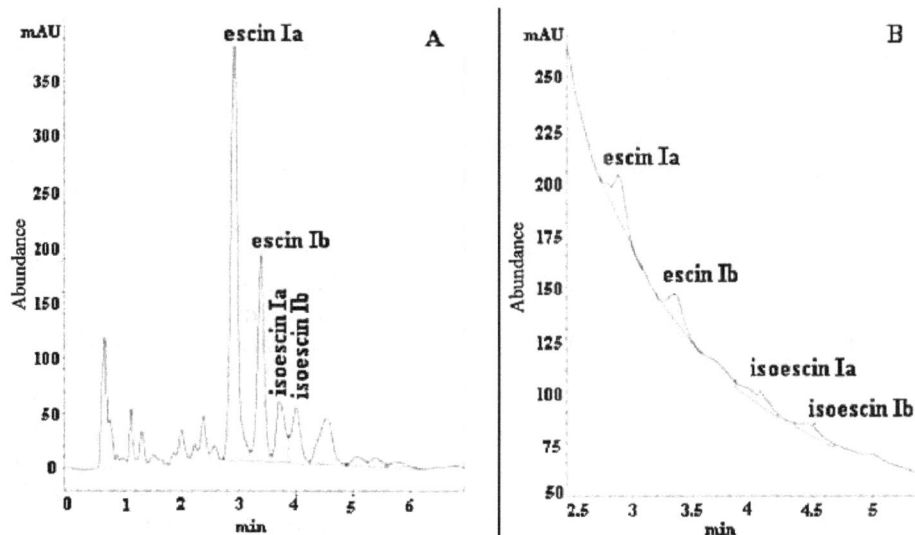

Figure 2. HPLC chromatograms of extracts of *Aesculus hippocastanum* L. endosperm (A); extracts of *Aesculus hippocastanum* L. skin, both harvested in 2014 (B). Please refer to text for HPLC conditions.

The presence of escins in the endosperm and the skin of *Aesculus hippocastanum* L. have been confirmed by TLC method. Spots were evaluated in comparison with the escin standards (the spot of purple color with R_f = 0.71). However, the color and the sizes of escins of the endosperm spots had much more intensity than spots of escins from the skin. This may indicate a greater accumulation of saponins in the seeds endosperm of *Aesculus hippocastanum* L.
The qualitative determination using TLC method showed the presence of escin Ia, escin Ib, isoescin Ia and isoescin Ib. The contents of escins in the skin and in the endosperm of *Aesculus hippocastanum* L. samples for the years 2012 and 2014 were compared. We can say that

Aesculus hippocastanum L. seed's skin has considerably less escins content (0.32 ± 0.012 g kg^{-1} and 0.19 ± 0.009 g kg^{-1}) than the seed's endosperm (52.05 ± 0.67 g kg^{-1} and 34.9 ± 0.51 g kg^{-1}), for the years of 2012 and 2014, respectively.

Also, it has been noticed that the content of escins in the skin and in the endosperm of seeds that were gathered in 2012 exceeds the content of escins in the skin and the endosperm of those stored till 2014.

Quantification of saponins content
The newly developed HPLC method has been applied for the determination the four saponins in different *Aesculus hippocastanum* L. extract samples (each sample was extracted twice and analysed thrice, n = 3). It is clear that among the four saponins, escin Ia is the most abundant saponin in *Aesculus hippocastanum* L. samples. Additionally, it is found that the contents of the four major saponins in the *Aesculus hippocastanum* L. samples are different. It is may be attributed to various factors such as geographical source, cultivation, harvest, storage and processing of the herb.

Conclusion
The presence of escins in the endosperm and skin of all samples of *Aesculus hippocastanum* L. have been confirmed by TLC method. The quantitative determination of four major saponins (escin Ia, escin Ib, isoescin Ia and isoescin Ib) has been conducted using HPLC method in the skin and endosperm of *Aesculus hippocastanum* L. samples for the years 2012 and 2014. The main site of localization of escins in *Aesculus hippocastanum* L. seeds is in its endosperm. Its content is decreased by more than 30% in endosperm and more than 40% in skin during storage for two years. Finally, the applicability of TLC means that the procedure is effectively portable and could be undertaken on site (e.g. in a motor vehicle situated near a plantation) for particularly rapid results.

Acknowledgments
This work is supported financially by a National Medical University (O.O.Bogomolets, Ukraine).

Conflict of Interest
The authors report no conflicts of interest.

References
1. Maria BMCF, Fabíola C, Juliana FS, Matheus FFP, Kátia CS, Lucymara FAL, et al. Evaluation of genotoxic and antioxidant activity of an *Aesculus hippocastanum* L. (Sapindaceae) phytotherapeutic agent. *Biomed Prev Nutr* 2013;3(3):261-6. doi: 10.1016/j.bionut.2012.10.014
2. Calixto JB. Twenty-five years of research on medicinal plants in latin america: A personal view. *J Ethnopharmacol* 2005;100(1-2):131-4. doi: 10.1016/j.jep.2005.06.004
3. Rietjens IM, Boersma MG, van der Woude H, Jeurissen SM, Schutte ME, Alink GM. Flavonoids and alkenylbenzenes: Mechanisms of mutagenic action and carcinogenic risk. *Mutat Res* 2005;574(1-2):124-38. doi: 10.1016/j.mrfmmm.2005.01.028
4. Bunkova R, Marova I, Nemec M. Antimutagenic properties of green tea. *Plant Foods Hum Nutr* 2005;60(1):25-9.
5. Leszek K, Andrzej MJ, Tomasz L, Paweł B, Małgorzata B, Maria R. Fine root parameters and mycorrhizal colonization of horse chestnut trees (*Aesculus hippocastanum* L.) in urban and rural environments. *Landscape Urban Plan* 2014;127:154-63. doi: 10.1016/j.landurbplan.2014.04.014
6. Dudek-Makuch M, Matlawska I. Flavonoids from the flowers of aesculus hippocastanum. *Acta Pol Pharm* 2011;68(3):403-8.
7. Yoshikawa M, Harada E, Murakami T, Matsuda H, Wariishi N, Yamahara J, et al. Escins-ia, ib, iia, iib, and iiia, bioactive triterpene oligoglycosides from the seeds of aesculus hippocastanum l.: Their inhibitory effects on ethanol absorption and hypoglycemic activity on glucose tolerance test. *Chem Pharm Bull (Tokyo)* 1994;42(6):1357-9.
8. Chinese Pharmacopoeia Commission. The Pharmacopoeia of the People's Republic of China. Beijing: Chemical Industry Press; 2005.
9. Natalya AP, Artem AM, Tamara DD. Study of biologically active substances of dry extract from the jeaves of ordinary horse chestnut with high-performance liquid chromatography. *Global J Pharmacol* 2013;7(3):321-4. doi: 10.5829/idosi.gjp.2013.7.3.1109
10. Gordana S, Blaženka J, Dragomir B. HPLC analysis of esculin and fraxin in horse-chestnut bark (*Aesculus hippocastanum* L.). *Croat Chem Acta* 1999;72(4):827-34.
11. Priscila A. De A, Michele CA, Hudson CP, Lidiane SD, Magda NL, Nádia RBR, et al. New HPLC method for quality control of β-escin in *aesculus hippocastanum* L. hydroalcoholic extract. *Lat Am J Pharm* 2013;32(7):1082-7.
12. Dudek-Makuch M, Matlawska I. Coumarins in horse chestnut flowers: Isolation and quantification by uplc method. *Acta Pol Pharm* 2013;70(3):517-22.
13. Biradar S, Dhumansure R, Patil M, Biradar K, Rao KS. Development and method validation of *Aesculus hippocastanum* extract. *Int Res J Pharm* 2012;3(7):324-7.
14. Dutra LS, Leite MN, Brandao MA, de Almeida PA, Vaz FA, de Oliveira MA. A rapid method for total beta-escin analysis in dry, hydroalcoholic and hydroglycolic extracts of aesculus hippocastanum l. By capillary zone electrophoresis. *Phytochem Anal* 2013;24(6):513-9. doi: 10.1002/pca.2425
15. Oszmianski J, Kalisz S, Aneta W. The content of phenolic compounds in leaf tissues of white (aesculus

hippocastanum l.) and red horse chestnut (aesculus carea h.) colonized by the horse chestnut leaf miner (cameraria ohridella deschka & dimic). *Molecules* 2014;19(9):14625-36.   doi: 10.3390/molecules190914625

16. Xu Y, Pan S. Effects of various factors of ultrasonic treatment on the extraction yield of all-trans-lycopene from red grapefruit (citrus paradise macf.). *Ultrason Sonochem*   2013;20(4):1026-32.   doi: 10.1016/j.ultsonch.2013.01.006

17. Xinsheng F, Jianhua W, Yingzi W, Xueke L, Hongying Z, Lixiang Z. Optimization of ultrasonic-assisted extraction of wedelolactone and antioxidant polyphenols from Eclipta prostrate L using response surface methodology. *Sep Purif Technol* 2014; 138(10):55-64. doi: 10.1016/j.seppur.2014.10.007

18. Jerman T, Trebše P, Vodopivec BM. Ultrasound-assisted solid liquid extraction (USLE) of olive fruit (Olea europaea) phenolic compounds. *Food Chem* 2010;123(1):175-82.   doi: 10.1016/j.foodchem.2010.04.006

19. Sun Y, Liu D, Chen J, Ye X, Yu D. Effects of different factors of ultrasound treatment on the extraction yield of the all-trans-beta-carotene from citrus peels. *Ultrason Sonochem* 2011;18(1):243-9. doi: 10.1016/j.ultsonch.2010.05.014

20. Xu Y, Pan S. Effects of various factors of ultrasonic treatment on the extraction yield of all-trans-lycopene from red grapefruit (citrus paradise macf.). *Ultrason Sonochem*   2013;20(4):1026-32.   doi: 10.1016/j.ultsonch.2013.01.006

17

Combined Activity of Colloid Nanosilver and *Zataria Multiflora Boiss* Essential Oil-Mechanism of Action and Biofilm Removal Activity

Maryam Shirdel[1], Hossein Tajik[1,2], Mehran Moradi[1]*

[1] *Department of Food Hygiene and Quality Control, Faculty of Veterinary Medicine, Urmia University, 1177, Urmia, West Azarbaijan, Iran.*

[2] *Department of Medicinal and Industrial Plant, Institute of Biotechnology, Urmia University, 1177 Urmia, Iran.*

Article info

Keywords:
· Antimicrobial
· Sanitizing
· Biofilm
· Essential oil
· Silver nanoparticle
· Combination

Abstract

Purpose: The aim of this study was to investigate antimicrobial and biofilm removal potential of *Zataria multiflora* essential oil (ZEO) and silver nanoparticle (SNP) alone and in combination on *Staphylococcus aureus* and *Salmonella* Typhimurium and evaluate the mechanism of action.

Methods: The minimum inhibitory concentration (MIC), and optimal inhibitory combination (OIC) of ZEO and SNP were determined according to fractional inhibitory concentration (FIC) method. Biofilm removal potential and leakage pattern of 260-nm absorbing material from the bacterial cell during exposure to the compounds were also investigated.

Results: MICs of SNP for both bacteria were the same as 25 µg/ mL. The MICs and MBCs values of ZEO were 2500 and 1250 µg/mL, respectively. The most effective OIC value for SNP and ZEO against *Salm.* Typhimurium and *Staph. aureus* were 12.5, 625 and 0.78, 1250 µg/ mL, respectively. ZEO and SNP at MIC and OIC concentrations represented a strong removal ability (>70%) on biofilm. Moreover, ZEO at MIC and OIC concentrations did a 6-log reduction of primary inoculated bacteria during 15 min contact time. The effect of ZEO on the loss of 260-nm material from the cell was faster than SNP during 15 and 60 min.

Conclusion: Combination of ZEO and SNP had significant sanitizing activity on examined bacteria which may be suitable for disinfecting the surfaces.

Introduction

Nanotechnology, the science of study and use of structures at nanoscale, is a promising tool for producing novel materials with biomedical applications. Silver nanoparticles (SNPs) has been extensively investigated in various scientific disciplines. Silver in the form of silver nitrate and silver sulfadiazine has been widely used to cure bacterial infections associated with burns. SNPs are considered as a potent antimicrobial, antifungal, antiviral and antiprotozoal compound and it is also reported to have anti-inflammatory activities.[1] Synthesis and use of SNPs as a new generation of antimicrobial agents would be a fascinating and economical tool to solve drug resistance. Microorganisms display different responses to nanoparticles which is related to differences in the bacterial structure and the composition of the cell wall.[1,2] Essential oils (EOs), as a plant secondary metabolites, are volatile aromatic compounds extracted from different parts of plants. For centuries, EOs have been used in medicine, perfumery, cosmetics and food. They are primarily used in medicine, but in the nineteenth-century, EOs have found their importance to impart aroma and taste ingredients.[3] Lamiaceae is a family of plant with more than 230 genera, which distributed nearly worldwide. It contains many well- known species with fairly similar properties in botanical characteristics and applications, including *Thymus vulgaris*, *Thymus caramanicus*, *Zataria multiflora*, *Ziziphora clinopodioides* and *Ziziphora tenuior*.[3-5] *Zataria multiflora* Boiss is an important medicinal plant, distributed in Iran, Afghanistan, and Pakistan. The main antimicrobial compounds of *Zataria multiflora* Boiss essential oil (ZEO) are thymol, carvacrol, and p-cymene. The plant also contains tannins, flavonoids, saponins and some bitter substances.[6] Among the phenolic compounds, thymol is the most characteristic chemical substance of ZEO which founds in leaves, flowers, and roots at various amounts.[6,7] ZEO displays inhibitory activity on both gram-negative and gram-positive bacteria.[8] The practical advantage of antimicrobial combinations has been comprehended for over 50 years. Combinations of two antimicrobial agents with a different mechanism of action, may enhance antimicrobial activity especially where resistance to a single agent develops by bacteria. Also, due to synergy or additive interaction, the combination of drugs allows utilizing lower antimicrobial concentration, reducing the harmful side effects and increasing treatment efficacy.[9] Tackling

*Corresponding author:** Mehran Moradi, Email: m.moradi@urmia.ac.ir

public health issues occur by the growing number of multidrug-resistant bacteria, proposes new antimicrobial formulation based on the combination of older antimicrobials with a rich source of new agents, such as natural products.[10] Simultaneous use of EOs and other antimicrobial compounds with great disinfectant properties has a high priority since using EOs in high concentrations make some unpleasant organoleptic changes in food and also on food contact surface when used as a sanitizing compound. Owing to the possible synergistic properties, combined use of EO with SNPs as a sanitizing mixture for food plant sanitation has been proposed.[11] The combined application of nanoparticles with EO has been reported.[2,12] To understand the combined antimicrobial and biofilm removal properties of SNP and ZEO, their effects on two important bacterial pathogens, *Staph aureus* and *Salm.* Typhimurium was investigated as a guideline for a possible application of formulated solution in sanitation schedule.

Materials and Methods
Silver nanoparticles solution (4000 µg/ mL with the particle size of 35 nm) was purchased from Pars Nano Nasb Co (Tehran, Iran) and sterilized by filtration through 0.22 µm filters before use. Peptone water, phosphate buffered saline (PBS), Luria-Bertani (LB) broth and agar, Agar-agar, and resazurin sodium were obtained from Sigma Chemical Co (St. Louis, MO., USA). All other chemicals were purchased from Merck (Darmstadt, Germany). The plant, *Zataria multiflora* Boiss, was purchased from local groceries. *Staph. aureus* ATCC 25923 and *Salm.* Typhimurium ATCC 14028 were obtained from the Department of Food Hygiene and Quality Control, Urmia University, Urmia, Iran.

Preparation of bacterial suspension
Staph. aureus and *Salm.* Typhimurium were grown at 37 ± 1 °C for 18 h by transferring 10 microliters of frozen stocks (at -20 °C) into 10 mL of LB broth. Bacterial suspensions were adjusted to ~8 $\log_{10}$ CFU mL^{-1} using visible-ultraviolet spectrophotometer (Amersham Pharmacia Biotech Inc., Buckinghamshire, UK) at 600 nm (optical density: ~0.1) and confirmed by plating and counting on LB agar after 24 h incubation at 37 ± 1 °C.

Essential oil extraction and quantification
The EO of *Zataria multiflora* Boiss (100 g) was extracted from dried aerial parts of plant using a Clevenger apparatus based on hydrodistillation procedure for 3 hours. The collected ZEO was dried over anhydrous Na_2SO_4, then filtrated and stored at 4 °C. The chemical composition of ZEOs was analyzed using a gas chromatograph (GC), as explained previously.[6]

Determination of Minimum inhibitory concentration (MIC) and minimum bactericidal concentrations (MBC)
The MICs and MBC of ZEO and SNP against both bacteria were determined in LB using broth microdilution assay in 96-wells polystyrene flat-bottomed microtitre plates based on CLSI guidelines.[13] Two-fold serial dilutions of ZEO were prepared in 0.1% peptone water containing 0.15% agar (to make a stable emulsion of EO in peptone water), whereas dilutions of SNP were made in 0.1% peptone water. The wells of a microplates with U-bottom were poured by 160 µL of LB and 20 µL of the bacterial suspension with $OD_{600} = 0.1$ to reach a suspension with 10^6 CFU/ mL in each well. Then, 20 µL either ZEO or SNP concentrations were added into the desired wells to achieve final concentrations of 312 to 5000 µg/ mL for ZEO and 62.5 to 2000 µg/mL for SNP. For every experiment, three controls, including LB alone, LB with bacteria and LB containing treatment agents without bacteria were used. The plate was mixed on a plate shaker at 250 rpm for 20 s and incubated at 37 ± 1 °C for 24 h. MICs were determined visually and by using 0.01% (w/v) resazurin sodium salt solution as explained previously. To determine MBCs, 10 µL from each well was inoculated into LB agar at 37 ± 1 °C for 24 h. The MBC was determined as the lowest concentration of antimicrobial agents that produces 99.99% inhibition in the initial population of microorganism. MBC: MIC ratio, which describes the relationship between the minimum *in vitro* bactericidal concentration and the MIC of antimicrobial agents, were also investigated.

Antimicrobial combination and interaction
Broth checkerboard micro-assay was carried out to evaluate the antagonistic, indifferent, additive and synergistic interactions of ZEO and SNP using the fractional inhibitory concentration (FIC) index method.[14] Eight different concentrations, 5 concentrations lower than MIC, two concentrations higher than MIC and one concentration as same as MIC of ZEO and SNP were used to design an 8 × 8 checkerboards of combinations. The microplates were prepared by dispensing 160 µL of LB and 20 µL of the logarithmic suspension of bacteria and 10 µL of different concentration of both antimicrobial agents into each well. Then, plates were kept in a plate shaker at 250 rpm for 20 s and incubated at 37 ± 1 °C for 24 h. MICs were determined visually and by resazurin reduction. MICs of the individual antimicrobials and all of the combinations were used to calculate Fractional inhibitory concentrations (FICs) of ZEO and SNP and FIC index using the following formula:

$$FIC \ of \ antibacterial \ \frac{MIC \ of \ antibacterial \ in \ combination}{MIC \ of \ antibacterial \ alone}$$

$$FIC \ index \ (FICI) = FIC_{ZEO} + FIC_{SNP}$$

If the FICI is < 0.5, the interaction is synergistic, if the FICI= 0.5-1, the interaction is additive, if the FICI= 1-4, the interaction is indifferent, and an FICI >4 is considered antagonistic. Optimal inhibitory combinations (OIC) is defined as the combinations producing an inhibitory effect by using the lowest concentration of one antimicrobial in combination with the other.[15]

Determination of the release of 260-nm absorbing material

260-nm absorbing material released into the supernatant was estimated according to the method described previously,[16] with some modifications. The bacterial suspension was prepared as described above. The procedure performed in 2 mL of harvested and washed cells (OD_{600nm} = 0.45) to which SNP and ZEO were added at final concentrations equivalent to their MICs and OIC and incubated in a shaker incubator (250 rpm at 37 °C). Two samples were taken at 15 and 60 min time points and centrifuged at 4000 g for 15 min and the absorbance was determined at 260 nm using PBS as blank. Controls containing bacterial supernatant without treatment agents and antibacterial compounds without bacteria were also prepared and analyzed.

Biofilm removal

Biofilm removal potential of both agents alone and in combination was assessed using 24-well flat-bottomed polystyrene microtiter plates according to the method explained previously with some modifications.[17] An aliquot of 200 µL of bacterial suspension with OD_{600} = 0.1 was dispensed into each well which was filled previously with 1800 µL of LB broth, using four repetitions per treatment to reach a suspension with 10^7 CFU/ mL per well. After incubation for 24 h at 37 ±1 °C, the planktonic cells in wells were then removed and the plates were washed three times with PBS and air-dried for 20 min at 23 ±2 °C. Then, 2000 µL of MIC, 2MIC and 4MIC concentrations of ZEO and SNP and their combinations (1/4 OIC, 1/2OIC, and OIC concentrations) were gently poured into the wells and incubated for 15 min at ambient temperature. The solutions were then removed and plates were washed three times with PBS and air-dried for 20 min at 23 ±2 °C. Following staining with 2 mL of 1% crystal violet (CV) (w/v) for 30 min, the contents of the wells were decanted and washed twice with tap water to remove the color excess and then allowed to air-dry for 30 min. The biomass of biofilms was quantified by solubilizing CV with 2 mL of acetic acid 33% and subsequent measuring optical absorbance (OD) at 540 nm. Wells containing LB broth and LB with bacteria without antibacterial were considered as negative and positive controls, respectively. Biofilm removal percentage was calculated as follow:

$$Reduction\ percentage = \frac{(C - B) - (T - B)}{(C - B)} \times 100$$

where C is OD_{540nm} of control wells, B is OD_{540nm} of negative controls and T is OD_{540nm} of treated wells.

Combined sanitizing activity

Sanitizing effects of ZEO and SNP combination were investigated by determining the growth of the microorganism in LB broth supplemented with different concentration of antimicrobials (1/4OIC, 1/2OIC, and OIC) to obtain optimal concentration for both compounds according to the method explained before with some modifications.[18] Bacterial cultures (1×10^7 CFU/ mL) (0.5 mL) were added to tubes containing 4.5 mL of antimicrobial agents in combination and then, tubes were incubated at 23± 2 °C for 15 min and bacterial growth was monitored by sampling (1mL) and counting the viable cells. After sampling, 1 mL aliquot were dispersed in a 9 mL neutralizing solution containing an equal volume of sodium thiosulphate 5% w/v and Tween-20 and remained for 10 min, to neutralize the subsequent activity of agents and then serial dilutions were prepared.

Statistical analysis

Each experiment was replicated in triplicate and carried out on three separate times and data were expressed as means ± S.E. Data were analyzed by analysis of variance (ANOVA, $P\leq0.05$) using GraphPad Prism version 5.00 for Windows, GraphPad Software, San Diego California USA (www.graphpad.com).

Results

ZEO chemical analysis

As shown in Table 1, 26 different components were identified in ZEO, representing 97.23%, of total EO. General chemical profile of ZEO was characterized by an abundance concentration of thymol (44%). In addition to thymol, carvacrol (14.04%) and p-cymene (11.15%), as main constituents, and traces of linalool, Υ-terpinene, and α-Pinene were also found in ZEO.

Antibacterial properties of ZEO and SNP

The inhibitory effects of ZEO and SNP alone and in combination against *Staph. aureus* and *Salm.* Typhimurium were investigated using microtiter plate assay. For *Staph. aureus*, the MIC values of ZEO and SNP were 1250 and 25 µg/mL and for *Salm.* Typhimurium the values were 2500 and 25 µg/mL, respectively. In all cases, MBC values were similar to MICs. The ZEO was found to be more effective on gram-positive than gram-negative bacteria whereas SNP displayed similar antibacterial activity on both bacteria. The MICs for SNP - ZEO combination were 0.78 and 12.5 µg/ mL against *Staph. aureus* and *Salm.* Typhimurium, respectively. ZEO-SNP combination inhibited *S. aureus* and *Salm.* Typhimurium at 625 µg/ mL. Based on the FICI scale (Table 2), the combination displayed a synergistic action on *Staph. aureus* (FICI=0.81) and *Salm.* Typhimurium (FICI= 0.75).

Loss of 260 nm absorbing material

Exposure of *Staph. aureus* and *Salm.* Typhimurium to ZEO at MIC concentrations over 15 min resulted in a significant increase in loss of 260 nm absorbing material from the bacterial cell compared with the control ($P<0.05$), indicating a stronger disruption of the cell membrane by ZEO (Figure 1, 2). Results also showed that the loss began before 15 min and continued up to 60 min. In general, loss of cytoplasmic materials by ZEO from both bacteria was faster than SNP. The leakage pattern of 260-nm absorbing material was directly linked to the sanitizing activity of both antimicrobial compounds. As shown in Figures 1 and 2, no significant release of 260 nm absorbing material with SNP- treated at MIC concentration over 15 min for both bacteria was found. Higher exposure time (60 min) significantly increased the cell leakage of *Salm*. Typhimurium, but not in case of *Staph. aureus*. Longer exposures (60 min) with OIC concentration of ZEO and SNP (Figures 1 and 2), caused 3 and 4-fold more gross membrane damage, in *Staph. aureus* and *Salm*. Typhimurium culture compared to the control sample, respectively.

Table 1. Chemical composition of ZEO.

Compounds	KI[a]	Area (%)	Compounds	KI	Area (%)
α-Thujene	931	0.15	linalool	1106	6.26
α-Pinene	639	3.66	Borneol	1163	0.19
Camphene	953	0.17	Terpinen-4-ol	1175	4.63
β-Pinene	980	1.55	Thymol methyl ether	1233	0.17
β-Mycrene	991	1.35	Bornyl acetate	1284	0.17
α-Phellandrene	1002	0.15	Thymol	1301	44
δ-3-Carene	1009	1	Carvacrol	1318	14.4
α-Terpinene	1016	1.74	Acetylthymol	1284	0.3
Cis-para-menth-2-en-1-o	1123	0.37	δ-Elemene	1340	0.24
p-Cymene	1028	11.15	Eugenol	1360	0.82
1,8-Cineole	1032	0.86	*Trans*-Caryophyllene	1423	2.78
Y-Terpinene	1060	0.08	Caryophyllene oxide	1583	0.93
α-Terpinolene	1087	0.08			
Total					**97.23%**

[a]Kovats indices calculated against *n*-alkanes on HP-5 column.

Table 2. Survival population (log CFU/ mL) of *Staph. aureus* and *Salm*. Typhimurium treated with ZEO and SNP alone and in combination during 15 min contact time at room temperature.

Microorganism*	Alone at MIC concentration		In combination		
	ZEO	SNP	OIC	1/2OIC	1/4OIC
Staph. aureus	0	$3.11 \times 10^5 \pm 0.08^a$	0	$3.11 \times 10^5 \pm 0.67^a$	$4.74 \times 10^5 \pm 0.41^a$
Salm. Typhimurium	0	$4.69 \times 10^5 \pm 0.19^b$	0	$3.90 \times 10^5 \pm 0.21^b$	$5.30 \times 10^5 \pm 0.33^b$

*Initial bacterial counts: 10^6 CFU mL^{-1}. Different letters for each column of indicate a statistically significant difference ($P < 0.05$).

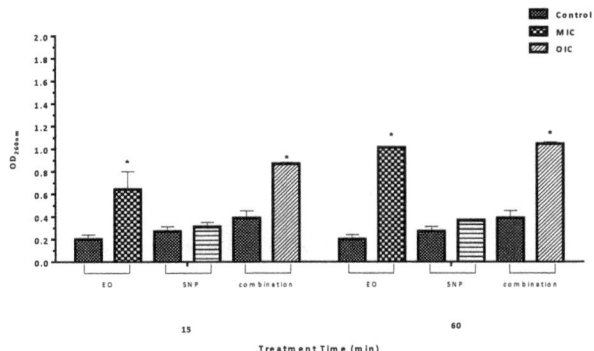

Figure 1. 260-nm absorbing material released from *Staph. aureus* cells after treatment with MIC concentration of silver nanoparticle (SNP), *Zataria multiflora* essential oil (EO) and their combination. Asterisks indicate significantly different values ($P<0.05$) when comparing optical density (OD) of control and each treatment at the same exposure time.

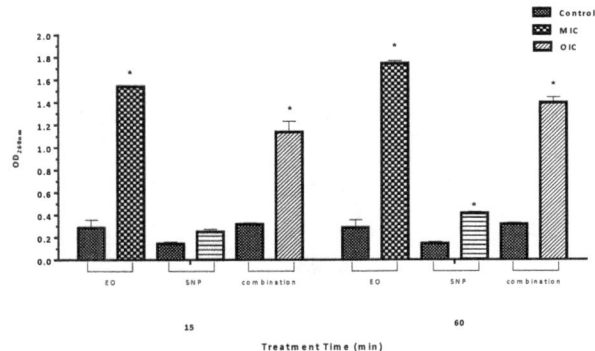

Figure 2. 260-nm absorbing material released from *Salm*. Typhimurium cells after treatment with MIC concentration of silver nanoparticle (SNP), *Zataria multiflora* essential oil (EO) and their combination. Asterisks indicate significantly different values ($P<0.05$) when comparing optical density (OD) of control and each treatment at the same exposure time.

Biofilm removal

As compared with *Salm.* Typhimurium (Figure 3b), higher removal of *Staph. aureus* biofilms were achieved at 15 min exposure time for SNP-ZEO (Figure 3a). Results demonstrated that biofilm of *Staph. aureus* is more sensitive to SNP - ZEO than *Salm.* Typhimurium. SNP at MIC, 2MIC, and 4MIC concentrations resulted in 93, 87 and 71.33% and 82, 79 and 58% removal of *Staph. aureus* and *Salm.* Typhimurium cells, respectively. For *Staph. aureus* and *Salm.* Typhimurium, 90.6%, and 89% bacteria were eliminated at a concentration of MIC for ZEO. Concerning the hydrophobicity property of ZEO, it can be observed in Figure 3, a reduction in the biofilm removal with increasing ZEO concentration supporting the use of surfactants could help in the disruption of such shortcoming.

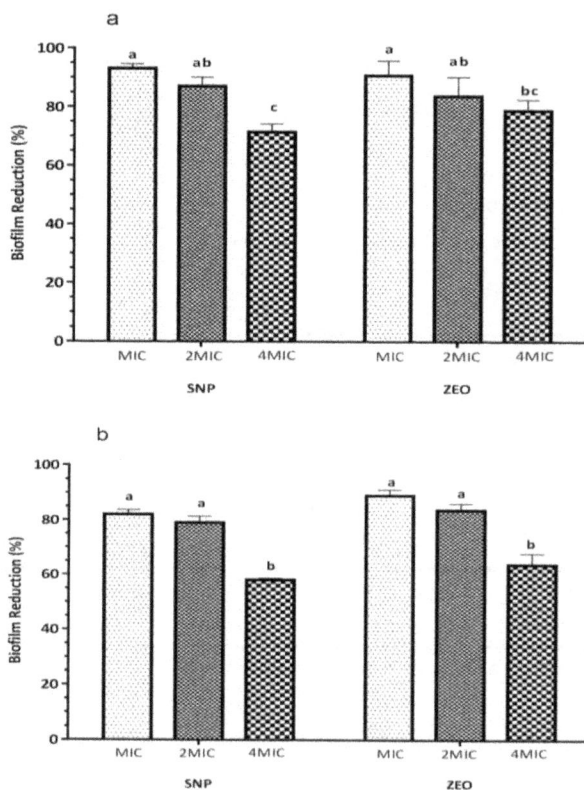

Figure 3. The effect of silver nanoparticle (SNP) and *Zataria multiflora* essential oil (ZEO) on removal one-day old biofilm of *Staph. aureus* (**a**) and *Salm.* Typhimurium (**b**) developed on polystyrene surface with 15 min contact time. Different letters for each concentration of antimicrobial indicate a statistically significant difference ($P < 0.05$).

Synergistic sanitizing activity

The purpose of this experiment was to achieve a best effective concentration of SNP and ZEO as a sanitizing solution. To assess the disinfectants efficiencies, MIC and OIC concentrations were determined. The reductions in the *Staph. aureus* and *Salm.* Typhimurium counts after 15 min exposure to MIC and various OIC concentrations were shown in Table 2. A reduction of 100% was achieved for both bacteria after 15 min exposure to ZEO.

A similar reduction was also found for OIC concentration. Whereas, less than 0.4 $\log_{10}$ CFU/ mL reduction was observed for the samples treated with SNP in alone.

As shown by 260 nm absorbing material measurements, SNP displayed an antimicrobial activity after a long time of exposure (at least after 1 h) compared with ZEO. In comparison with *Staph. aureus*, *Salm.* Typhimurium had higher resistance to SNP. Additionally, no significant reduction ($P < 0.05$) was observed in the microbial counts of 1/2OIC and 1/4OIC with SNP treated samples.

Discussion

The components identified in ZEO (Table 1) in this study was similar to previous works. According to Saedi Dezaki et al. (2007),[19] the major components of ZEO were thymol (41.81%), carvacrol (28.85%), and *p*-cymene (5.63-13.16%). In the study of Saei-Dehkordi, et al. (2010),[7] a variation of the major components, thymol (27.5-64.87%), carvacrol (2.7-22.39), *p*-cymene (8.36%) and linalool (0-7.92%) of ZEO were observed, due to the collection of plant material from five main phytogeographic grown towns in Iran. Factors such as growth phase and geographic origin of plant, method of plant drying and processing affect EO content and chemical compositions.[7]

In our study, the antibacterial properties of ZEO was not different to the results reported from other studies, apart from some detected variable bacterial susceptibilities that may cause the differences in the chemical composition of ZEOs and the bacterial strains used by others. The hydrophobic property of most EOs could increase their permeability and accumulation in the bacterial cell membranes.[6,7]

Silver ions and silver-based compounds are widely known as highly toxic to 16 major species of bacteria due to their multiple mechanisms of action. Zarei et al. (2014) reported the MIC values of SNP against *Listeria monocytogenes*, *S.* Typhimurium, *Escherichia coli* O157:H7 and *Vibrio parahaemolyticus* in the range of 3.12- 6.25 μg mL^{-1} according to microdilution method in Tryptic soy broth.[20] The small size and high ratio of surface to volume in SNPs, allow them to more effectively contact with microorganisms and induce their antimicrobial activities.[21] It has been shown that antibacterial efficacy of SNP varies between different prepared SNPs. Given the fact that factors such as the type of bacteria, the media of inoculation, type and the size of nanoparticle and the method of preparation must be considered when comparing the antibacterial activity of different nanoparticles.[1]

The additive or partial synergy effect is a type of interaction in which the combined effect is equal to the sum of the effects of the individual agents. As shown previously,[22] SNP interaction with EO is a bacteria-dependent phenomenon. The synergistic properties of SNP with ZEO on *Staph. epidermidis* and *Staph. aureus* (FICI= 0.5-1) has been demonstrated, but no synergistic effects were found against Methicillin-resistant *Staph.*

aureus and *Ps. aeruginosa* (FICI value of 3 and 1.25, respectively).

The MBC: MIC ratio ≥ 8 is considered as an indicator of bacteriostatic activity.[23] In the current study, MIC/MBC of both SNP and ZEO were 1:1, suggesting a bactericidal effect on *Staph. aureus* and *Salm. Typhimurium*. It was demonstrated that oregano EO reveals a synergistic activity with common antibiotics such as gentamicin against some potential pathogens,[24] additive activity in combination with another antibiotic such as amoxicillin and polymyxin on Extended-Spectrum Beta-Lactamase (ESBL)-producing *E.coli*,[25] and synergistic with other EO obtained from *Thymus vulgare* and *Rosmarinus officinalis*.[26]

Measuring the loss of 260-nm absorbing material from the bacteria is an indicator of cell leakage which could be used to understand the mechanism of action of antimicrobial compounds. The presence of materials with an absorbance at 260 nm in the supernatant of bacterial solution indicates a loss of nucleic acids from the cell. Based on the results of this study (Figures 1 and 2), the higher values determined by the measurements at 260 nm are an indication for the leakage of bacterial contents which subsequently confirms the physical damages of bacterial cell walls by ZEO.[4] However, the reductions in the efficacy of SNP may be best explained by bacterial blocking caused by higher concentrations of SNP, which could reduce the contact surface of nanoparticles with bacteria and its antibacterial efficacy.

SNP can cause agglomeration after adding to the nutritious media such as LB and as shown previously,[2] treatment of *Staph. aureus* with a combination of EO and SNP, induced a reduction in cell density, exopolysaccharide, morphology changes, and cell destruction. However, membrane permeability created by EO might allow the small molecules of SNP to enter the cell.

Researchers are aware of the importance of biofilms in causing diseases and drug resistance, therefore finding a safe and effective method for biofilm removal is of great importance. Natural agents are considered as a safe way to remove biofilms. Although the research on SNP interaction with biofilm is still in its early phases, we currently know that removal of biofilm by SNP could occur in three steps: transportation to the vicinity of the biofilm, attachment, and penetration within the biofilm.[27] It has been shown that eradication of biofilms by SNP is not a concentration-dependent process, rather it occurs in a time-dependent manner.[28] The main compounds of ZEO are thymol, a monoterpene phenolic derivative, and its phenol isomer, carvacrol. Both of them contribute to antimicrobial and antioxidant properties of Lamiaceae family.[4] Additionally, hydrophobic characteristics of these ingredients allow the penetration of ZEO into outer exopolysaccharide and inner layers of biofilms.[29] In our study, by decreasing the OIC concentration from 1/2OIC to 1/4OIC (Figure 4), the biofilm removal properties were significantly decreased ($P<0.05$) from 64 % to 43.33 % for *Staph. aureus* (Figure 4) whereas OIC

concentration, removed 76% of biofilm mass. For *Salm. Typhimurium* (Figure 4) the values were 96.46%, 81.50% and 68 % for OIC, 1/2OIC and 1/4OIC concentrations, respectively. It means that combined use of SNP and ZEO boosted biofilm removal potential of both antibacterial compounds against different pathogens. According to Gurunathan et al. (2014), the combined use of NPs and antibiotic such as ampicillin exhibit antibiofilm activity on Gram-positive and Gram-negative bacteria by 55 and 70%, whereas combining those NPs with vancomycin revealed a 75 and 55% reduction of biofilm of Gram-positive and Gram-negative bacteria.[1] It is worth mentioning that, differences in the method used to evaluate biofilm removal activity and differences in the sensitivity of different bacteria, the age of biofilm and type of surface which biofilm developed could cause different results in the biofilm removal percentage in previous studies.

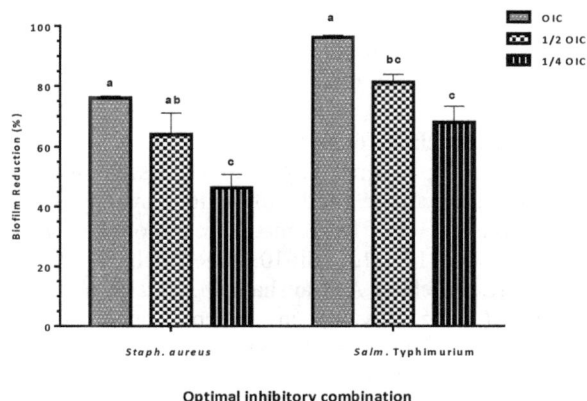

Figure 4. The effect of silver nanoparticle (SNP) and *Zataria multiflora* essential oil (ZEO) combination on removal one-day old biofilm of *Staph. aureus* and *Salm.* Typhimurium developed on polystyrene surface with 15 min contact time. Different letters for each concentration of antimicrobial indicate a statistically significant difference ($P < 0.05$).

Conclusion

The results of our study demonstrated that SNP and ZEO have synergistic antibacterial activities against *Staph. aureus,* and *Salm.* Typhimurium. It was also shown that the antimicrobial and biofilm removal properties of SNP and ZEO were affected by the type of microorganisms and concentrations of both compounds. ZEO displayed a fast antimicrobial activity. Both antimicrobials represented considerable biofilm removal activity on both bacteria. The combination of SNP and ZEO was additive, which means significant antibacterial and antibiofilm activity could achieve by use of agents at concentrations without compromising their antibacterial effects. The best concentrations for SNP- ZEO sanitizing solution were 12.5 µg/ mL for SNP and 625 µg/ mL for ZEO. Our results highlighted the powerful combination activity of SNP and ZEO which accelerated antibacterial activity, alleviated undesirable sensorial property of ZEO and reduced the concentration of both compounds.

Acknowledgments
This study was funded by a grant from Faculty of Veterinary Medicine and Institute of Biotechnology, Urmia University. The authors would like to thank Dr. Mahmoudian for his assistance.

Conflict of Interest
The authors declare no conflict of interest related to this work.

References

1. Gurunathan S, Han JW, Kwon DN, Kim JH. Enhanced antibacterial and anti-biofilm activities of silver nanoparticles against gram-negative and gram-positive bacteria. *Nanoscale Res Lett* 2014;9(1):373. doi: 10.1186/1556-276X-9-373
2. Scandorieiro S, de Camargo LC, Lancheros CA, Yamada-Ogatta SF, Nakamura CV, de Oliveira AG, et al. Synergistic and additive effect of oregano essential oil and biological silver nanoparticles against multidrug-resistant bacterial strains. *Front Microbiol* 2016;7:760. doi: 10.3389/fmicb.2016.00760
3. Hyldgaard M, Mygind T, Meyer RL. Essential oils in food preservation: Mode of action, synergies, and interactions with food matrix components. *Front Microbiol* 2012;3:12. doi: 10.3389/fmicb.2012.00012
4. Sajed H, Sahebkar A, Iranshahi M. Zataria multiflora boiss. (shirazi thyme)--an ancient condiment with modern pharmaceutical uses. *J Ethnopharmacol* 2013;145(3):686-98. doi: 10.1016/j.jep.2012.12.018
5. Shokri H, Sharifzadeh A. Zataria multiflora boiss.: A review study on chemical composition, anti-fungal and anti-mycotoxin activities, and ultrastructural changes. *J HerbMed Pharmacol* 2017;6(1):1-9.
6. Moradi M, Tajik H, Razavi Rohani SM, Mahmoudian A. Antioxidant and antimicrobial effects of zein edible film impregnated with Zataria multiflora Boiss. Essential oil and monolaurin. *LWT - Food Sci Technol* 2016;72:37-43. doi: 10.1016/j.lwt.2016.04.026
7. Saei-Dehkordi SS, Tajik H, Moradi M, Khalighi-Sigaroodi F. Chemical composition of essential oils in zataria multiflora boiss. From different parts of iran and their radical scavenging and antimicrobial activity. *Food Chem Toxicol* 2010;48(6):1562-7. doi: 10.1016/j.fct.2010.03.025
8. Sharififar F, Moshafi MH, Mansouri SH, Khodashenas M, Khoshnoodi M. In vitro evaluation of antibacterial and antioxidant activities of the essential oil and methanol extract of endemic Zataria multiflora Boiss. *Food Control* 2007;18(7):800-5. doi: 10.1016/j.foodcont.2006.04.002
9. Desbois AP, Lang S, Gemmell CG, Coote PJ. Surface disinfection properties of the combination of an antimicrobial peptide, ranalexin, with an endopeptidase, lysostaphin, against methicillin-resistant Staphylococcus aureus (MRSA). *J Appl Microbiol* 2010;108(2):723-30. doi: 10.1111/j.1365-2672.2009.04472.x
10. Bassetti M, Righi E. New antibiotics and antimicrobial combination therapy for the treatment of gram-negative bacterial infections. *Curr Opin Crit Care* 2015;21(5):402-11. doi: 10.1097/mcc.0000000000000235
11. Gutierrez J, Barry-Ryan C, Bourke P. The antimicrobial efficacy of plant essential oil combinations and interactions with food ingredients. *Int J Food Microbiol* 2008;124(1):91-7. doi: 10.1016/j.ijfoodmicro.2008.02.028
12. Taghizadeh M, Solgi M. The application of essential oils and silver nanoparticles for sterilization of bermudagrass explants in in vitro culture. *Int J Hort Sci Technol* 2014;1(2):131-40.
13. Clinical and laboratory standards institute. Performance standards for antimicrobial susceptibility testing; twentieth informational supplement. Document M100-S22. Wayne, Pa, USA: CLSI; 2012.
14. Moody JA. Synergism testing: Broth microdilution checkerboard and broth microdilution methods. In: Isenberg HD, editor. Clinical microbiology procedures handbook. Washington, DC: American Society for Microbiology; 2003. PP. 1-28.
15. Dong X, Chen F, Zhang Y, Liu H, Liu Y, Ma L. In vitro activities of rifampin, colistin, sulbactam and tigecycline tested alone and in combination against extensively drug-resistant acinetobacter baumannii. *J Antibiot (Tokyo)* 2014;67(9):677-80. doi: 10.1038/ja.2014.99
16. Rhayour K, Bouchikhi T, Tantaoui-Elaraki A, Sendide K, Remmal A. The mechanism of bactericidal action of oregano and clove essential oils and of their phenolic major components on escherichia coli and bacillus subtilis. *J Essent Oil Res* 2003;15(5):356-62. doi: 10.1080/10412905.2003.9698611
17. Mahdavi M, Jalali M, Kasra Kermanshahi R. The effect of nisin on biofilm forming foodborne bacteria using microtiter plate method. *Res Pharm Sci* 2007;2(2):113-8.
18. Phongphakdee K, Nitisinprasert S. Combination inhibition activity of nisin and ethanol on the growth inhibition of pathogenic gram negative bacteria and their application as disinfectant solution. *J Food Sci* 2015;80(10):M2241-6. doi: 10.1111/1750-3841.13015
19. Saedi Dezaki E, Mahmoudvand H, Sharififar F, Fallahi S, Monzote L, Ezatkhah F. Chemical composition along with anti-leishmanial and cytotoxic activity of *Zataria multiflora*. *Pharm Biol* 2016;54(5):752-8. doi: 10.3109/13880209.2015.1079223
20. Zarei M, Jamnejad A, Khajehali E. Antibacterial effect of silver nanoparticles against four foodborne pathogens. *Jundishapur J Microbiol* 2014;7(1):e8720. doi: 10.5812/jjm.8720

21. Perez-Diaz M, Alvarado-Gomez E, Magana-Aquino M, Sanchez-Sanchez R, Velasquillo C, Gonzalez C, et al. Anti-biofilm activity of chitosan gels formulated with silver nanoparticles and their cytotoxic effect on human fibroblasts. *Mater Sci Eng C Mater Biol Appl* 2016;60:317-23. doi: 10.1016/j.msec.2015.11.036

22. Sheikholeslami S, Mousavi SE, Ahmadi Ashtiani HR, Hosseini Doust SR, Mahdi Rezayat S. Antibacterial activity of silver nanoparticles and their combination with zataria multiflora essential oil and methanol extract. *Jundishapur J Microbiol* 2016;9(10):e36070. doi: 10.5812/jjm.36070

23. Parhi AK, Zhang Y, Saionz KW, Pradhan P, Kaul M, Trivedi K, et al. Antibacterial activity of quinoxalines, quinazolines, and 1,5-naphthyridines. *Bioorg Med Chem Lett* 2013;23(17):4968-74. doi: 10.1016/j.bmcl.2013.06.048

24. Honorio VG, Bezerra J, Souza GT, Carvalho RJ, Gomes-Neto NJ, Figueiredo RC, et al. Inhibition of *Staphylococcus aureus* cocktail using the synergies of oregano and rosemary essential oils or carvacrol and 1,8-cineole. *Front Microbiol* 2015;6:1223. doi: 10.3389/fmicb.2015.01223

25. Rosato A, Piarulli M, Corbo F, Muraglia M, Carone A, Vitali ME, et al. *In vitro* synergistic antibacterial action of certain combinations of gentamicin and essential oils. *Curr Med Chem* 2010;17(28):3289-95.

26. Si H, Hu J, Liu Z, Zeng ZL. Antibacterial effect of oregano essential oil alone and in combination with antibiotics against extended-spectrum β-lactamase-producing *Escherichia coli*. *FEMS Immunol Med Microbiol* 2008;53(2):190-4. doi: 10.1111/j.1574-695X.2008.00414.x

27. Ikuma K, Decho AW, Lau BL. When nanoparticles meet biofilms-interactions guiding the environmental fate and accumulation of nanoparticles. *Front Microbiol* 2015;6:591. doi: 10.3389/fmicb.2015.00591

28. Khameneh B, Zarei H, Fazly Bazzaz BS. The effect of silver nanoparticles on staphylococcus epidermidis biofilm biomass and cell viability. *Nanomed J* 2014;1(5):302-7. doi: 10.7508/nmj.2015.05.003

29. Vazquez-Sanchez D, Cabo ML, Rodriguez-Herrera JJ. Antimicrobial activity of essential oils against staphylococcus aureus biofilms. *Food Sci Technol Int* 2015;21(8):559-70. doi: 10.1177/1082013214553996

18

Role of Essential Oil of *Mentha Spicata* (Spearmint) in Addressing Reverse Hormonal and Folliculogenesis Disturbances in a Polycystic Ovarian Syndrome in a Rat Model

Mahmood Sadeghi Ataabadi[1], Sanaz Alaee[1]*, Mohammad Jafar Bagheri[2], Soghra Bahmanpoor[2]

[1] *Department of Reproductive Biology, School of Advanced Medical Sciences and Technologies, Shiraz University of Medical Sciences, Shiraz, Iran.*
[2] *Department of Anatomy, School of Medicine, Shiraz University of Medical Sciences, Shiraz, Iran.*

Article info

Keywords:
· PCOS
· *Mentha spicata*
· Folliculogenesis
· Rat

Abstract

Purpose: Given the antiandrogenic effects of spearmint, in this study we evaluated the effects of its essential oil on polycystic ovarian syndrome in a rat model.

Methods: Female rats were treated as follows: Control, normal rats which received 150 mg/kg spearmint oil or 300 mg/kg spearmint oil, or sesame oil; and PCOS-induced rats which received 150 mg/kg spearmint oil or 300 mg/kg spearmint oil, or sesame oil. Then the animals were killed and the levels of LH, FSH, testosterone and ovarian folliculogenesis were evaluated.

Results: Spearmint oil reduced body weight, testosterone level, ovarian cysts and atretic follicles and increased Graafian follicles in PCOS rats.

Conclusion: Spearmint has treatment potential on PCOS through inhibition of testosterone and restoration of follicular development in ovarian tissue.

Introduction

Polycystic ovary syndrome (PCOS) is an endocrine disorder associated with hyperandrogenism and elevated level of oxidative stress and, often, obesity, abnormal menstrual cycle, insulin resistance and oligomenorrhea or anovulation.[1]

An impressive number of plant species is traditionally used for treatment of fertility-related diseases.[2] Currently in Iran, *Mentha spicata* (spearmint) essential oil is produced commercially and used orally as a carminative and antispasmodic agent. This herbal plant is also recommended for alleviating hirsutism and menstrual pain.

It is confirmed that spearmint tea has antiandrogen properties and significantly decreases testosterone level and hirsutism in women with PCOS.[3,4] It also has antioxidant, anticancer, anti-inflammatory and antidiabetic properties,[5] but the effects of spearmint oil on PCOS have not been determined. In the current study, we evaluated the effects of spearmint oil on an animal model of PCOS.

Materials and Methods

Preparation of *Mentha spicata* essential oil

Purified *Mentha spicata* essential oil was purchased from Barij Essence Pharmaceutical Company, Mashhad Ardehal, Kashan, Iran and according to the manufacturer's data sheet contained 57.02% carvone, 24.63% limonene, 2.7% pulegone, 1.8% menthol and 0.34% cineole.

Animals

Mature Wistar albino female rats were obtained from the animal house of Shiraz University of Medical Sciences, Shiraz, Iran. Rats were kept in temperature-controlled rooms with constant humidity and 12 hr/12 hr light/dark cycle, with free access to standard diet and water. The study protocol was approved by the Animal Ethical Committee of Shiraz University of Medical Sciences.

Rats with two normal estrus cycles were weighed and treated as follows: Group I (control): Received 1 ml distilled water orally for 20 days; Group II: Received letrozole; Group III: Received letrozole and then received spearmint oil (150 mg/kg); Group IV: Received letrozole and then received spearmint oil (300 mg/kg); Group V: Received letrozole and then received sesame oil; Group VI: Received spearmint oil (150 mg/kg); Group VII: Received spearmint oil (300 mg/kg); and Group VIII: Received sesame oil. PCOS induction was carried out by treating rats in groups II, III, IV and V daily with letrozole orally (1 mg/kg) for 28 days and confirmed by observation of persistent estrus phase and a high number of ovarian cysts in ovarian histological sections. Spearmint oil was dissolved in sesame oil and administered to rats orally for 20 days.

*Corresponding author: Sanaz Alaee, Email: alaee@sums.ac.ir

After treatment duration, animals were weighed, killed by ether, blood sample was taken from the heart and the ovarian tissues were removed.

Hormonal assay
Blood samples were centrifuged at 3000 rpm and Serum concentrations of testosterone (Padtan Elm Company, Tehran, Iran), LH and FSH (Hangzhao Eastbiopharm Co., Ltd., Hangzhao, China) were measured with their specific kits.

Histological analysis
Ovaries were removed, fixed and sections of 5μm thickness were cut and stained with hematoxylin and eosin. The number of primordial, primary, secondary, Graafian and atretic follicles, corpus lutea and cysts were counted in ovarian sections using a light microscope (Olympus, Tokyo, Japan).

Statistical analysis
Statistical analysis was performed using SPSS 16 software (IBM, Armonk, USA). For analysis of data, the One-Way ANOVA test was used followed by the Tukey test to compare the means. P value of <0.05 was considered statistically significant.

Results and Discussion
The body weight, level of LH and FSH, testosterone and the number of primordial, primary, secondary, Graafian and atretic follicles and corpus lutea was not different among control and rats which received spearmint oil or sesame oil ($p>0.05$).

The weight of animals in the PCOS-induced group and in the PCOS-induced groups that received spearmint oil (150 mg/kg) and sesame oil was significantly higher than that of the control group ($p=0.006$, $p=0.004$ and $p<0.001$, respectively), but in PCOS-induced rats that had received the high dose of spearmint oil (300 mg/kg) the weight was significantly lower in comparison both to PCOS-induced rats ($p=0.005$) and to PCOS-induced groups that received spearmint oil (150 mg/kg) and sesame oil ($p=0.003$ and $p< 0.001$)(Table 1). Therefore, spearmint has no effects on body weight in normal condition, which was observed by other studies using spearmint extract,[6] but in PCOS condition spearmint serves to control body weight.

Table 1. Body weight and the level of LH, FSH and testosterone of control, PCOS and PCOS rats which received spearmint oil

Groups	Weight at the beginning (g)	Weight at the end (g)	LH (ng/dl)	FSH (ng/dl)	Testosterone (mIU/ml)
(I) Control	161.33 ± 7.50	203.50 ± 14.05*	22.26±1.76	16.96±3.76	0.14 ± 0.02
(II) PCOS	149.00 ± 8.12	230.00±17.81	24.56±1.98	13.62±0.65	3.04 ± 0.69 †
(III) PCOS+ Spearmint (150mg/kg)	151.85 ± 6.46	235.57±12.36	21.88±4.13	13.61±1.64	0.20 ± 0.11
(IV) PCOS+ Spearmint (300mg/kg)	153.50 ± 7.23	205.00±10.70**	21.45±2.63	15.40±3.86	0.12 ± 0.01
(V) PCOS +Sesame oil	157.83 ± 12.87	244.16±10.90	25.85±3.49	14.50±0.88	0.14 ± 0.02

Data are shown as mean±SD.
$P<0.05$ is considered statistically significant.
* Significant differences between control and group II, group III and group V
** Significant differences between group IV and group II, III and V
† Significant differences between group II and other groups

The level of testosterone in PCOS-induced groups that received spearmint oil was significantly lower than that of the PCOS-induced group ($p<0.001$) (Table 1). Studies have shown attenuation of testosterone in PCOS women after receiving spearmint teas.[3,4]

The number of primordial follicles in PCOS-induced rats and also in PCOS-induced rats that received either of two doses of spearmint oil and sesame oil was significantly lower than in the control group ($p=0.016$, $p=0.046$, $p=0.001$ and $p=0.002$, respectively). There was no significant change in the number of primary follicles among these groups ($p>0.05$).

The number of secondary follicles was significantly lower in the PCOS-induced group compared with the control group ($p=0.043$).

There were no Graafian follicles in the PCOS-induced group and in PCOS-induced groups that received the lower dose of spearmint (150 mg/kg) or sesame oil. However, in the PCOS-induced group that received the higher dose of spearmint, Graafian follicles were observed ($p>0.05$). The number of atretic follicles was significantly higher in the PCOS-induced group compared with the control group ($p< 0.001$), but in the two PCOS-induced groups that received spearmint oil, the number of atretic follicles decreased significantly in comparison to the PCOS-induced group ($p=0.008$ and $p=0.011$). The number of corpus lutea was significantly lower in the PCOS-induced group compared with control group ($p=0.003$), but it was insignificantly higher in the PCOS-induced groups that received spearmint oil in comparison to the PCOS-induced group ($p>0.05$). In PCOS-induced groups that received spearmint oil or sesame oil, the number of ovarian cysts was significantly lower than in the PCOS-induced group ($p< 0.001$). In the PCOS-induced group which received high doses of spearmint oil, no cysts were observed (Table 2).

It is demonstrated that in PCOS condition, obesity, insulin resistance and hyperglycemia all correlate with a high level of oxidative stress, inducing a hyperandrogenemic environment in the ovary. Although locally produced androgens serve as substrate for estrogen production in folliculogenesis, an excessive level of androgens overrides follicular development, resulting in follicular atresia, disturbed follicular development and anovulation.[7]

Elevated visceral adiposity and hyperinsulinemia are observed in PCOS women, resulting in increased androgen production of the ovaries and adrenal gland. Reducing body weight of anovulatory obese women decreases insulin resistance, testosterone concentration and restores ovulation.[8]

Table 2. The number of primordial, primary, secondary, Graafian and atretic follicles, corpus lutea and cysts in ovarian tissue of control, PCOS and PCOS rats which received spearmint oil

Groups	Primordial follicle	Primary follicle	Secondary follicle	Graafian follicle	Atretic Follicles	Corpus Luteum	Cysts
(I) Control	8.41 ± 5.48 *	8.72 ± 7.76	6.33± 2.57	0.16 ± 0.38	2.66 ± 2.26	7.25 ± 3.64	0.00
(II) PCOS	2.83 ± 2.99	2.66 ± 2.16	1.33 ± 1.21**	0.00	15.83±9.96†	1.33±1.03**	10.50±4.50§
(III) PCOS+Spearmint(150 mg/kg)	3.20 ± 3.76	4.20 ± 3.70	2.20 ± 3.03	0.00	2.60 ± 2.30	4.80 ± 3.56	0.20 ± 0.44
(IV) PCOS+Spearmint(300 mg/kg)	2.14 ± 2.11	5.28 ± 2.98	2.85 ± 2.11	0.14 ± 0.03	4.00 ± 4.43	4.28 ± 2.42	0.00
(V) PCOS+Sesame oil	2.000 ± 1.67	2.500±2.05	2.00 ± 1.20	0.00	10.16 ± 8.49	2.83 ± 2.22	1.66 ± 2.25

Data are shown as mean±SD.
$P<0.05$ is considered statistically significant.
* Statistically significant differences between control and other groups
** Significant differences between group II and control groups
† Significant differences between group II and control, group III and group IV
§ Significant differences between group II and other groups

According to our results, spearmint oil decreases body weight in the PCOS condition, and since it has antiandrogenic potential, its administration leads to decrease of androgen production. Studies show that spearmint leaves decrease cholesterol and, in type II diabetes, decrease oxidative stress.[9] Additionally, phenolic compounds of spearmint leaf extract significantly enhance the antioxidant defense system and reduce body weight and levels of glucose and cholesterol in diabetic male rats.[10,11]

In the current study, no Graafian follicle was observed in PCOS-induced rats and only the administration of the higher dose of spearmint resulted in the production of these follicles in the ovarian tissue. Furthermore, administration of spearmint decreased the number of atretic follicles and ovarian cysts in PCOS-induced rats, a circumstance which is also associated with the antioxidant and antiandrogenic effects of spearmint oil. Moreover, the attenuated level of corpus lutea in PCOS-induced rats increased in PCOS rats that received spearmint oil, which reflects the higher rate of ovulation in these groups.

Therefore, spearmint oil by reduction of weight and testosterone and having antioxidant potential can restore follicular maturation and induce ovulation, which, respectively, was observed in the lower number of atretic follicles and higher number of Graafian follicles and corpus lutea in the PCOS-induced rats that received spearmint oil.

Conclusion
Spearmint can be administered as a potential agent for treatment of PCOS, but further research is needed to examine the effects of this herbal plant on all parameters related to fertility.

Acknowledgments
We thank Shiraz University of Medical Sciences for the ethical approval and financial support of this research (grant number:93-01-74-8667).

Conflict of Interest
The authors declare that there are no conflicts of interest.

References
1. Victor VM, Rovira-Llopis S, Banuls C, Diaz-Morales N, Martinez de Maranon A, Rios-Navarro C, et al. Insulin resistance in pcos patients enhances oxidative stress and leukocyte adhesion: Role of myeloperoxidase. *PLoS One* 2016;11(3):e0151960. doi: 10.1371/journal.pone.0151960
2. Monsefi M, Ghasemi A, Alaee S, Aliabadi E. Effects of anethum graveolens l. (dill) on oocyte and fertility of adult female rats. *J Reprod Infertil* 2015;16(1):10-17.
3. Grant P. Spearmint herbal tea has significant anti-androgen effects in polycystic ovarian syndrome. A randomized controlled trial. *Phytother Res* 2010;24(2):186-8. doi: 10.1002/ptr.2900
4. Akdogan M, Tamer MN, Cure E, Cure MC, Koroglu BK, Delibas N. Effect of spearmint (mentha spicata labiatae) teas on androgen levels in women with hirsutism. *Phytother Res* 2007;21(5):444-7. doi: 10.1002/ptr.2074
5. Raut JS, Karuppayil SM. A status review on the medicinal properties of essential oils. *Ind Crop Prod* 2014;62:250-64. doi.10.1016/j.indcrop.2014.05.055
6. Nozhat F, Alaee S, Behzadi K, Azadi Chegini N. Evaluation of possible toxic effects of spearmint

(mentha spicata) on the reproductive system, fertility and number of offspring in adult male rats. *Avicenna J Phytomed* 2014;4(6):420-9.

7. Pan JX, Zhang JY, Ke ZH, Wang FF, Barry JA, Hardiman PJ, et al. Androgens as double-edged swords: Induction and suppression of follicular development. *Hormones (Athens)* 2015;14(2):190-200. doi: 10.14310/horm.2002.1580

8. Moran LJ, Noakes M, Clifton PM, Tomlinson L, Galletly C, Norman RJ. Dietary composition in restoring reproductive and metabolic physiology in overweight women with polycystic ovary syndrome. *J Clin Endocrinol Metab* 2003;88(2):812-9. doi: 10.1210/jc.2002-020815

9. Rajeshwari CU, Preeti M, Andallu B. Efficacy of mint (*Mentha spicata L.*) leaves in combating oxidative stress in type 2 diabetes. *Int J Life Sci* 2012;1(2):28-34.

10. Al-Rekabi EA. Anti-oxidant and hepatoprotective activity of phenolic compounds of leaves extracts from *mentha longifolia* and *mentha spicata* in diabetic male rats. *World J Pharm Res* 2015;4(6):346-54.

11. Al-Fartosi KG, Radi H, Al-Rekabi EA. Lipid Profile of Diabetic Male Rats Treated with Phenolic Compounds of Leaves Extracts from *Mentha longifolia* and *Mentha spicata*. *Int J Pharm Biol Med Sci* 2014:3(2):26-31.

19

Evaluation of NPP1 as a Novel Biomarker of Coronary Artery Disease: A Pilot Study in Human Beings

Amir Hooshang Mohammadpour[1,2] , Saeed Nazemi[3], Fatemeh Mashhadi[2], Atefeh Rezapour[2], Mohammad Afshar[4,5], Sepideh Afzalnia[3], Afsaneh Mohammadi[3], Hamid Reza Mashreghi Moghadam[6], Maryam Moradian[7], Seyed Mohammad Hasan Moallem[8], Saeed Falahaty[2], Azadeh Zayerzadeh[2], Sepideh Elyasi[1,2]*

[1] Pharmaceutical Research Center, Mashhad University of Medical Sciences, Mashhad, Iran.
[2] Department of Clinical Pharmacy, School of Pharmacy, Mashhad University of Medical Sciences, Mashhad, Iran.
[3] Research and Education Department, Razavi Hospital, Mashhad, Iran.
[4] Department of Anatomy, Birjand University of Medical Sciences, Birjand, Iran.
[5] Medical Toxicology Research Center, Mashhad University of Medical Sciences, Mashhad, Iran.
[6] Birjand Cardiovascular Disease Research Center; Department of Cardiology, Birjand University of Medical Sciences, Birjand, Iran.
[7] Department of Pediatric Cardiology, Rajaie Cardiovascular Medical and Research Center, Tehran, Iran.
[8] School of Medicine, Mashhad University of Medical Sciences, Mashhad, Iran.

Article info

Keywords:
· Coronary Artery Calcification
· ENPP1
· Biomarker
· Inorganic pyrophosphate
· Glycoprotein 1- nucleotides

Abstract

Purpose: Coronary artery calcification (CAC) is utilized as an important tool for global risk assessment of cardiovascular events in individuals with intermediate risk. Ecto phosphodiesterase/nucleotide phosphohydrolase-1(ENPP1) converts extracellular nucleotides into inorganic pyrophosphate and it is a key regulator of tissue calcification that adjusts calcification in tissues like vascular smooth muscle cells. The main purpose of this clinical study was to find out the correlation between ENPP1 serum concentration and CAC in human for the first time.

Methods: In this study 83 patients (16 diabetic patients and 67 non-diabetic patients) with coronary artery disease who fulfilled inclusion and exclusion criteria, entered the study. For all patients a questionnaire consisting demographic data and traditional cardiovascular risk factors were completed. Computed tomography (CT)-Angiography was carried out to determine coronary artery calcium score and enzyme-linked immunosorbent assay (ELISA) method was used for measuring ENPP1 serum concentrations.

Results: There was a reverse significant correlation between ENPP1 serum concentration and total CAC score and also CAC of right coronary artery (RCA) ($P<0.05$) in non-diabetic patients.

Conclusion: On the basis of our results, ENPP1 serum concentration may be a suitable biomarker for coronary artery disease at least in non-diabetic patients. However, more studies with higher sample size are necessary for its confirmation.

Introduction

Vascular calcification is a life threatening complication of cardiovascular disease and an independent risk factor for high morbidity and mortality.[1] It is an inevitable process particularly in the advanced stages of atherosclerosis which can cause the plaque rupture. Coronary artery calcification (CAC) is a surrogate marker for subclinical atherosclerosis and recently determined as strong predictor that comforts the prediction of future cardiovascular events particularly in intermediate risk subjects. It is determined by electron beam-computed tomography (EBCT).[2] Increased coronary artery calcium score (CACS) correlates with the risk of cardiovascular disease.[3] Recent studies have provided impetus to shift from cellular interaction based calcification models to models emphasizing on the important role of extracellular matrix in calcification. Adenosine triphosphate (ATP) and other nucleotides and nucleosides play different biochemical roles depending on differential tissue expression, cell distribution, and substrate availability and their presence in either the intracellular or extracellular compartment. Ecto-nucleotidases classified to four families including ecto-nucleotide pyrophosphate / phosphor - diesterase (ENPP) family. ENPP1 is a member of ENPP family that expresses in different tissues including cartilage, kidney, heart, parathyroid and skeletal muscle, and to a greater extent in vascular smooth muscle cells (VSMCs), osteoblasts and chondrocytes.[4-6] NPP1 is known to play vital roles in calcium/phosphate regulation, and repression of soft tissue mineralization, and maintaining skeletal

*Corresponding author: Sepideh Elyasi, Email: Elyasis@mums.ac.ir

structure and function. NPP1 hydrolyses ATP to produce either inorganic pyrophosphate (PP$_i$) plus adenosine monophosphate (AMP) or inorganic phosphate (P$_i$) plus adenosine diphosphate (ADP) in a two stage process via either ADP or a phosphate bound intermediate.[7-9] PP$_i$ is a central regulator of calcification in the extracellular matrix. In extracellular, PP$_i$ draw ups gene expression and cellular differentiation, which have main physiologic effects on chondrogenesis and expression of osteopontin. PP$_i$ strongly inhibits the nucleation and advancement of hydroxyapatite (HA) and other basic calcium phosphate crystals.[7,10,11] Therefore, through generating PPi, NPP1 is a key regulator of tissue calcification and bone development and can be effective in prevention of pathologic tissue calcification.

According to this, we evaluated the ENPP1 as a diagnostic biomarker in human to determine the extent of coronary artery calcification.

Materials and Methods
Patients
Eighty-three patients, who aged higher than 40 years old with diagnosis of coronary artery disease by angiography which was performed by the cardiologist, were enrolled in this study between November 2015 and March 2016. This test is the best way to detect coronary artery disease (CAD) in the arteries, over 51% of which are blocked by atherosclerotic plaques and useful in detecting the vessels responsible for advanced CAD. However, it does not provide information about the artery wall and atherosclerosis may not be diagnosed that has not yet captured the duct.[12] patients with >50% coronary stenosis of at least one artery were considered as CAD+ and included in study. Patients were recruited from Cardiology ward of Razavi Hospital, Mashhad, Iran. This study was accepted by ethics committee of Mashhad University of Medical Sciences (code: 931459). All patients signed the consent form prior to entry in the study. All patients signed the consent form prior to entry in the study.

Patients with calcium and phosphor metabolic disorder or receiving medications which are effective on calcium and/or phosphate and immunosuppressant or antioxidant medications, intake of folic acid and methotrexate, malignancies, heart failure, hypo or hyper parathyroidisim, renal insufficiency, history of osteoarticular disorders and chronic inflammatory diseases, and acute infection during the study were excluded from the study. A questionnaire containing demographic data, laboratory data, drug and medical and familial history of cardiovascular risk factors was completed for all patients.

Determination of ENPP1 serum concentration and CAC
Twenty milliliter of whole blood was collected from patients and centrifuged at 2500 rpm for 10 min. Two milliliter serum were isolated and divided into 4 micro sets of 0.5 ml. The serum was stored at -70 °C until required for analysis. Routine biochemical measurements

such as plasma glucose, total cholesterol (TC), triglycerides, low density lipoprotein Cholesterol (LDL-c), high-density lipoprotein cholesterol (HDL-c), and serum calcium and phosphorus level were carried out by routine laboratory methods. Serum level of soluble ENPP1 was measured with an enzyme-linked Immunosorbant assay (ELISA) -kit (Zellbio, Germany); each assay was calibrated using ENPP1 standard curve following the manufacturer's instructions. Coronary Artery Calcification score of left main coronary artery (LMCA), left anterior descending (LAD) and circumflex (CX) and right coronary artery (RCA) was determined by high resolution B mode ultrasonography in radiology department of Razavi Hospital. CAC measurement is now considered a potentially useful test for improving coronary risk assessment in selected intermediate-risk asymptomatic patients in whom high CAC scores signify increased cardiovascular risk beyond that predicted by conventional cardiovascular risk factors alone. Agatston score is a semi-automated tool to calculate a score based on the extent of coronary artery calcification detected by an unenhanced low-dose CT scan which is routinely performed in patients undergoing cardiac CT. Due to an extensive body of search, it allows for an early risk stratification as patients with a high Agatston score (>160) have an increased risk for a major adverse cardiac event. Although it does not allow for the assessment of soft non-calcified plaques, it has shown a good correlation with contrast enhanced CT coronary angiography.[13,14]

However, it should be defined that when the pretest probability of coronary artery disease is low (eg, asymptomatic screening setting), a CAC score of zero is associated with low risk of coronary artery disease and low risk of near-term coronary events but in older asymptomatic patients with risk factors, CAC=0 is associated with a moderate increased risk of events and in patients with clinical signs and symptoms associated with an intermediate-to-high risk of coronary disease, CAC=0 is often associated with myocardial ischemia on provocative testing and with a high risk of near-term coronary events.[15]

Statistical Analysis
Data recruited from the standard forms were gathered and then analyzed with SPSS version 16.0 (Systat Software, Inc., Chicago, IL). For descriptive assessment, mean ± standard deviations of continuous variables were provided. For nominal variables, number and percentages were reported. Correlation between Serum Concentration of ENPP1 with CAC was analyzed using spearman correlation test. Chi-squared test and t test were applied for continuous and nominal data, where appropriate. Results were considered significant at p<0.05.

Results
Characteristics of the study Population
The study population consists of 83 patients, male (77%) and female (23%). The mean age of population was

56.80±10.73 years. Patients' characteristics, laboratory tests including biochemical parameters, and traditional cardiovascular risk factors and mean ENPP1 serum level are summarized in Table 1. Moreover, these factors are defined in diabetic and non-diabetic patients separately and female/male ratios, positive family history of CAD and hypertension prevalence were significantly different between these two groups.

Table 1. patients characteristic, laboratory data, traditional cardiovascular risk factors and mean ENPP1 serum level of patients

Patients characteristic	All patients (n=83) (Mean±SD)	Diabetic patients (n=16) (Mean±SD)	Non-diabetic patients (n=67) (Mean±SD)	P value
Age (year)	57.13±10.7	56.4±10.52	57.74±10.65	0.95[1]
BMI (kg/m^2)	28.36±4.78	28.46±3.8	27.99±5.46	0.43[1]
Female/male ratio	0.29	0.54	0.32	0.005*[2]
Laboratory tests	**Mean±SD**			
HDL-C (mg/dl)	41.92±9.97	40.76±9.14	45.24±15.68	0.66[1]
LDL-C (mg/dl)	90.81±29.14	95.88±34.56	88.69±28.04	0.06[1]
Total cholesterol (mg/dl)	163.30±33.32	165.76±38.28	164±33.81	0.09[1]
FBS (mg/dl)	104.56±24.00	141.2±44.05	97.57±14.71	0.005*[1]
Traditional risk factors	**Frequency (%)**			
Hypertension (%)	45.88	60	45.34	0.005*[2]
Dyslipidemia (%)	63.52	65	61.62	0.63[2]
Positive family history (%)	51.76	47.62	62.79	0.005*[2]
Diabetes (%)	20.58	100	0	-
Current Smoking (%)	35.29	33.33	23.25	0.66[2]
Concentration of ENPP1 (pg/mL)	106.4214±78.54876	132.62±100.5	100.26±71.97	0.14[1]

BMI: Body Mass Index, HDL-C: High Density Lipoprotein-Cholesterol, LDL-C: Low Density Lipoprotein-Cholesterol, FBS: Fast Blood Sugar, ENPP1: Ecto-nucleotide pyrophosphate/phosphor-di-esterase
[1] independent sample T test [2]chi square
* P value<0.05 is considered significant

Correlation between ENPP1 serum level and Coronary Artery Calcification agatson score

There was a reversed significant correlation between ENPP1 serum level and total coronary artery calcification score and CAC score of RCA in non-diabetic patients (P<0.05) but, there was no significant correlation between ENPP1 serum level and CAC score of LMCA, LAD and CX.(p>0.05) (Table 2)

Table 2. Correlation between ENPP1 serum concentration with LAD, RCA, LMCA, and CX coronary artery calcification score

Coronary artery Calcium score	Mean ±SD	P value Spearman Correlation Test	Correlation coefficient
Total calcification of coronary vessels (agatson score)	357.29±590.81	0.004	-0.121
Calcification in coronary LAD (agatson score)	184.60±304.46	0.345	0.044
Calcification in coronary RCA (agatson score)	63.37±101.86	0.00	-0.22
Calcification in coronary CX (agatson score)	44.86±99.00	0.416	-0.264
Calcification in coronary LMCA (agatson score)	34.11±116.00	0.494	-0.107

CAC: Coronary Artery Calcification, LAD: Left Anterior Descending, RCA: Right Coronary Artery LMCA: Left Main Coronary Artery, CX: Circumflex

Moreover, based on Rumberger method we divided patients based on their total CAC to three groups; mild (CAC lower than 25th of range), moderate (between 25th and 75th of range) and severe (≥75th of CAC range). Fifty-four percent of the patients were in mild group and 44.4% and 1.6% were in moderate and severe groups, respectively. There was no significant difference between ENPP1 serum level of these groups (P>0.05).

Discussion

In this study, the correlation of the ENPP1 serum level with CAC was evaluated for the first time in human. As mentioned in results, there was a significant reversed correlation between ENPP1 serum level and total and RCA CAC score in non-diabetic patients (P<0.05) but no significant correlation with CAC score of LAD, LM and CX (P ≥0.05). Several In vitro and In vivo studies have been conducted on the relationship between coronary artery calcification and serum ENPP1 level previously but they were only limited to the examination of genetic disorders and gene mutations of ENPP1 in infants and evaluation of the relationship between serum levels of ENPP1 and calcification of atherosclerotic plaques in diabetic patients.

Based on previous studies, it is entirely apparent that the calcification is suppress by ENPP1 by means of PP$_i$ that it is a potent inhibitor of hydroxyl apatite (HA) crystal formation in mineralized competent of tissues.

NPPs can convert AMP into adenosine and P_i, although conflicting reports suggest that AMP competitively inhibits NPP activity. PPi is hydrolyzed by tissue-nonspecific alkaline phosphatase (TNAP) into inorganic phosphate (Pi), which co-crystallizes with calcium into HA and thereby promotes bone formation. Thus, PPi has a dual role as it can both suppress and promote HA crystal deposition, depending on the expression ratio and catalytic activities of NPP1 and TNAP. The distorted balance of Pi/PPi ultimately leads to pathological calcification.[16-19] In another study, NPP1-deficient mice showed reduced levels of extracellular PPi, causing pathological calcification of cartilage and soft tissues, such as arterial smooth muscle walls and also abnormal bone development.[16,17] So, according to the previous studies, it is clear that NPP1 and PP_i physiologically work to prevent calcification of arteries and certain other soft tissues.[20,21] This study was the first clinical study that evaluated the relationship between serum concentrations of ENPP1 and coronary artery calcification in patients with chronic heart ischemia. According to the results mentioned above, there was a significant reversed relationship between the coronary artery calcification and this biomarker in non-diabetic patients.

A study was conducted in 2010 by Jeong et al. which assessed the relationship between coronary artery calcification and ENPP1 gene expression levels in 140 diabetic patients. None of patients had history of cardiovascular disease and no relationship was found between coronary artery calcification and ENPP1 gene expression levels.[22] In present study 16 diabetic patients and 67 non-diabetic patients were included and no relationship was found between total coronary artery calcification score and serum concentrations of ENPP1. However, after exclusion of diabetic patients a significant relationship was observed (P = 0.004). Nowadays type 2 diabetes prevalence is increasing steadily all over the world. One of the criteria for type 2 diabetes, is insulin resistance in different body tissues such as skeletal muscle, liver and fat tissues that occurs due to impaired peripheral receptor signaling of insulin. In several studies it has been observed that ENPP1, which is connected directly to the insulin receptor α, impairs receptor function and then reduces the signaling cascade, in a wide variety of tissues such as skeletal muscle and liver.[23] In some other studies has been observed that the expression level of ENPP1 in patients with insulin resistance has been increased and also it is mentioned that regulatory increased ENPP1level in rat liver, induces insulin resistance and glucose tolerance.[24-26] In a multicenter clinical study conducted in Italy and America in 2005, it is observed that increased expression of ENPP1 is associated with a higher prevalence of diabetes and myocardial infarction.[27] So, in this research, we excluded patients with type 2 diabetes and it was found that the level of serum ENPP1 is affected by type 2 diabetes and there is a significant negative relationship between the ENPP1 serum levels and the total calcification score of coronary arteries in non-diabetic patients with cardiovascular disease.

This significant negative correlation was also found by CAC of RCA but not the other coronary arteries. It may be due to non-uniform distribution of other vessels' calcium scores resulting from small sample size. So, limited number of patients included in this study is the major limitation of this study.

Conclusion

In this study, the correlation of the ENPP1 serum level with CAC was clinically evaluated for the first time in patients with coronary artery disease. There was a reverse significant correlation between ENPP1 serum level and total CAC and CAC of RCA in non-diabetic patients (P<0.05), but there was no significant correlation between ENPP1 serum level patients and LAD, LM and CX (P >0.05). Further studies are recommended in this field with higher sample size.

Acknowledgments

This study is part of a research thesis for a Pharm.D. degree at Mashhad University of Medical Sciences.
The authors are thankful for the funding of this study by the Research Council of Mashhad University of Medical Sciences.

Conflict of Interest

The authors have no conflicts of interest.

References

1. Santos RD, Nasir K, Carvalho JA, Raggi P, Blumenthal RS. Coronary calcification and coronary heart disease death rates in different countries, not only the influence of classical risk factors. *Atherosclerosis* 2009;202(1):32-3. doi: 10.1016/j.atherosclerosis.2008.04.017

2. Budoff MJ, Achenbach S, Blumenthal RS, Carr JJ, Goldin JG, Greenland P, et al. Assessment of coronary artery disease by cardiac computed tomography: A scientific statement from the american heart association committee on cardiovascular imaging and intervention, council on cardiovascular radiology and intervention, and committee on cardiac imaging, council on clinical cardiology. *Circulation* 2006;114(16):1761-91. doi: 10.1161/circulationaha.106.178458

3. Abedin M, Tintut Y, Demer LL. Vascular calcification: Mechanisms and clinical ramifications. *Arterioscler Thromb Vasc Biol* 2004;24(7):1161-70. doi: 10.1161/01.atv.0000133194.94939.42

4. Nitschke Y, Weissen-Plenz G, Terkeltaub R, Rutsch F. Npp1 promotes atherosclerosis in apoe knockout mice. *J Cell Mol Med* 2011;15(11):2273-83. doi: 10.1111/j.1582-4934.2011.01327.x

5. Terkeltaub RA. Inorganic pyrophosphate generation and disposition in pathophysiology. *Am J Physiol Cell Physiol* 2001;281(1):C1-c11. doi: 10.1152/ajpcell.2001.281.1.C1

6. Johnson K, Terkeltaub R. Inorganic pyrophosphate (ppi) in pathologic calcification of articular cartilage. *Front Biosci* 2005;10:988-97.

7. Bollen M, Gijsbers R, Ceulemans H, Stalmans W, Stefan C. Nucleotide pyrophosphatases/phosphodiesterases on the move. *Crit Rev Biochem Mol Biol* 2000;35(6):393-432. doi: 10.1080/10409230091169249

8. Stefan C, Jansen S, Bollen M. Modulation of purinergic signaling by npp-type ectophosphodiesterases. *Purinergic Signal* 2006;2(2):361-70. doi: 10.1007/s11302-005-5303-4

9. Goding JW, Terkeltaub R, Maurice M, Deterre P, Sali A, Belli SI. Ecto-phosphodiesterase/pyrophosphatase of lymphocytes and non-lymphoid cells: Structure and function of the pc-1 family. *Immunol Rev* 1998;161:11-26.

10. Terkeltaub R. Physiologic and pathologic functions of the NPP nucleotide pyrophosphatase/phosphodiesterase family focusing on NPP1 in calcification. *Purinergic Signal* 2006;2(2):371-7. doi: 10.1007/s11302-005-5304-3

11. Addison WN, Azari F, Sorensen ES, Kaartinen MT, McKee MD. Pyrophosphate inhibits mineralization of osteoblast cultures by binding to mineral, up-regulating osteopontin, and inhibiting alkaline phosphatase activity. *J Biol Chem* 2007;282(21):15872-83. doi: 10.1074/jbc.M701116200

12. Longo DL, Fauci AS, Kasper DL, Hauser SL, Jameson J, Loscalzo J, editors. Harrison's Principles of Internal Medicine. 18th ed. New York, NY: McGraw-Hill; 2012.

13. van der Bijl N, Joemai RM, Geleijns J, Bax JJ, Schuijf JD, de Roos A, et al. Assessment of agatston coronary artery calcium score using contrast-enhanced ct coronary angiography. *AJR Am J Roentgenol* 2010;195(6):1299-305. doi: 10.2214/ajr.09.3734

14. Arad Y, Spadaro LA, Goodman K, Newstein D, Guerci AD. Prediction of coronary events with electron beam computed tomography. *J Am Coll Cardiol* 2000;36(4):1253-60.

15. Greenland P, Bonow RO. How low-risk is a coronary calcium score of zero? The importance of conditional probability. *Circulation* 2008;117(13):1627-9. doi: 10.1161/circulationaha.108.767665

16. Hessle L, Johnson KA, Anderson HC, Narisawa S, Sali A, Goding JW, et al. Tissue-nonspecific alkaline phosphatase and plasma cell membrane glycoprotein-1 are central antagonistic regulators of bone mineralization. *Proc Natl Acad Sci U S A* 2002;99(14):9445-9. doi: 10.1073/pnas.142063399

17. Johnson K, Polewski M, van Etten D, Terkeltaub R. Chondrogenesis mediated by PPi depletion promotes spontaneous aortic calcification in NPP1-/- mice. *Arterioscler Thromb Vasc Biol* 2005;25(4):686-91. doi: 10.1161/01.ATV.0000154774.71187.f0

18. Ciancaglini P, Yadav MC, Simao AM, Narisawa S, Pizauro JM, Farquharson C, et al. Kinetic analysis of substrate utilization by native and TNAP-, NPP1-, or PHOSPHO1-deficient matrix vesicles. *J Bone Miner Res* 2010;25(4):716-23. doi: 10.1359/jbmr.091023

19. Harmey D, Hessle L, Narisawa S, Johnson KA, Terkeltaub R, Millan JL. Concerted regulation of inorganic pyrophosphate and osteopontin by akp2, enpp1, and ank: An integrated model of the pathogenesis of mineralization disorders. *Am J Pathol* 2004;164(4):1199-209. doi: 10.1016/s0002-9440(10)63208-7

20. Okawa A, Nakamura I, Goto S, Moriya H, Nakamura Y, Ikegawa S. Mutation in npps in a mouse model of ossification of the posterior longitudinal ligament of the spine. *Nat Genet* 1998;19(3):271-3. doi: 10.1038/956

21. Mackenzie NC, Zhu D, Milne EM, van 't Hof R, Martin A, Darryl Quarles L, et al. Altered bone development and an increase in FGF-23 expression in ENPP1(-/-) mice. *PLoS One* 2012;7(2):e32177. doi: 10.1371/journal.pone.0032177

22. Jeong DJ, Lee DG, Kim HJ, Cho EH, Kim SW. ENPP1 K121Q genotype not associated with coronary artery calcification in korean patients with type 2 diabetes mellitus. *Korean Diabetes J* 2010;34(5):320-6. doi: 10.4093/kdj.2010.34.5.320

23. Seo HJ, Kim SG, Kwon OJ. The K121Q polymorphism in ENPP1 (PC-1) is not associated with type 2 diabetes or obesity in korean male workers. *J Korean Med Sci* 2008;23(3):459-64. doi: 10.3346/jkms.2008.23.3.459

24. Grarup N, Urhammer SA, Ek J, Albrechtsen A, Glumer C, Borch-Johnsen K, et al. Studies of the relationship between the enpp1 k121q polymorphism and type 2 diabetes, insulin resistance and obesity in 7,333 danish white subjects. *Diabetologia* 2006;49(9):2097-104. doi: 10.1007/s00125-006-0353-x

25. Meyre D, Bouatia-Naji N, Vatin V, Veslot J, Samson C, Tichet J, et al. Enpp1 K121Q polymorphism and obesity, hyperglycaemia and type 2 diabetes in the prospective desir study. *Diabetologia* 2007;50(10):2090-6. doi: 10.1007/s00125-007-0787-9

26. McAteer JB, Prudente S, Bacci S, Lyon HN, Hirschhorn JN, Trischitta V, et al. The ENPP1 K121Q polymorphism is associated with type 2 diabetes in european populations: Evidence from an updated meta-analysis in 42,042 subjects. *Diabetes* 2008;57(4):1125-30. doi: 10.2337/db07-1336

27. Bacci S, Ludovico O, Prudente S, Zhang YY, Di Paola R, Mangiacotti D, et al. The K121Q polymorphism of the ENPP1/PC-1 gene is associated with insulin resistance/atherogenic phenotypes, including earlier onset of type 2 diabetes and myocardial infarction. *Diabetes* 2005;54(10):3021-5.

20

Changes of Insulin Resistance and Adipokines Following Supplementation with *Glycyrrhiza Glabra L*. Extract in Combination with a Low-Calorie Diet in Overweight and Obese Subjects

Mohammad Alizadeh[1], Nazli Namazi[1,2]*, Elham Mirtaheri[1]*, Nafiseh Sargheini[3], Sorayya Kheirouri[4]

[1] *Nutrition Research Center, Faculty of Nutrition, Tabriz University of Medical Sciences, Tabriz, Iran.*
[2] *Diabetes Research Center, Endocrinology and Metabolism Clinical Sciences Institute, Tehran University of Medical Sciences, Tehran, Iran.*
[3] *Molecular Biomedicine, University of Bonn, Bonn, Germany.*
[4] *Department of Nutrition, Tabriz University of Medical Sciences, Tabriz, Iran.*

Article info

Keywords:
· Calorie restricted diet
· Licorice
· Adipokine
· Insulin Resistance
· Obesity

Abstract

Purpose: Adipose tissue is a highly active endocrine organ which plays a key role in energy homeostasis. The aim of this study was to determine the effects of dried licorice extract along with a calorie restricted diet on body composition, insulin resistance and adipokines in overweight and obese subjects.

Methods: Sixty-four overweight and obese volunteers (27 men, 37 women) were recruited into this double-blind, placebo-controlled, randomized, clinical trial. Participants were randomly allocated to the Licorice (n=32) or the placebo group (n=32), and each group received a low-calorie diet with either 1.5 g/day of Licorice extract or placebo for 8 weeks. Biochemical parameters, anthropometric indices, body composition and dietary intake were measured at baseline and at the end of the study.

Results: A total of 58 subjects completed the trial. No side effects were observed following licorice supplementation. At the end of the study, waist circumference, fat mass, serum levels of vaspin, zinc-α2 glycoprotein, insulin and HOMA-IR were significantly decreased in the intervention group, but only the reduction in serum vaspin levels in the licorice group was significant when compared to the placebo group (p<0.01).

Conclusion: Supplementation with dried licorice extract plus a low-calorie diet can increase vaspin levels in obese subjects. However, the anti-obesity effects of the intervention were not stronger than a low-calorie diet alone in the management of obesity.

Introduction

Adipose tissue is a highly active endocrine organ, which plays a key role in energy homeostasis, response to hormonal signals, metabolic regulation and adipokine secretion.[1] Current evidence suggests that adipose tissue secrets more than 50 signaling molecules and hormones, called adipokines.[1,2] Adipokines are involved in the regulation of thermogenesis, appetite, glucose metabolism, insulin sensitivity and other endocrine functions.[3] One adipokine is vaspin, a visceral adipose tissue-derived hormone which can be considered to be a new link between obesity and metabolic complications such as insulin resistance, type 2 diabetes and atherosclerosis.[4] Several studies have indicated an association between vaspin and body mass index (BMI); but the findings are contradictory. [5]

Zinc-alpha 2 glycoprotein (ZAG-2) is another adipokine which plays a main role in the mobilization and utilization of lipids.[5] It also can control fat mass (FM) and energy expenditure, induce lipolysis and act as a hormone-regulating lipid in glucose metabolism.[6] Some studies found an inverse relationship between ZAG, body mass index (BMI) and waist circumference (WC). It has also been suggested that ZAG may simulate adiponectin to protect against inflammation and the complications of obesity.[7]

Prior studies have indicated that some medicinal herbs, such as *Nigella sativa*,[8] green tea[9] and *Glycyrrhiza glabra*[10,11] are involved in the regulation of hormones and weight. *Glycyrrhiza glabra L.* (Fabaceae family), generally known as Mulaithi or Licorice, is a medicinal herb which is widely grown in the Mediterranean region and Southwest Asia. It contains various components with pharmacological properties, including glycyrrhizin, glabridin, flavonoids, beta-Glycyhrritinic acid, chalcones, isoflavones and triterpenoid saponins.[12,13] Licorice root is frequently used in traditional medicine, particularly for gastric and duodenal ulcers, dyspepsia and allergenic reactions. Human and animal models have not

*Corresponding authors: Nazli Namazi, Elham Mirtaheri, Email: nazli.namazi@yahoo.com , Email: e.mirtaheri@yahoo.com

demonstrated any toxic or serious side effects of licorice consumption.[14]

It has been suggested that licorice root can alter body composition[10,11,15] and reduce insulin resistance.[16-18] However, there are limited clinical trials with contradictory results on the effects of licorice on obesity.[10,15,19] To the best of our knowledge, no clinical trials have evaluated the effects of licorice supplement with a low-calorie diet on the management of obesity and hormonal regulation. Accordingly, the primary aim of this study was to determine the effects of dried licorice extract together with a calorie restricted diet on anthropometric indices, body composition, insulin resistance and adipokines in overweight and obese subjects. The secondary aim was to evaluate the effects of licorice along with a low calorie diet on blood pressure and liver enzymes.

Material and Methods

Participants

In this double-blind randomized placebo-controlled clinical trial, 64 overweight and obese volunteers (27 men, 37 women) were recruited. Subjects were chosen by advertisement and dietitian referral from March to September 2012 at Tabriz University of Medical Sciences. A total of 64 subjects were enrolled based on FM variable in a previous study,[10] with α-value of 0.05, power of 90% and considering a 20% loss to follow up. Inclusion criteria were as follows: age 30-60 yrs old and BMI>25 kg/m.[2] The following were used as exclusion criteria cardiovascular disease, liver, thyroid and kidney disorders, diabetes, smoking, pregnancy or lactation of having taken any anti-obesity, vitamin and mineral supplements or herbal drugs in the 3 months prior to the study. Subjects who consumed any medications for hypertension or had Systolic Blood Pressure (SBP) ≥140 mmHg and Diastolic Blood Pressure (DBP) ≥ 90 mmHg were also excluded.

At the beginning of the trial, general characteristics including age, medication history and any family history of obesity were collected using a questionnaire.

Study Design and Intervention

Eligible participants were randomly allocated to the licorice (n=32) or placebo groups (n=32). Randomization was facilitated by random number table with a permuted block size of two. The participants were stratified for sex, age and BMI. All of the participants received a low-calorie diet; created by an expert dietitian who designed individualized diets with a 500 kcal deficit from the participates' energy requirements. The calories provided by the diets consisted of 55% carbohydrate, 15% protein and 30%. The intervention and placebo groups took 0.5 g/day (3 times a day 30 min before each meal) of dried licorice extract and placebo (corn starch), respectively for 8 consecutive weeks. To maintain blinding, a subject with no clinical involvement in the study performed the allocation. The patients and investigators remained blinded to the treatment assignment until data analysis.

Visits occurred every 20 days and supplements were distributed among the volunteers based on the allocation code after the randomization. Participants received a phone call every week to minimize withdrawal and ensure their adherence to the study protocol. The subjects were asked to maintain their usual physical activity level during the trial.

Licorice extract characteristics

The dried hydroalcoholic extract of licorice root (ethanol 70: water 30% v/v) was prepared by the Darook pharmacological company (Esfahan-Iran). It contained lowered Glycyrrhizin (<0.01%).

Measurements

Anthropometric indices, body composition, dietary intake, physical activity, blood pressure and biochemical parameters were measured at baseline and at the end of the study. Weight, height and WC were measured using standard methods. Assessment of dietary intake and physical activity levels were measured as explained in our previous study.[12]

Body composition measurements

BMI was calculated by dividing the weight in kilograms to the square of the height in meters. Body composition was measured using TANITA Bioelectrical Impedance Analysis (BC-418 MA, 50 kHz) after 12-14 hours fasting. We measured the amounts of FM and fat free mass (FFM) with an accuracy of ±0.1 kg. Previous studies reported a significant correlation between TANITA and Dual Energy X-Ray absorptiometry (DEXA) test for the measurement of body composition.

Biochemical measurements

At the baseline and at the end of the trial, 10 mL of venous blood was collected after 12-14h fasting. The serum was separated from whole blood by centrifugation at 2500 rpm for 10 min. Serum levels of Fasting blood sugar (FBS) was measured on the day of sampling using Auto analyzer (Abbot Model Aclyon 300 USA) by commercially enzymatic kit (Pars Azmoon, Iran). The remaining serum samples were kept at -20 °C until measurement. Enzyme-linked immunosorbent assay (ELISA) method was used to determine insulin (Pars Azmoon, Iran), vaspin (Orgenium, Fenland) and ZAG-alpha 2 (Orgenium, Fenland) concentrations. Based on FBS and insulin levels, insulin resistance was evaluated using the homeostasis model assessment-insulin resistance (HOMA-IR) formula as follows:

HOMA-IR = fasting glucose (mg/dL) ×fasting insulin (μU/mL) /405[20]

Blood pressure measurement

Blood pressure was measured after 10 minutes rest in seated and relaxed position using a Microlife AG-30 mercury sphygmomanometer on the left arm. It was repeated after 5 min and the average of the two measurements was reported.

Statistical analysis

Data were analyzed using SPSS software version 13.0 (SPSS Inc., Chicago, IL, USA). The normality of the data distribution was evaluated by the one-sample Kolmogorov-Smirnov test. The results were expressed as mean±SD for variables with normal distribution, median (25th, 75th percentiles) for variables with non-normal distribution, and percentage (%) for qualitative variables. The Chi square test was used for the comparison of qualitative variables. Independent t tests (for baseline measurements) and analysis of covariance (ANCOVA) were used to compare quantitative variables between groups, controlling for confounding factors. The Mann-Whitney U test was used for comparison variables with non-normal distribution between two groups. Pair t-test was also used for within- group comparison. $p<0.05$ was considered statistically significant.

Results

As presented in Figure 1, of the 64 participants, 58 subjects completed the study (intervention group, n=29; placebo group, n=29). The power of the study at the end of the study was 85%. Participants did not report any serious side effects for taking licorice supplement, except one who reported gastrointestinal problems and discontinued the study.

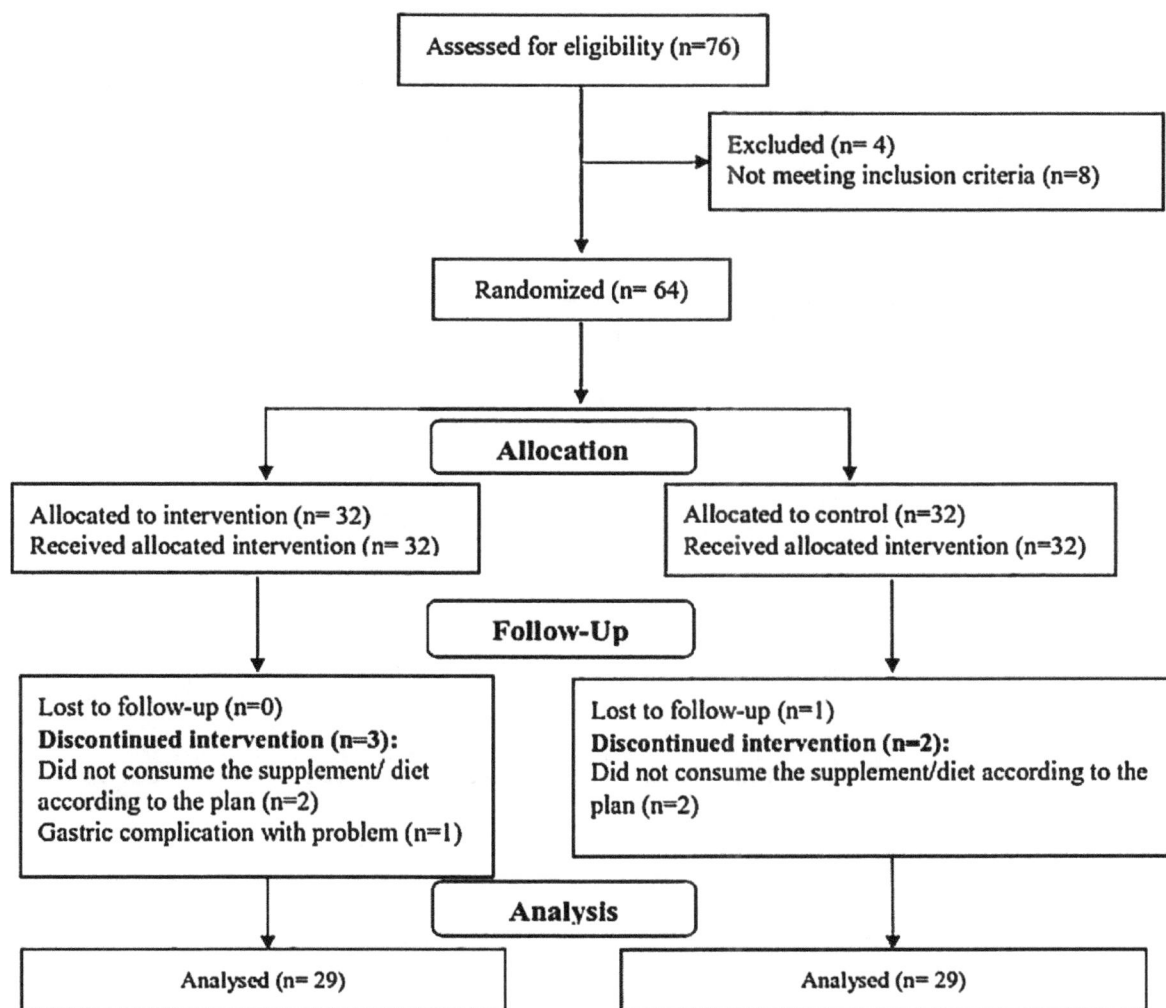

Figure 1. Flowchart of the study

There were no significant differences between the two study groups (except in height) at the baseline (Table 1). Table 3 shows anthropometric indices and body composition at baseline and at the end of the study. No significant differences were observed in the licorice and placebo groups at the start of the study. In the licorice group, a slight reduction (-2.3%) was observed in BMI at the end of the trial, but it was not significant within or between the groups (ANCOVA; adjusted for height and baseline value). FM decreased significantly at the end of the study in both groups when compared to the baseline (-7.2 vs. -6.5%; p<0.01). However, a comparison of licorice and placebo groups did not indicate any significant reduction in FM after the intervention (p=0.6). In both the licorice and placebo groups, FFM slightly increased (0.3%; p=0.8) and significantly decreased (-1.3%; p<0.01), respectively, but inter group comparisons did not show any significant differences in FFM at the end of the trial (p=0.7).

Table 1. Baseline characteristics of the study participants

	Variables	Licorice group (n=29)	Placebo group (n=29)
-	Age (year)	36.0 ± 11.9*	33.6 ± 4.8
Sex (n(%))	Male	13 (44.8)	14 (48.2)
	Female	16 (55.2)	15 (51.8)
-	Weight(kg)	87.6 ± 15.5	81.9 ± 11.0
	Height(cm)	161.9 ± 8.3	158.4 ± 5.8
Physical activity (n(%))	Sedentary	18 (62.0)	16 (55.1)
	Moderate	11 (38.0)	13 (44.9)

* Mean± SD

No adverse effects were observed on blood pressure (Table 2) and biochemical tests (Table 3) (p>0.05 for all variables). In this present study, the licorice supplement contained less than 0.01% Glycyrrhizin, so no significant changes were observed in SBP and DBP after 8 weeks of the intervention.

Biochemical parameters are presented in Table 3. At baseline there were no significant differences between the two study groups in biochemical parameters, except in fasting blood sugar (FBS) levels. Serum levels of FBS was not affected by the intervention (p=0.8). However, comparison between the two groups indicated that, insulin concentrations and HOMA-IR decreased in both the groups after 8 weeks of the intervention, and that significant reductions in insulin and insulin resistance were only observed in the licorice group when compared to baseline (ANCOVA, adjusted for changes in weight, energy intake changes, and baseline values). Further, no significant reduction of the two factors were observed between the two groups (p<0.05 for both variables).

Furthermore, levels of fat-derived hormones (vaspin and ZAG) also changed significantly following the licorice supplementation plus weight-loss diet when compared to baseline (-27.8 and 32.2%, respectively). Comparison of the licorice and placebo groups indicated that only the changes in serum levels of vaspin was significant at the end of the study (-27.8 vs. -4.2%, respectively).

Table 2. Comparison of anthropometric indices and body composition between Licorice and placebo groups at baseline and at the end of the trial

-	Variable	Licorice group (n=29)	Placebo group (n=29)	P-value** (Between groups)
BMI (Kg/m²)	Baseline	33.6±4.8*	32.7±3.7	0.4†
	End	32.8±4.8	32.3±3.5	0.2‡‡
	Pre to post P-value‡	0.3	0.6	
Waist circumference (cm)	Baseline	106.9±13.4	108.9±10.4	0.5†
	End	101.3±10.9	102.4±10.1	0.7
	Pre to post P-value‡	<0.01	<0.01	-
FM (Kg)	Baseline	31.7±8.3	30.6±6.7	0.5†
	End	29.4±10.6	28.6±6.3	0.6
	Pre to post P-value‡	<0.01	<0.01	-
FFM (Kg)	Baseline	55.9±10.7	51.3±8.0	0.04†
	End	56.1±12.0	50.6±5.1	0.7
	Pre to post P-value‡	0.8	<0.01	-
SBP (mmHg)	Baseline	110.2±10.1	110.5±10.5	0.4†
	End	109.0±10.0	110.0±10.4	0.8
	Pre to post P-value‡	0.2	0.2	-
DBP (mmHg)	Baseline	70.3±7.0	70.3±8.0	0.9†
	End	70.1±9.0	70.2±10.0	0.4
	Pre to post P-value‡	0.2	0.8	-

FM: Fat Mass; FFM: Fat Free Mass; SBP: Systolic Blood Pressure; DBP: Diastolic Blood Pressure
* Mean± SD
** ANCOVA (adjusted for energy intake changes and baseline values)
† Independent t-test
‡ Paired t-test
‡‡ ANCOVA (adjusted for height and baseline values)

Discussion

The present study highlights that licorice extract supplementation concurrently with a low-calorie diet, sufficiently attenuates serum levels of vaspin hormone in overweight and obese subjects with no significant side effects. The findings also revealed that a low-calorie while taking licorice supplementation was no more efficacious than a low-calorie diet alone on the management of obesity.

Table 3. Comparison of biochemical parameters between Licorice group and placebo group at baseline and at the end of trial

-	Variable	Licorice group (n=29)	Placebo group (n=29)	P-value (Between groups)**
FBS (mg/dL)	Baseline	98.5± 7.8*	93.2 ± 7.1	0.02†
	End	97.5 ± 7.3	93.5± 6.5	0.8
	Pre to post P-value‡	0.4	0.7	-
Vaspin (ng/mL)	Baseline	24.4±9.3	21.1±4.9	0.13†
	End	17.6±3.7	20.2±5.4	<0.01
	Pre to post P-value‡	0.01	0.1	-
ZAG (μg/mL)	Baseline	86.1±40.0	92.3±34.8	-
	End	113.9±57.5	101.3±40.2	0.5†
	Pre to post P-value‡	<0.01	0.4	0.4
Insulin (μU/mL)	Baseline	9.5 (5.3, 12.2)	9.5 (7.2, 13.5)	0.7†
	End	7.1 (5.0, 8.5)	9.2 (4.7, 11.0)	0.2
	Pre to post P-value‡	0.02	0.1	-
HOMA-IR	Baseline	2.3 (1.3, 3.0)	2.2 (1.3, 3.0)	0.8‡‡
	End	1.5 (1.2, 2.0)	2.0 (1.1, 2.5)	0.3
	Pre to post P-value‡	<0.01	0.4	-
AST (U/L)	Baseline	16.6±3.9	17.8±4.0	0.09†
	End	16.0±2.4	17.0±5.3	0.07
	Pre to post P-value‡	0.4	0.7	-
ALT (U/L)	Baseline	15.5±2.7	16.6±7.8	0.2†
	End	15.0±6.4	16.0±7.5	0.3
	Pre to post P-value‡	0.7	0.9	-

FBS: Fasting blood sugar; ZAG: Zinc alpha2 glyco protein; AST: Aspartate transaminase; ALT:Alanine aminotransferase
* Mean± SD
** ANCOVA (adjusted for weight changes, energy intake changes and baseline values)
† Independent t-test for variables with normal distribution and Mann-Whitney U test for variables with non-normal distribution
‡ Paired t-test
‡‡ ANCOVA (adjusted for FBS at baseline)

There are limited clinical trials with contradictory findings on the effects of licorice supplementation on anthropometric indices and body composition. Our findings were in accordance with two studies; Bell et al. reported that Glavonoid™ (Licorice Flavenoid Oil (LFO)) did not reduce body weight, FM and WC in overweight and grade I-II obese subjects after 8 weeks.[19] Moreover, Hajiaghamohammadi et al. reported that 2 g/day aqueous licorice extract did not reduce BMI in patients with non-alcoholic fatty liver disease after 8 weeks.[21] Our results were in opposition to Tominaga et al.'s study; who found that 300 and 1800 mg/day supplementation with Kaneka Glavonoid rich oil ™ (LFO) suppressed weight gain in overweight subjects with unhealthy lifestyle after 12 weeks. However, weight and BMI was increased at the end of the study in the placebo group. In addition, supplementation with 900 mg/day LFO decreased visceral fat in overweight subjects. They suggested that the reduction in FM was helpful in weight maintenance.[10] In another study in the U.S population, Tominaga et al. indicated that 300 mg/day LFO decreased WC and visceral fat after 12 weeks.[22]

Based on Armanina et al's., study, 3.5 g/day Licorice supplement decreased FM with no changes in BMI in normal weight subjects after 8 weeks.[15] Aoki et al. also indicated that adding 1 and 2% LFO to diet of obese mice for 8 weeks significantly slowed down weight gain and decreased abdominal white adipose tissue.[11] Differences in results of these studies may be due to differences in energy intake, physical activity level, dose and type of licorice (extract, oil), the duration of the intervention, BMI range and ethnic group. In our study, we compared the efficacy of licorice supplement concurrent with a calorie-restricted diet vs. a calorie-restricted diet alone. Based on evidence, differences between two groups were not significant at the end of the trial. It seems that licorice plus a weight loss diet prevents a reduction in FFM. However, they were not significant between the two intervention groups.

In this study, licorice extract with a calorie-restricted diet did not decrease serum levels of FBS, insulin concentrations, ZAG and HOMA-IR; but the intervention decreased serum levels of vaspin after 8 weeks. Limited clinical trials have evaluated the effects of licorice on glycemic status. In line with our study, Tominaga et al. found that 1800 mg/day LFO did not change FBS and insulin concentrations in overweight subjects after 12 weeks.[10] However, Luan et al. indicated that 10 µMg of glabridin, a main component of licorice, decreased insulin levels and insulin resistance in women with polycystic ovary syndrome after 12 months.[16] Zhao et al. demonstrated that 300 mg/day of licorice flavonoid decreased FBS and insulin levels in type 2 diabetic rats after 5 weeks,[17] and on Wu et al.'s study demonstrated that 40 mg/kg/day glabridin decreased FBS and insulin resistance in diabetic mice after 28 days.[18]

In our study, as no significant changes were observed in serum levels of FBS and insulin, insulin resistance did not change following the supplementation with Licorice extract. Reduction in body weight and fat mass are two main factors involve in improving insulin resistance in overweight and obese subjects. However, Licorice extract did not reduce these two anthropometric indices considerably. Therefore, no changes in insulin resistance might be due to this issue. In the current trial, we used the index of HOMA-IR to examine insulin resistance. There are several indices to assess this parameter.[23] Using different indices based on their different components can affect the results. Moreover, observing no changes in insulin resistance can be partially explained by the type of supplement. The aforementioned studies have examined licorice flavonoid, while our study assessed whole licorice extract. Different dosages, types of supplement, amounts of flavonoid, changes in weight, BMI at baseline, duration of the intervention, and methods for insulin resistant estimation are possible factors that can lead to different findings.

In our study, due to mineralcorticoid actions and vasopresser effects of Glycyrrihizin,[24,25] Glycyrrihizinhas been reduced to <0.01%. This could be attributed to the observation that the supplementation did not lead to any significant reduction in FBS and insulin concentrations. Furthermore, patient medical history, baseline BMI, dosages and form of licorice or its pure component and the duration of intervention can affect the final findings of each study.

To the best of our knowledge, our study was the first to evaluate the effects of supplementation with licorice extract on vaspin and ZAG hormone levels. Vaspin is an adipokine with insulin- sensitizing effects, and may be involved in obesity-associated diseases including type 2 diabetes, insulin resistance, atherosclerosis and cardiovascular disease. Therefore, it may be a possible target in the pharmaco-therapeutic treatment of obesity and its complications.[5,26] Handisurya et al. reported that

weight loss following gastric bypass decreased BMI and vaspin hormones in morbidly obese subjects after 12 months. They declared that visceral adipose tissue was the predominant localization for vaspin gene expression, and vaspin secretion decreased due to significant reductions in BMI after gastric bypass.[27] Based on Chung et al,. study lifestyle modification with orlistat decreased BMI and vaspin levels after 12 weeks. They hypothesized that weight loss (BMI reduction $\geq$ 2%) leads to a reduction in vaspin levels.[28] In this study, it seems that a larger reduction in BMI (-2.3%) in the licorice group compared to the placebo group might have resulted in a reduction in vaspin levels. However, due to the absence of adequate studies on the effects of licorice on vaspin levels, the underlying mechanisms are not clear. The results of our study contradict those of Koiuo et al. regarding changes in vaspin. They found that a calorie-restricted diet with orlistat or sibutramine decreased weight with no changes in vaspin concentrations after 6 months.[29] This discrepancy could be due to differences in the type of intervention, study duration and the rate of weight and BMI reduction.

Zinc-alpha 2 glycoprotein is an adipokine secreted from white and brown adipose tissues. Some studies have reported its possible effects on obesity and metabolic syndrome.[5,6] The expression of ZAG is regulated by TNF-alpha and PPAR-γ; thus, it may participate in lipid metabolism, enhance energy expenditure and skeletal muscle glucose transporters, inhibit of enzymes in lipogenesis pathways and stimulate adiponectin hormone expression.[30] In this study, there were no significant differences between the two groups. It seems that a greater reduction in weight or FM is needed to change levels of ZAG.

The main side effects of licorice are hypertension and hypokalemic-induced secondary disorders.[31] Glycyrrhizin plays a key role in occurring these side effects.[31] Therefore, in the present study we used a kind of licorice extract with reduced glycyrrhizin. Accordingly, except one who reported stomachache no side effects were reported.

This had some limitations. Firstly, the effects of licorice supplementation without calorie restricted diet were not evaluated. Secondly, the duration of the intervention was short and thirdly gene expressions of hormones were not measured. For future studies, we suggest that higher dosages and different forms (oil, pure components of licorice such as glabridin and flavonoids) of licorice extract are evaluated for their effect on the management of obesity.

Conclusion

We conclude that supplementation with dried licorice extract plus a low-calorie diet can increase vaspin levels in obese subjects, with no changes in insulin resistance and body composition. Overall, the effects of the intervention was not stronger than a low-calorie diet alone in the management of obesity.

Acknowledgments
We are grateful to the participants for their cooperation. The authors also would like to thank the Nutrition Research Center, Tabriz University of Medical Sciences for funding the project.

Conflicts of Interest
Authors declare no conflicts of interest

References
1. Galic S, Oakhill JS, Steinberg GR. Adipose tissue as an endocrine organ. *Mol Cell Endocrinol* 2010;316(2):129-39. doi: 10.1016/j.mce.2009.08.018
2. Bluher M. Adipose tissue dysfunction in obesity. *Exp Clin Endocrinol Diabetes* 2009;117(6):241-50. doi: 10.1055/s-0029-1192044
3. Poulos SP, Hausman DB, Hausman GJ. The development and endocrine functions of adipose tissue. *Mol Cell Endocrinol* 2010;323(1):20-34. doi: 10.1016/j.mce.2009.12.011
4. Auguet T, Quintero Y, Riesco D, Morancho B, Terra X, Crescenti A, et al. New adipokines vaspin and omentin. Circulating levels and gene expression in adipose tissue from morbidly obese women. *BMC Med Genet* 2011;12:60. doi: 10.1186/1471-2350-12-60
5. Bluher M. Vaspin in obesity and diabetes: Pathophysiological and clinical significance. *Endocrine* 2012;41(2):176-82. doi: 10.1007/s12020-011-9572-0
6. Gong FY, Zhang SJ, Deng JY, Zhu HJ, Pan H, Li NS, et al. Zinc-alpha2-glycoprotein is involved in regulation of body weight through inhibition of lipogenic enzymes in adipose tissue. *Int J Obes (Lond)* 2009;33(9):1023-30. doi: 10.1038/ijo.2009.141
7. Cabassi A, Tedeschi S. Zinc-alpha2-glycoprotein as a marker of fat catabolism in humans. *Curr Opin Clin Nutr Metab Care* 2013;16(3):267-71. doi: 10.1097/MCO.0b013e32835f816c
8. Mahdavi R, Alizadeh M, Namazi N, Farajnia S. Changes of body composition and circulating adipokines in response to nigella sativa oil with a calorie restricted diet in obese women. *J Herb Med* 2016; 6 (2):67-72.DOI: 10.1016/j.hermed.2016.03.003
9. Chan CC, Koo MW, Ng EH, Tang OS, Yeung WS, Ho PC. Effects of chinese green tea on weight, and hormonal and biochemical profiles in obese patients with polycystic ovary syndrome--a randomized placebo-controlled trial. *J Soc Gynecol Investig* 2006;13(1):63-8. doi: 10.1016/j.jsgi.2005.10.006
10. Tominaga Y, Mae T, Kitano M, Sakamoto Y, Ikematsu H, Nakagawa K. Licorice flavonoid oil effects body weight loss by reduction of body fat mass in overweight subjects. *J Health Sci* 2006;52(6):672-83. doi: 10.1248/jhs.52.672
11. Aoki F, Honda S, Kishida H, Kitano M, Arai N, Tanaka H, et al. Suppression by licorice flavonoids of abdominal fat accumulation and body weight gain in high-fat diet-induced obese c57bl/6j mice. *Biosci Biotechnol Biochem* 2007;71(1):206-14.
12. Mirtaheri E, Namazi N, Alizadeh M, Sargheini N, Karimi S. Effects of dried licorice extract with low-calorie diet on lipid profile and atherogenic indices in overweight and obese subjects: A randomized controlled clinical trial. *Eur J Integr Med* 2015;7(3):287-93. doi: 10.1016/j.eujim.2015.03.006
13. Ahn J, Lee H, Jang J, Kim S, Ha T. Anti-obesity effects of glabridin-rich supercritical carbon dioxide extract of licorice in high-fat-fed obese mice. *Food Chem Toxicol* 2013;51:439-45. doi: 10.1016/j.fct.2012.08.048
14. Parvaiz M, Hussain K, Khalid S, Hussnain N, Iram N, Hussain Z, et al. A review: Medicinal importance of glycyrrhiza glabra L.(fabaceae family). *Global J Pharmacol* 2014;8(1):8-13. doi: 10.5829/idosi.gjp.2014.8.1.81179
15. Armanini D, De Palo CB, Mattarello MJ, Spinella P, Zaccaria M, Ermolao A, et al. Effect of licorice on the reduction of body fat mass in healthy subjects. *J Endocrinol Invest* 2003;26(7):646-50. doi: 10.1007/bf03347023
16. Luan B-G, Sun C-X. Effect of glabridinon on insulin resistance, c-reactive protein and endothelial function in young women with polycystic ovary syndrome. *Bangladesh J Pharmacol* 2015;10(3):681-7. doi: 10.3329/bjp.v10i3.23648
17. Zhao H, Wang Y, Wu L, Yongping MA. Effect of licorice flavonoids on blood glucose, blood lipid and other biochemical indicators in type 2 diabetic rats. *China J Physiol* 2012;1:30–3.
18. Wu F, Jin Z, Jin J. Hypoglycemic effects of glabridin, a polyphenolic flavonoid from licorice, in an animal model of diabetes mellitus. *Mol Med Rep* 2013;7(4):1278-82. doi: 10.3892/mmr.2013.1330
19. Bell ZW, Canale RE, Bloomer RJ. A dual investigation of the effect of dietary supplementation with licorice flavonoid oil on anthropometric and biochemical markers of health and adiposity. *Lipids Health Dis* 2011;10:29. doi: 10.1186/1476-511x-10-29
20. Dai CY, Huang JF, Hsieh MY, Hou NJ, Lin ZY, Chen SC, et al. Insulin resistance predicts response to peginterferon-alpha/ribavirin combination therapy in chronic hepatitis c patients. *J Hepatol* 2009;50(4):712-8. doi: 10.1016/j.jhep.2008.12.017
21. Hajiaghamohammadi AA, Ziaee A, Samimi R. The efficacy of licorice root extract in decreasing transaminase activities in non-alcoholic fatty liver disease: A randomized controlled clinical trial. *Phytother Res* 2012;26(9):1381-4. doi: 10.1002/ptr.3728
22. Tominaga Y, Kitano M, Mae T, Kakimoto S, Nakagawa K. Effect of licorice flavonoid oil on visceral fat in obese subjects in the united states.

Nutrafoods 2014;13(1):35-43. doi: 10.1007/s13749-014-0002-9

23. Park SE, Park CY, Sweeney G. Biomarkers of insulin sensitivity and insulin resistance: Past, present and future. *Crit Rev Clin Lab Sci* 2015;52(4):180-90. doi: 10.3109/10408363.2015.1023429

24. Zadeh JB, Kor ZM, Goftar MK. Licorice (glycyrrhiza glabra linn) as a valuable medicinal plant. *Int J Adv Biol Biom Res* 2013;1(10):1281-8.

25. Shimoyama Y, Hirabayashi K, Matsumoto H, Sato T, Shibata S, Inoue H. Effects of glycyrrhetinic acid derivatives on hepatic and renal 11beta-hydroxysteroid dehydrogenase activities in rats. *J Pharm Pharmacol* 2003;55(6):811-7. doi: 10.1211/002235703765951429

26. Russell ST, Tisdale MJ. Antidiabetic properties of zinc-alpha2-glycoprotein in ob/ob mice. *Endocrinology* 2010;151(3):948-57. doi: 10.1210/en.2009-0827

27. Handisurya A, Riedl M, Vila G, Maier C, Clodi M, Prikoszovich T, et al. Serum vaspin concentrations in relation to insulin sensitivity following rygb-induced weight loss. *Obes Surg* 2010;20(2):198-203. doi: 10.1007/s11695-009-9882-y

28. Chung HK, Chae JS, Hyun YJ, Paik JK, Kim JY, Jang Y, et al. Influence of adiponectin gene polymorphisms on adiponectin level and insulin resistance index in response to dietary intervention in overweight-obese patients with impaired fasting glucose or newly diagnosed type 2 diabetes. *Diabetes care* 2009;32(4):552-8. doi: 10.2337/dc08-1605

29. Koiou E, Tziomalos K, Dinas K, Katsikis I, Kalaitzakis E, Delkos D, et al. The effect of weight loss and treatment with metformin on serum vaspin levels in women with polycystic ovary syndrome. *Endocr J* 2011;58(4):237-46.

30. Stejskal D, Karpisek M, Reutova H, Stejskal P, Kotolova H, Kollar P. Determination of serum zinc-alpha-2-glycoprotein in patients with metabolic syndrome by a new elisa. *Clin Biochem* 2008;41(4-5):313-6. doi: 10.1016/j.clinbiochem.2007.11.010

31. Nazari S, Rameshrad M, Hosseinzadeh H. Toxicological effects of glycyrrhiza glabra (licorice): A review. *Phytother Res* 2017;31(11):1635-50. doi: 10.1002/ptr.5893

21

Green Synthesis of Carbon Dots Derived from Walnut Oil and an Investigation of Their Cytotoxic and Apoptogenic Activities toward Cancer Cells

Elham Arkan[1], Ali barati[1], Mohsen Rahmanpanah[2], Leila Hosseinzadeh[2]*, Samaneh Moradi[2], Marziyeh Hajialyani[2]

[1] *Nano Drug Delivery Research Center, Kermanshah University of Medical Sciences, Kermanshah, Iran.*
[2] *Pharmaceutical Sciences Research Center, Faculty of Pharmacy, Kermanshah University of Medical Sciences, Kermanshah, Iran.*

Article info

Keywords:
· Apoptogenic Activity
· Carbon Quantum Dots
· Human Carcinoma Cell Lines
· Walnut Oil

Abstract

Purpose: This paper introduces a green and simple hydrothermal synthesis to prepare carbon quantum dots (CQDs) from walnut oil with a high quantum yield. In addition, cytotoxic and apoptogenic properties of the CQDs were analyzed on human cancer cell lines.

Methods: The optical properties and morphological characteristic were investigated by the TEM, XRD, FT-IR, UV-vis and photoluminescence (PL).The cytotoxic potential of walnut CQDs was evaluated on PC3, MCF-7 and HT-29 human carcinoma cell lines using the MTT methods. The mechanism of action was studied by investigating the mode of cell death using the activation of caspase-3 and 9 as well as mitochondrial membrane potential (MMP). Cellular uptake of the CQDs was detected by fluorescence microscope. CQDs had an average size of 12 nm and a significant emission at 420 nm at an excitation wavelength of 350 nm was recorded.

Results: The prepared CQDs possessed a good fluorescent quantum yield of 14.5% with quinine sulfate (quantum yield 54%) as a reference and excellent photo as well as pH stabilities. The walnut CQDs were proved to be an extremely potent cytotoxic agent, especially against MCF-7 and PC-3 cell lines. Induction of apoptosis by CQDs was accompanied by an increase in the activation of caspase-3. Caspase-9 activity did not increase after exposure to the CQDs. Additionally; the MMP did not show any significant loss.

Conclusion: The results of our study can corroborate the cytotoxic and apoptotic effect of walnut CQDs in the PC3 and MCF-7 cancer cell lines.

Introduction

Carbon-based materials have some properties such as good flexibility, high strength and stability and excellent electrical and thermal conductivity. Carbon fibers, fullerene, porous materials, carbon nanotubes and carbon quantum dots are some of the members in the carbon-based family.[1] Carbon quantum dots (CQDs) are taken into account as a new class of nano-carbonaceous materials with photoluminescence properties discovered by Xu et al. (2004).[2,3]

It now seems that priority of the CQDs rather than semiconductor quantum dots and organic dyes is due to their high optical and chemical stability and biocompatibility.In addition, they have low metabolic degradation, bright fluorescence, low toxicity, suitable water solubility and low photo-degradation.[4,5] These advantages suggest that the CQDs can be used as a non-toxic replacement for semiconductor quantum dots. Laser irradiation,[6] ultrasonic treatment,[7] hydrothermal treatment,[8] and electrochemical oxidation,[9] are methods

developed for the preparation of the CQDs. Some of these methods have some defects such as complicated process, expensive material and equipment required and low reported yields. However, using a cost-effective and high-yield method for large scale fluorescent CQDs preparation is important. Hydrothermal method is one of the proper approaches for the production of carbon dots that can produce them from different sources of carbon including organ molecules and carbohydrates.[10]

Furthermore, the most important advantages of the CQDs is that they have many hydroxyl and carboxyl groups on their surface.[11] The mentioned groups can be beneficial for therapeutic agents conjugation and biological effects in the fields of multicolor bio-labeling and bio-imaging,[12] and catalysis.[13]Moreover, there have been several studies about anticancer effects of the CQDs.[14] Natural products are the useful sources which could be used in the preparation of CQDs.[15] Chi-Lin Li et al. used Ginger for production of CQDs and observed

*Corresponding author: Leila Hosseinzadeh, Email: lhoseinzadeh@kums.ac.ir

that the obtained CQDs selectively inhibited the growth of the HepG2 cells.[14] In addition, the suppressor activity of green tea-derived CQDs was shown against two human breast carcinoma cell lines.[16]

The present study aims to produce CQDs by a facile, green, and low-cost hydrothermal method using walnut (*Jungleregia*) oil, as the precursor. It must be noted that there are several investigations on the anti-proliferative effects of the different parts (leaf, seed, root and green husk) of this medicinal plant.[17,18] Next, the cytotoxic effects of the CQDs were investigated on three human cancer cell lines: PC3, MCF-7 and HT-29 cells. Moreover, the molecular mechanisms, in which CQDs exert the cytotoxic effect, were also assessed on the most sensitive cell lines.

Materials and Methods

Hydrazine and ammonium bromide were purchased from Merck (Germany). 3-(4,5-dimethylthiazol-2yl)-2,5-diphenyltetrazoliumbromide (MTT), rhodamine, caspase 9 substrate and Caspase-3 Detection assay Kit were purchased from Sigma Aldrich (St Louis, MO, USA). Cell culture medium, penicillin–streptomycin, and fetal bovine serum (FBS) were obtained from Gibco (Gibco, Grand Island, NY, USA).

Synthesis of Carbon Dots

In the present study, CQDs were produced using hydrothermal methods as follows.

The oil was separated from walnut and passed through Whatman filter paper to eliminate large particles. The oil was then centrifuged for 15 min at 6000 rpm for five times. Then, 30 ml of the clear walnut oil was transferred into a 100 mL Teflon-lined stainless steel laboratory autoclave and heated in an oven at temperature of 220°C for 24 h, and cooled to room temperature. The brownish solution was centrifuged at 14000 rpm for 15 min for three times to remove large or agglomerated particles and the supernatant containing CQDs was further purified using a 0.2 μm membrane.

Quantum yield

The relative fluorescence quantum yield of resultant CQDs were evaluated at an excitation wavelength of 320 nm and the following equation was used :

$$Q_x = Q_r \left(\frac{I_x}{I_r} \right) \left(\frac{A_r}{A_x} \right) \left(\frac{\eta_x^2}{\eta_r^2} \right)$$

Where, r and x reflect the standard reference and the sample of interest respectively, Q is the quantum yield, I is the integrated emission spectra, η is the refractive index of the solvent, and A is the absorbance. In order to avoid self-absorption effect, the absorbance was kept below 0.1 quinine sulfate in 0.1 M H2SO4 because lead to avoid self-absorption effects. Quinine sulfate had known quantum yield of 0.54 that was selected as standard reference.

Cell culture

PC3, human prostate cancer cell line, was obtained from Pasteur Institute (Tehran, Iran). The PC3 was established in 1979 from bone metastasis of grade IV of prostate cancer in a 62-year-old Caucasian male. This cell line is useful to evaluate prostatic cancer cells response to anti-cancer drugs.[19] MCF-7 human breast cancer cells are used widely for research on chemotherapy agents for breast cancer.[20] HT-29 is a human colorectal adenocarcinoma cell line with epithelial morphology. This cell line was established in 1964 from the primary tumor of a 44-year-old Caucasian female with colorectal adenocarcinoma.[21] The cells were cultured in Dulbecco's modified Eagle's medium (DMEM-F12) with 5% (v/v) fetal bovine serum, 100 U/mL penicillin, and 100 mg/mL streptomycin. The medium was changed 2-3 days and was sub-cultured when the cell population density reached to 70–80% confluence.

Assay of inhibitory effects of CQDs on the growth of human carcinoma cell lines

The inhibitory effects of walnut CQDs on the growth of PC3, MCF-7, and HT-29 cells were evaluated by MTT assay. Briefly, the cells were suspended in a mixture of DMEM-F12 and 10% bovine serum, 100 units/mL of penicillin and 100 μg/mL of streptomycin at a concentration of 1×10^5 cells/mL. The cell suspension was pipetted into a 96-well plate (100 μL /well) and was permitted to adhere in a humidified incubator containing 5% CO2 at 37 °C. 24 hours after seeding, the cells were treated with different concentrations (0-10 μg/mL) of CQDs dissolved in DMSO. After 24 h, the medium was replaced by 100 μL of 0.5 mg/mL of MTT in growth medium and were incubated at 37°C for 3 hrs. Next, the supernatants were removed carefully and DMSO (100 μL) was added to each well to dissolve formazan crystals. Then, the absorbance of each well at 570 nm was determined using an Elisa plate reader (Synergy-2 of BioTek Instruments Inc., Winooski, VT, USA). For each compound the IC50 value was calculated by plotting the log 10 of the viability percentage versus concentration .

Cellular uptake of CQDs

The cellular uptake of CQDs was evaluated in MCF-7 and PC-3 cells. Briefly, the cells were seeded in 12-well plates at a density of 5.0×10^5 cells/well. After 24 h the cells were treated with the fresh medium containing the IC50 concentration of CQDs and followed by incubation for 4 h at 37°C in a 5% CO2/95% air atmosphere. Fluorescence images were taken at 100 magnifications under a fluorescence microscope (Micros AUSTR1A) with imaging system. The cells without any CQDs treatment were used as a comparative control.

Assessment of Mitochondrial Membrane Potential (MMP)

Rhodamine 123 florescent dye, a cell permeable cationic dye, was used in MMP assay. Depolarization of MMP during cell apoptosis results in the loss of rhodamine 123 from the mitochondria and a decrease in intracellular florescence ntensity.[22] At the end of treatment, cells were incubated with rhodamine 123 for 30 min at 37 °C. The fluorescence intensity was measured at an excitation wavelength of 488 nm and an emission wavelength of 520 nm using a florescence microplate reader (BioTek, H1M, USA).

Measurement of caspase-3 and caspase-9 activities

The caspases activities were determined based on the manual of the sigma Caspase-3 assay kit. Briefly, cells were detached and lysed with lysis buffer containing protease inhibitors. The lysed cells centrifuged for 10 min at 14000 rpm. Next, the supernatant was transferred to a tube and mixed with caspase-3 and caspase-9 substrates. After 1 h incubation at 37°C, the absorbance of the chromophore p-nitroanilide was detected by a microplate reader at 405 nm. As a control, non-treated cells were analyzed and the data were expressed by percentage of control.

Statistical analysis

All data were analyzed using one-way ANOVA using Graph Pad Prism software (GraphPad software, San Diego, CA, USA). Differences between the mean$\pm$ SEM (standard error of the mean) of samples were considered significant at $P < 0.05$. The IC_{50} values were generated from the MTT results using GraphPad Prism software.

Results and Discussion

Characterization of CQDs

In the FTIR spectra of the CQDs, the spread band observed at 3200-3500 cm^{-1} belonged to C–OH and N–H stretching vibrations. Also, one at 2800-2950 cm^{-1} was assigned to the C–H stretching vibrations (Figure 1-a). The bending vibrations of the N–H could appear at 1400 cm^{-1}. Peaks appearing at approximately 1600 and 1280 cm^{-1} indicated the presence of C=O and C–NH–C stretching vibration, respectively. The band at approximately 1066 cm^{-1} presented the existence of C–O (hydroxyl, ester, epoxide or ether) groups.

The TEM images (Figure 1-b) showed that the CQDs were spherical as well as monodisperse and had a narrow size distribution. The average diameter of the CQDs was 12.3 ± 2.7 nm.

The XRD pattern of the prepared CQDs (Figure 1-c) displayed a broad peak centered at approximately $2\theta=20°$, indicating a graphitic nature with highly disordered carbon atoms.

The elementary composition of the prepared CQDs was confirmed by elemental analysis. The results for the presented atoms were: C 37.26 wt.%; N 2.25 wt.%; H 4.07 wt.%; S 0.97 wt.% and O (calculated) 55.45 wt.%. We also showed the diluted walnut oil and walnut CQDs in hexane under room light (Figure 1-d) and UV light (365 nm) (Figure 1-e).

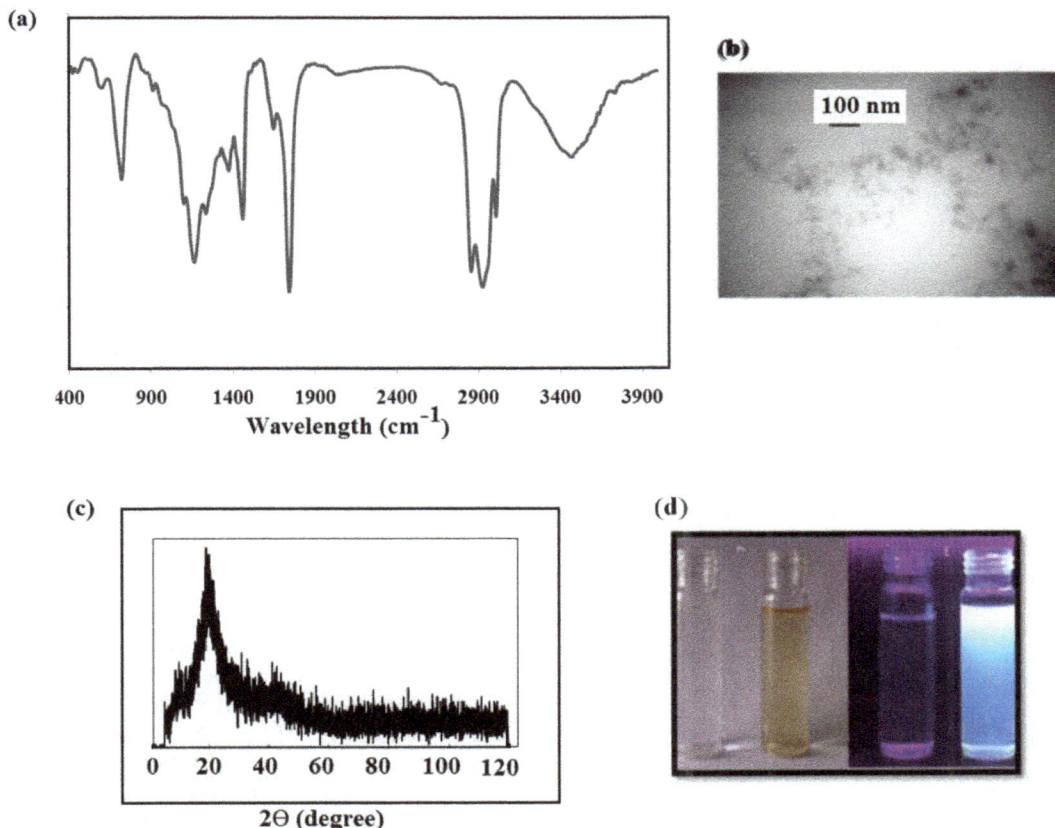

Figure 1. (a) FTIR spectra, (b) TEM images at different magnifications 100 nm of CQDs and (c) XRD pattern of CQDs prepared from walnut oil. The photographs of prepared CQDs in solution under visible light (d) and 365 nm UV lamp light (e).

Optical Properties of the CQDs

The optical properties of the CQDs were investigated by photoluminescence (PL) and excitation spectra of the prepared CQDs at room temperature.

In the UV–Vis spectrum corresponding to the CQDs, a sharp peak at220 nm and a broad peak at 270 nm (Figure 2-a) were shown. The observed peaks could be assigned to π–π^* and n–π^* transitions of C=C and C=O bonds. Increasing the peak at 270 nm conformed the addition of more C=O bonds to the CQD structures. The PL recorded at the excitation wavelengths ranging from 320 to 440 nm indicated a generic excitation-dependent property (Figure 2-b). The maximum PL appeared at the excitation of 360 nm with the maximum at 430 nm. The quantum yield of the CQDs was estimated to be 14.5 at an excitation wavelength of 340 nm and in the presence of quinine sulfate as a standard reference. The results showed a strong and stable PL, which was found excitation-dependent.

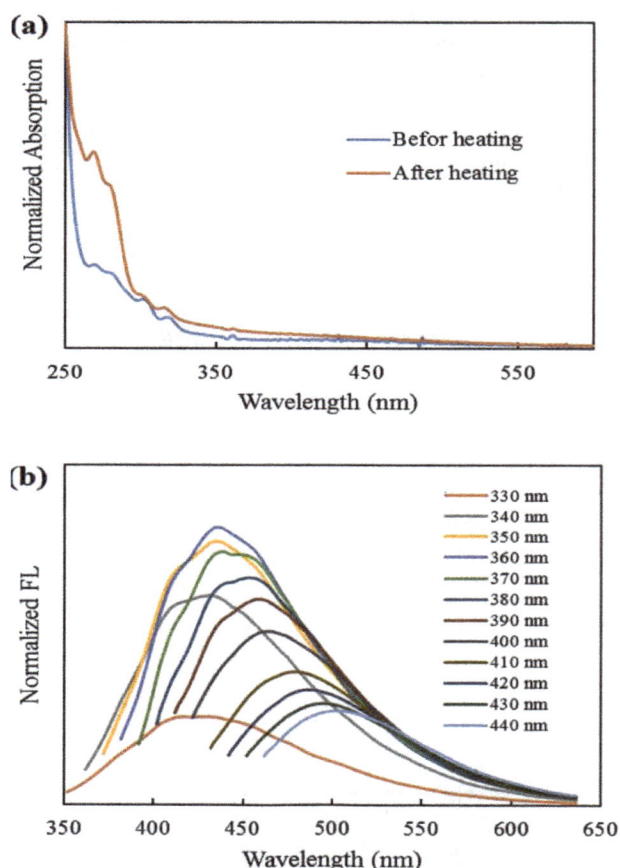

(a)

(b)

Figure 2.(a) UV–Vis absorption spectrum before and after converting the walnut oil to CQDs (b) UV-vis absorption and PL emission spectra of the prepared CQDs from walnut oil.

Inhibition of Cell Viability

MTT assay was performed in order to examine the possible anti-proliferative effect of CQDs on PC3, MCF7 and HT-29 cell lines. Complete dose-response curves were generated and IC_{50} values were calculated against three human carcinoma cell lines. Walnut CQDs have

proved to be an outstandingly potent cytotoxic agent, especially against PC3 and MCF7 cell lines as confirmed by its IC_{50} value. As shown in Figure 3, exposure to the CQDs for 24 hrs resulted in a concentration-dependent decrease in cell viability, with the approximate IC_{50} of 1.25 ± 0.062 µg/cc, 5 ± 1.03µg/cc , and >10 µg/cc in MCF-7, PC-3 and human carcinoma cell lines, respectively.

The synthesized CQDs decreased the cell proliferation by 50% in the MCF-7 and PC-3 cancer cells at the concentrations of 1.25µg/mL and 5µg/mL, respectively. These values are below20 µg/mL, indicating that the CQDs potentially present an interesting cytotoxic activity toward the PC3 and MCF-7, and human carcinoma cell lines.[23,24]

As mentioned before, the different parts (leaf, seed, root and green husk) of walnut (*Jungle regia*) have shown cytotoxic effect against human carcinoma cell line. Wei *et al.* showed the inhibitory effect of the *J. regia* leaf extract on the growth of PC-3 cells (IC_{50}= 48.4 µg/mL) through apoptosis. Furthermore, the cell cycle phase distribution altered after exposure to the mentioned extract in the PC-3 cell line.[25] In the another study, Carvalho *et al.* evaluated the anti-proliferative effect of walnut leaf, green husk and seed methanolic extracts on renal carcinoma cell lines, A498 and 769P as well as Caco-2, human epithelial colorectal adenocarcinoma cells. Their results revealed that walnut extracts exert the slight inhibitory effect on the growth of cells.[26]

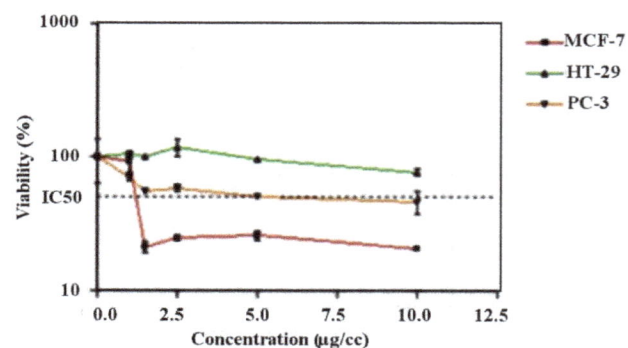

Figure3. Cytotoxic effects of CQDs in human carcinoma cell lines. PC-3, MCF-7 and HT29 cells were incubated with different concentrations of CQDs for 24 h. The cell proliferation inhibition was determined by MTT assay as described under materials and methods. Data are presented as mean ± S.E.M (n=3)

Cellular Uptake of CQDs

In an attempt to assess whether walnut CQDs are able to enter the cells, we performed fluorescence microscopy imaging of the cells incubated with the CQDs (Figure 4). As shown in Figure 4-a, after the treatment, we observed bright fluorescence intensity spread all over the cells incubated with the CQDs. In addition, as Figures 4-b and 4-c show, the intracellular fluorescence of the CQDs increased the dose dependently after exposure to different concentrations of the CQDs in PC3 and MCF-7 cell line, respectively.

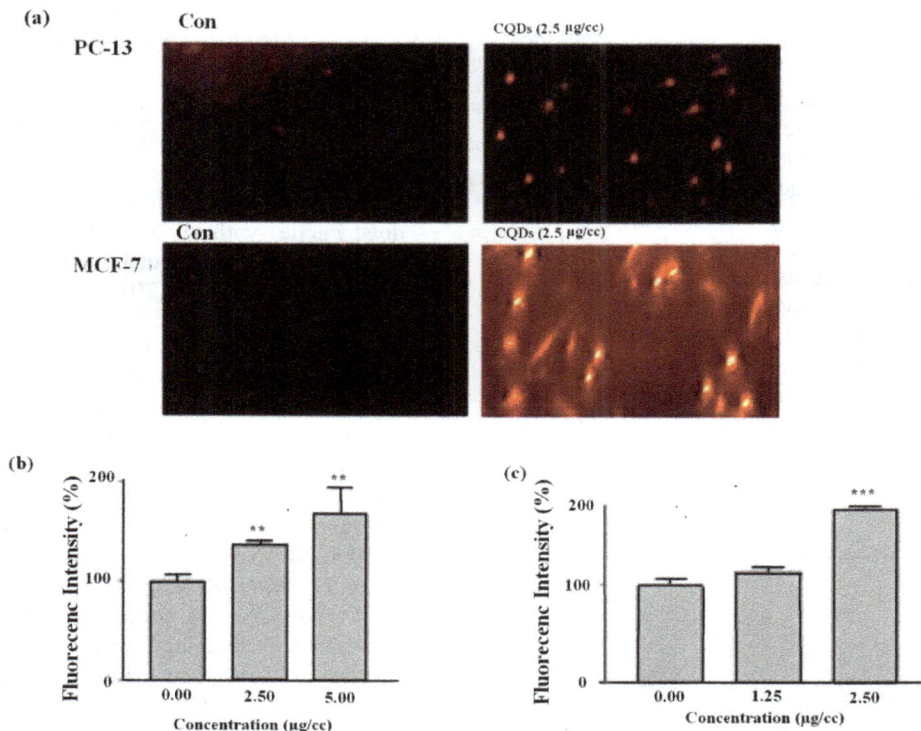

Figure 4.(a) Fluoroescence microscope images demonstrating the intracellular distribution in PC3 and MCF-7 cell lines.CQDs accumulation in (b) PC3 and (c) MCF-7 cells after 4 h exposure to different concentrations of CQDs. Data are presented as mean ± S.E.M (n=3). **$P< 0.01$, ***$P< 0.001$ versus control.

The apoptotic potentials of the CQDs: Effects of CQDs on Caspases – 3 and 9 activities and MMP

Apoptosis has been accepted as a preferable mode of action of the antitumor drug,[27] and considerable effort is directed toward the development of potential medicines inducing apoptosis in the malignant cells. Therefore, we investigated the apoptotic potentials of the CQDs on the most sensitive cell lines using some apoptosis- related parameters. Activation of caspases is well-known to play an essential role in the initiation and progression of programmed cell death. From this family, caspase-3 is an executioner caspase that proteolytically cleave many proteins playing a central role in apoptotic cell death.[28] It serves as a target for different signaling pathways of the programmed cell death. In order to indicate the type of cell death involved in our experiments, the activity of caspase-3 and caspase-9 was examined in PC-3 and MCF-7 cells. The obtained results showed the dose-dependent alteration of the caspase-3 activity and exposure to the CQDs caused increasing the caspase-3 activity of both MCF-7 and PC3 cell lines (Figures 5-a, 5-b). The drugs used in chemotherapy, induce apoptosis through death receptor pathway (extrinsic) or at the mitochondria by stimulating the intrinsic pathway.[29] Thepermeabilization of the mitochondrial membrane during mitochondria dependent pathway, causes bioenergetics failure and permits the release of a small hem protein, cytochrome c (Cyt c), to the cytosol, leading to caspase-9 activation.[28] To determine which

apoptotic pathway is activated by the CQDs, the activation of caspase-9 was examined. As Figure 4-b shows, 24h treatment with the CQDs was not able to increase the activation of caspase- 9 in the MCF-7 and PC-3 cell lines.

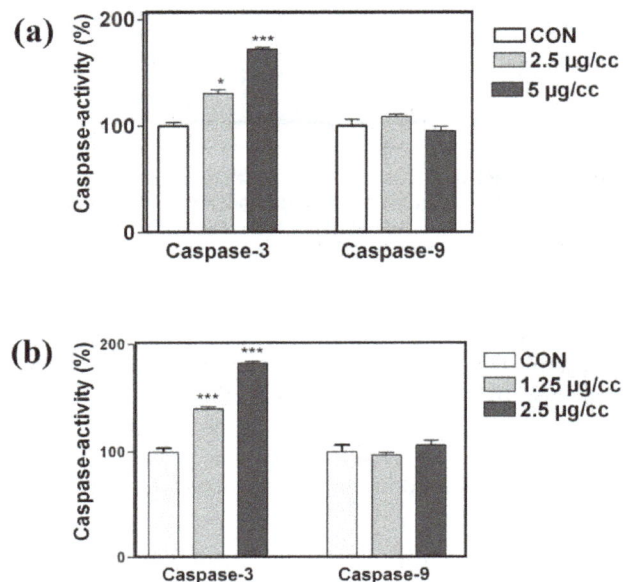

Figure 5. Involvement of activation of caspases in the induction of apoptosis by walnut CQDs in PC3 and MCF-7 cancer cells. Cells were incubated with CQDs for 24 h and cell lysates were assayed using microplate reader for activation caspases. Significant differences were compared with the control. Data are presented as mean ± S.E.M. *$P< 0.05$,**$P< 0.01$, versus control.

The involvement of the mitochondrial pathway in the CQD-mediated apoptotic cell death was also examined by measuring the MMP in the PC-3 and MCF-7 cells. As shown in Figure 5, when cells were treated with the CQDs for 24 h at 37°C, no decrease in the retention of rhodamine 123 was observed at the used concentrations (Figure 6). These results suggest that the mitochondrial pathway probably does not cause a substantial role in the CQD-induced apoptosis. In the recent study, a novel bio-peptide isolated from walnut residual protein and its anti-proliferative ability was evaluated against human carcinoma cell line. Results indicated that the isolated bio-peptide was able to inhibit cancer cells growth selectively through inducing apoptosis and could be used for cancer treatment.[30]

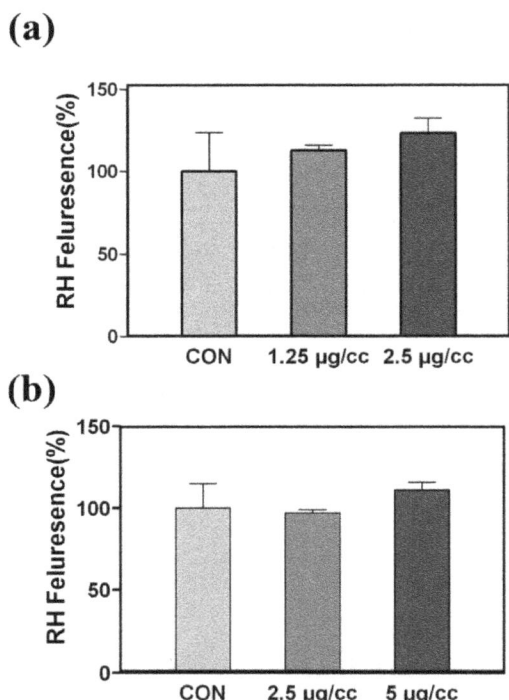

(a)

(b)

Figure 6. Effect of CQDs on MMP collapse.(a) MCF-7 and (b) PC3 cells were treated with different concentrations of CQDs for 24 h. Graphs show the change in MMP as represented by the mean florescence intensity (MFI) of rhodamine 123.

Conclusion
It can be concluded that walnut carbon quantum dots have cytotoxic and apoptotic potential on prostate and breast cancer cells. Therefore, these CQDs may be considered an economical and easily accessible source of effective agents used in cancer chemotherapy.

Acknowledgments
The authors gratefully acknowledge the research council of Kermanshah University of Medical Sciences for the financial support. This work was performed in partial fulfillment of the requirement for pharm.D of Mohsen Rahmanpanah, in faculty of pharmacy, Kermanshah University of Medical Sciences, Kermanshah, Iran.

Conflict of Interest
The authors declare no conflict of interests.

References
1. Zhang R, Chen W. Nitrogen-doped carbon quantum dots: Facile synthesis and application as a "turn-off" fluorescent probe for detection of Hg2+ ions. *Biosens Bioelectron* 2014;55:83-90. doi: 10.1016/j.bios.2013.11.074
2. Li Y, Zhang X, Luo J, Huang W, Cheng J, Luo Z, et al. Purification of CVD synthesized single-wall carbon nanotubes by different acid oxidation treatments. *Nanotechnology* 2004;15(11):1645. doi: 10.1088/0957-4484/15/11/047
3. Baker SN, Baker GA. Luminescent carbon nanodots: emergent nanolights. *Angew Chem Int Ed Engl* 2010;49(38):6726-44. doi: 10.1002/anie.200906623
4. Yang ST, Wang X, Wang H, Lu F, Luo PG, Cao L, et al. Carbon dots as nontoxic and high-performance fluorescence imaging agents. *J Phys Chem C Nanomater Interfaces* 2009;113(42):18110-4. doi: 10.1021/jp9085969
5. Dong Y, Pang H, Yang HB, Guo C, Shao J, Chi Y, et al. Carbon-Based Dots Co-doped with Nitrogen and Sulfur for High Quantum Yield and Excitation-Independent Emission. *Angew Chem Int Ed Engl* 2013;52(30):7800-4. doi: 10.1002/anie.201301114
6. Sun YP, Zhou B, Lin Y, Wang W, Fernando KA, Pathak P, et al. Quantum-sized carbon dots for bright and colorful photoluminescence. *J Am Chem Soc* 2006;128(24):7756-7. doi: 10.1021/ja062677d
7. Li H, He X, Liu Y, Huang H, Lian S, Lee ST, et al. One-step ultrasonic synthesis of water-soluble carbon nanoparticles with excellent photoluminescent properties. *Carbon* 2011;49(2):605-9. doi: 10.1016/j.carbon.2010.10.004
8. Qu S, Wang X, Lu Q, Liu X, Wang L. A Biocompatible Fluorescent Ink Based on Water-Soluble Luminescent Carbon Nanodots. *Angew Chem* 2012;124(49):12381-4. doi: 10.1002/ange.201206791
9. Li H, He X, Kang Z, Huang H, Liu Y, Liu J, et al. Water-soluble fluorescent carbon quantum dots and photocatalyst design. *Angew Chem Int Ed Engl* 2010;49(26):4430-4. doi: 10.1002/anie.200906154
10. Barati A, Shamsipur M, Arkan E, Hosseinzadeh L, Abdollahi H. Synthesis of biocompatible and highly photoluminescent nitrogen doped carbon dots from lime: Analytical applications and optimization using response surface methodology. *Mater Sci Eng C Mater Biol Appl* 2015;47:325-32. doi: 10.1016/j.msec.2014.11.035
11. Yang C, Ogaki R, Hansen L, Kjems J, Teo BM. Theranostic carbon dots derived from garlic with efficient anti-oxidative effects towards macrophages. *RSC Adv* 2015;5(118):97836-40. doi: 10.1039/C5RA16874K

12. Qu K, Wang J, Ren J, Qu X. Carbon Dots Prepared by Hydrothermal Treatment of Dopamine as an Effective Fluorescent Sensing Platform for the Label-Free Detection of Iron(III) Ions and Dopamine. *Chemistry* 2013;19(22):7243-9. doi: 10.1002/chem.201300042

13. Zhao S, Lan M, Zhu X, Xue H, Ng TW, Meng X, et al. Green Synthesis of Bifunctional Fluorescent Carbon Dots from Garlic for Cellular Imaging and Free Radical Scavenging. *ACS Appl Mater Interfaces* 2015;7(31):17054-60. doi: 10.1021/acsami.5b03228

14. Li CL, Ou CM, Huang CC, Wu WC, Chen YP, Lin TE, et al. Carbon dots prepared from ginger exhibiting efficient inhibition of human hepatocellular carcinoma cells. *J Mater Chem B* 2014;2(28):4564-71. doi: 10.1039/C4TB00216D

15. Mehta VN, Jha S, Basu H, Singhal RK, Kailasa SK. One-step hydrothermal approach to fabricate carbon dots from apple juice for imaging of mycobacterium and fungal cells. *Sens Actuators B Chem* 2015;213:434-43. doi: 10.1016/j.snb.2015.02.104

16. Hsu PC, Chen PC, Ou CM, Chang HY, Chang HT. Extremely high inhibition activity of photoluminescent carbon nanodots toward cancer cells. *J Mater Chem B* 2013;1(13):1774-81. doi: 10.1039/C3TB00545C

17. Shah TI, Sharma E, Shah GA. Anti-proliferative, cytotoxicity and anti-oxidant activity of Juglans regia extract. *Am J Cancer Prev* 2015;3(2):45-50. doi: 10.12691/ajcp-3-2-4

18. Salimi M, Majd A, Sepahdar Z, Azadmanesh K, Irian S, Ardestaniyan MH, et al. Cytotoxicity effects of various Juglans regia (walnut) leaf extracts in human cancer cell lines. *Pharm Biol* 2012;50(11):1416-22. doi: 10.3109/13880209.2012.682118

19. Shokoohinia Y, Hosseinzadeh L, Alipour M, Mostafaie A, Mohammadi-Motlagh HR. Comparative evaluation of cytotoxic and apoptogenic effects of several coumarins on human cancer cell lines: osthole induces apoptosis in p53-deficient H1299 cells. *Adv Pharmacol Sci* 2014;2014:847574. doi: 10.1155/2014/847574

20. Osborne CK, Hobbs K, Trent JM. Biological differences among MCF-7 human breast cancer cell lines from different laboratories. *Breast Cancer Res Treat* 1987;9(2):111-21. doi: 10.1007/BF01807363

21. Cohen E, Ophir I, Shaul YB. Induced differentiation in HT29, a human colon adenocarcinoma cell line. *J Cell Sci* 1999;112(Pt 16):2657-66.

22. Perry SW, Norman JP, Barbieri J, Brown EB, Gelbard HA. Mitochondrial membrane potential probes and the proton gradient: a practical usage guide. *BioTechniques* 2011;50(2):98-115. doi: 10.2144/000113610

23. Lee CC, Houghton P. Cytotoxicity of plants from Malaysia and Thailand used traditionally to treat cancer. *J Ethnopharmacol* 2005;100(3):237-43. doi: 10.1016/j.jep.2005.01.064

24. Geran RI, Greenberg NH, McDonald MM, Schumacher AM, Abbott BJ. Protocols for screening chemical agents and natural products against animal tumour and other biological systems. *Cancer Chemother Rep* 1972;3:17-9.

25. Li W, Li DY, Wang HD, Zheng ZJ, Hu J, Li ZZ. Juglans regia Hexane Extract Exerts Antitumor Effect, Apoptosis Induction and Cell Circle Arrest in Prostate Cancer Cells in vitro. *Trop J Pharm Res* 2015;14(3):399-405. doi: 10.4314/tjpr.v14i3.7

26. Carvalho M, Ferreira PJ, Mendes VS, Silva R, Pereira JA, Jeronimo C, et al. Human cancer cell antiproliferative and antioxidant activities of Juglans regia L. *Food Chem Toxicol* 2010;48(1):441-7. doi: 10.1016/j.fct.2009.10.043

27. Milner AE, Palmer DH, Hodgkin EA, Eliopoulos AG, Knox PG, Poole CJ, et al. Induction of apoptosis by chemotherapeutic drugs: the role of FADD in activation of caspase-8 and synergy with death receptor ligands in ovarian carcinoma cells. *Cell Death Differ* 2002;9(3):287-300. doi: 10.1038/sj.cdd.4400945

28. Elmore S. Apoptosis: a review of programmed cell death. *Toxicol Pathol* 2007;35(4):495-516. doi: 10.1080/01926230701320337

29. Ahmadi F, Derakhshandeh K, Jalalizadeh A, Mostafaie A, Hosseinzadeh L. Encapsulation in PLGA-PEG enhances 9- nitro-camptothecin cytotoxicity to human ovarian carcinoma cell line through apoptosis pathway. *Res Pharm Sci* 2015;10(2):161-8.

30. Ma S, Huang D, Zhai M, Yang L, Peng S, Chen C, et al. Isolation of a novel bio-peptide from walnut residual protein inducing apoptosis and autophagy on cancer cells. *BMC Complement Altern Med* 2015;15:413. doi: 10.1186/s12906-015-0940-9

22

Evaluation of Volatile Profile, Fatty Acids Composition and in vitro Bioactivity of *Tagetes minuta* Growing Wild in Northern Iran

Farshid Rezaei, Rashid Jamei*, Reza Heidari

Department of Biology, Faculty of Science, University of Urmia, West Azerbaijan, Iran.

Article info

Keywords:
· *Tagetes minuta*
· GC-MS analysis
· Antioxidant capacity
· Fatty acid
· HPLC-UV

Abstract

Purpose: The aim of the present study was to investigate the chemical properties of wild *Tagetes minuta* L. (family Astreacea) collected from Northern Iran during the flowering period concerning the chemical combination of the essential oil along with its antioxidant properties and composition of fatty acids.

Methods: The essential oil of the plant was extracted by a Clevenger approach and analyzed using gas chromatography-mass spectroscopy (Capillary HP-5ms GC/MS Column). Fatty acid contents of this species as a result of hexane extraction were analyzed by means of gas chromatography (GC-FID) while their phenolic contents were analyzed by high performance liquid chromatography (HPLC-UV). In this research also the total polyphenolic (TPC) and total flavonoid (TFC) content was determined spectrophotometrically while the antioxidant activity was evaluated using the DPPH (2,2'-diphenyl-1-picrylhydrazyl) bleaching method.

Results: GC/MS analysis of the essential oil identified monoterpenoid fractions (52.13%) as the main components and among them dihydrotagetone (23.44%) and spathulenol (10.56%) were the predominant compounds. The evaluation of fatty acid content revealed that saturated acids were prevailing compounds and the major components are: palmitic (30.74±0.4%) and capric (24.15±0.5%) acids. Chromatographic separation of its phenolic contents indicated that this herb contain sinapic acid derivatives rather than hydroxybenzoic acid derivatives. Also the essential oil showed an effective antioxidant capacity (TPC=153.27±0.9 mg/g, TFC=63.79±0.1 mg/g, IC_{50} = 29.31±0.8 µg/ml).

Conclusion: The results proved that the plant could be used for nutritional and pharmaceutical purposes.

Introduction

Tagetes minuta from sunflower (Asteraceae - Helenieae) family is a species native to South America but is now a widespread weed in most parts of the world.[1] *T. minuta* is reported to contain a number of bioactive metabolites of high medicinal, industrial and nutritional value.[2,3] The majority of published studies of *T. minuta* focused on the chemodiversity of volatile oils, flavonoids and thiophenes.[4] Etheric oils are a source of bioactive and valuable molecules that are used in many fields such as aromatherapy, cosmetic, pharmaceutical, nutrition, agronomic and perfume industries.[5] The essential oil compositions of *T. minuta* has been studied previously in Iran and other parts of the world.[6-11] From these findings, it could be seen that the variation in Tagetes oil depends on several environmental as well as genetic factors.[12,13] In addition, according to different activities of various bioactive compounds, these differences between components of the essential oil will be important in pharmaceutical and nutritional uses.[14] All these scientific facts, make a thorough evaluation necessary of the native "Tagetes oil" at regional level. Scientific evidence suggests that vegetable oils as another important class of phytochemicals play a vital role in a healthful diet.[15] They provide energy and essential fatty acids (linoleic and linolenic acids), which are necessary for good health. The oils are also crucial to the absorption of the fat-soluble vitamins A, D, E, and K.[15] The amount of unsaturated fats is one of the most important parameter of different edible vegetable oils.[16] On the other hand, the influence of common environment and genes on the fatty acid composition of plants has been demonstrated by several researchers.[17,18] Previously published investigations on *Tagetes* species have demonstrated strong antioxidant properties.[19,20] Phenol and related compounds occur in food products, especially those of plant origin and are known to be responsible for the antioxidant activities. These secondary metabolites are the subject of increasing scientific interest because of their importance in human health.[21] In recent years, a number of researchers have reported that environmental factors (soil type, sun exposure and rainfall) can widely affect phenolic compounds of the foods.[21] However,

*Corresponding author: Rashid Jamei, Email: r.jamei@urmia.ac.ir

since the biosynthesis of volatile compounds are affected by geographical variation and there is no report on the composition of the essential oil of *T.minuta* from North of Iran, also no study has been carried out previously on phenolic and fatty acid compounds of this plant grown in Iran, therefore this work was carried out; to identification and compare volatile constituents by GC-MS; to analyze the phenolic acids by HPLC and finally; to investigate quantification of fatty acids in the oil extracted of *Tagetes minuta* by GC which may be used as initial materials for medical purposes and use in relevant industries.

Material and Methods
Plant material
Tagetes minuta L. plant was collected in early-autumn of 2015 from Roodbar (latitude: 37° 44' 20" N ; longitude: 40° 96' 44 " E and 180 m above sea level) in Province of Guilan (Noth of Iran). In this time the plant is in full swing, which can be used for the extraction of essential oil. Plant identification was carried out by botanist, Guilan Agricultural Research Center (GARC), Dr. Morady and a voucher specimen of the plant has been deposited (no. 5543). The material was aired for a few days in a well-ventilated and protected from direct sunlight.

Essential oil isolation
Air-dried aerial parts (flowering stage - 50g) were subjected to hydrodistillation for 3 h using a Clevenger-type apparatus (British type) to extract essential oils. The oil samples obtained were dehydrated over anhydrous sodium sulfate and kept in a cool and dark place until further analyses.

GC-MS analysis
The analysis of volatile organic compounds isolated from *T.minuta* was performed using a complete HP/Agilent 6890/5973 GC-MS system with a FID detector (Palo Alto, USA). The GC column specified for the methods was a capillary HP-5MS column (5% phenylmethylsiloxane, 30 m X 0.25 mm i.d., coating thickness 0.25 μm). The injector temperature was set at 250 °C and helium carrier gas flow was adjusted to 1 ml/min. The samples pass through the interface heated to 200 °C into the mass spectrometer operated at 70 eV, which is scanned from 30-300 amu. The electron multiplier voltage was increased to near 3000 V, and the injection volume was 1 μl. GC oven temperature ranged from 70° to 240 °C at l0 °C /min. Qualitative identification for separated constituents was achieved using MS data libraries (Wiley7n.1 and NIST 2008), by comparison of their retention time (RT) obtained on HP-5MS column and then verified by (RI, HP-5MS) with those published in the literature.[22]

Crude oil extraction and GC analysis
Fatty acid methyl esters (FAMEs) were prepared using 2 mol/l NaOH in methanol and n-heptane. The oil samples

were analyzed for chemical components using GC equipped with Flame Ionization Detector (GC-FID, model 6890 N, Agilent Technologies, USA) and DB-Wax capillary column having 30 meter length (30 m, 0.25 mm i.d., 0.25 μm film thickness). It was also fitted to a injector with Agilent tapered liner (4mm id). A fixed quantity of oil (1 μl) was injected into the column after dilution. Oven temperature ranged between 100-230 °C. The temperature of the FID injection system was 250 °C and that of FID detector was 280 °C. Nitrogen carrier gas flow was adjusted to 1.8 ml/min. The identification of individual component was made by running standards (Sigma, Chemical Co.St. Louis). The area under individual peak being calibrated into percent area by integrator itself, gives the percentage of individual component in the sample.

HPLC-UV separations
Methanol extract (80%) and essential oil of the plant were evaluated in this study. The main Polyphenol standards were used for separation and characterisation of phenolic compounds in the aromatic herb. The analysis of phenolic acids was performed with a HPLC system Knauer-Germany equipped with UV-Vis detector according to the method proposed the authors.[23] The filtered samples were injected on Eurospher 100–5 C_{18} column (25 cm X 4.6 mm; 5 μm) from Agilent Technologies. In this experiment, the mobile phase for the HPLC-UV system was composed of deionized water/acetic acid (2% v/v) as solvent A and acetonitrile as solvent B at flow rate 0.8 ml/min. The gradient used in the evaluation was as follows: from 0 to 5 min isocratic 85% A flow, from 5 to 19 min a linear gradient of 85% A to 100% B. In this process, fifteen minutes of equilibration (85% A) is required before another injection. The column temperature was maintained at 25°C and the injection volume was 20 μl. Peaks were detected at 280 nm. Finally, phenolic compounds were determined according to their UV spectra, relative retention times and comparison with reference curves.

Determination of total phenolic content (TPC)
Total phenolic concentration (TPC) in the bioactive extracts namely the methanol extracts and essential oils were estimated spectrophotometrically (WPA Biowave S2100) by the Folin–Ciocalteu (FC) assay described perviously with slight modification.[24] In this study the TPC was expressed as milligrams of gallic acid equivalents (GAE) per gram dry weight of samples. Briefly, an aliquot of (20 μl) the samples were transferred into a test tube and 1 ml reactive FC (previously diluted 10-fold) was added and mixed. Afterward, 0.8 ml of 7.5% sodium carbonate solution was added to the mixture and mixed gently. After incubation for 30 min in the dark and at ambient temperature (25 °C), the absorbance was read at 765 nm of wave length against blank by using a UV–Visible spectrophotometer. TPC values were calculated from a standard curve plotted with known concentration of

gallic acid and all determinations were done in triplicate. (The calibration equation for Gallic acid: y =0.0421 x - 0.0232, R^2 =0.998).

Determination of total flavonoid contents (TFC)
Quantification of flavonoids was based on a procedure described by Shin et al. consisting of a spectrophotometric test at 510 nm.[25] Methanolic solution of extracts and EOs (20 µl) were mixed with 1 ml of distilled water and 0.075 ml of a 5% Sodium nitrite solution. After 5 min, 0.15 ml of 10% aluminium chloride solution was added. It was left at room temperature for 6 min and 0.5 ml of sodium hydroxide (1 mol/l) was added. Then the absorbance of each mixture was measured immediately at 510 nm with a double beam UV/Visible spectrophotometer. The calibration curve was plotted by preparing quercetin solutions in methanol. (The calibration equation for quercetin: y = 0.0779 x - 0.0136, $R^2 = 0.9979$).

DPPH (2,2'-diphenyl-1-picrylhydrazyl) method
The free-radical scavenging activity was measured by the decrease in absorbance of methanolic solution of DPPH.[26] Briefly, 10 µl of the samples were added to 2 ml of methanolic DPPH (0.0023 mol/l) solution, and allowed to react at room temperature. After 30 min the absorbance values were measured at 520 nm and converted into the percentage antioxidant activity using the following formula:

% inhibition of DPPH radical = 100 − 100 (AS ÷ A0)

where A0 is absorbance of the blank and AS is absorbance of the sample at 520 nm. Also the IC$_{50}$ of the plant was obtained by plotting the percent DPPH remaining at the steady state (60 min) of the reaction against the corresponding antioxidant level. The IC$_{50}$ is the concentration of antioxidant to quench 50% DPPH under the experimental conditions.

Statistical analysis
Statistical analysis was carried out using SPSS software version 17 (one-way ANOVA and $p < 0.05$). All the samples were done in triplicate, except those for GC-MS method which were analyzed once; The results are expressed as mean values and standard deviation (SD).

Results and Discussion
Chemical composition of the essential oil
The results of GC-MS analyses of Tagetes oil is reported in Table 1 for the first time from Northern Iran. The volatile oil (orange-yellow color) obtained by hydrodistillation method of the aerial parts of Tagetes minuta showed an average yield of 0.77% (according to dry material weight). The different chemical constituents of the plant were identified and listed in order of their increasing retention times on the HP-5MS column. A total of twenty-four chemical compounds were separated and detected, representing 92.32% of the total oil. Most of the volatile compounds analyzed during this work

contain mainly 9 monoterpenes (52.13%) and 15 sesquiterpenes (40.19%).The oil profile exhibits dihydrotagetone (23.44%) as the most abundant compound. The other main compounds were spathulenol (10.56%), caryophyllene oxide (6.35%), alpha-atlantone (4.76%) and isoaromadendrene epoxide (3.11%), respectively. In fact, the essential oil tested was rich in monoterpenoids. The oil of T. minuta L. has been evaluated in some parts of the country by a number of investigators who have recognized α-terpineol (20.8%), β-ocimene (17.6%)[6] and dihydrotageton (45.9%), trans-ocimenone (27.0%), cis-β-ocimene (11.9%)[8] and limonene (13.0%), piperitenone (12.2%), α-terpinolene (11.0%)[7] as the major components in this species. A review and analysis of the literature revealed that no oil of any Tagetes minuta has been found in which spathulenol and caryophyllene oxide were the main ingredients so its identification of potential significance in Iran. Also according to the Articles, no isoaromadendrene epoxide and neophytadiene were reported of the oil. On the other hand, the main chemical substance essential oil obtained from Tagetes oil in England was dihydrotagetone (54.1%).[10] As high amount of dihydrotagetone found in the oil our plant (23.44%). The main constituents identified in another studies in South Africa and Saudi Arabia were cis-β-ocimene and 5 octyn-4-one 2,7-dimethyl (50.9%, 11.52% respectively).[9,10] On comparison to this reports, the findings of our study indicated the diversity of volatile terpenes and their percentage which can be attributed to ecological, climatic and genetically factors. Here it is worth noting that despite this variations, the main constituents of T. minuta oil growing wild in north of Iran are oxygenated monoterpenoids (41.75%) that can be a valuable for further research especially medicinal properties.

Analysis of fatty acids
In this study, the fatty acid composition of the T.minuta were obtained by hexane extraction and analyzed using a GC–FID for the first time from Iran. The fatty acid profiles of the vegetable oil tested are presented in Table 2. A total of 12 fatty acids were detected and quantified. The amount of fatty acid contents of the extracted oil decreased in the order of: saturated fatty acids (SFA) > polyunsaturated fatty acids (PUFA) > monounsaturated fatty acids (MUFA) ranging from 89.35%, 7.63% and 3.02%, respectively. Palmitic acid (16:0) was the most abundant fatty acid in all the samples. In addition to palmitic acid (30.74 ± 0.4%), other abundant fatty acids extracted from the vegetable oil were capric acid (24.15±0.5%), luric acid (16.58±0.7%), myristic acid (11.02±0.4%) and linoleic acid (5.75±0.5%) respectively. The remaining fatty acids were minor in concentrations (Table 2). Of course, in the evaluation linoleic acid (5.75%) and linolenic acid (1.86%) showed considerable amounts. However, comparing between the fatty acid profiles obtained from current study with fatty acids previous reported on this plant some differences

were observed.[17] For example, Ahmad et al. reported that the major constituents of the seed oil were linoleic (51.95%), palmitic (21.64%) and oleic (16.23%) acids.[17] The differences seem to be associated with genetic factors as well as environmental conditions. However, these findings proved that the plant sources of beneficial fatty acids such as palmitic, louric and linoleic acids. Scientific research has shown that linolenic acid is related to a lower risk of heart patients.[27]

Table 1. Chemical composition of the volatile oil of *T.minuta*

Compounds	RI*	Percent
Sabinen	972	0.8
Limonene	1032	2.38
β-Ocimene	1050	7.2
Dihydrotagetone	1052	23.44
trans-Tagetone	1139	5.76
Camphor	1145	2.05
Z-Tagetone	1148	3.5
Z-ocimenone	1229	4.2
Bornyl acetate	1287	2.8
β-Caryophyllene	1418	1.17
α-Humulene	1455	1.06
Germacrene D	1483	1.29
Caryophyllene oxide	1582	6.35
(E)-Nerolidol	1564	0.94
Viridiflorol	1593	0.9
Spathulenol	1576	10.56
Carotol	1596	0.7
Isoaromadendrene epoxide	1602	3.11
E-sesqui-lavandulol	1610	1.76
β-Atlantone	1668	1.42
α-Bisabolol	1682	0.63
α-Atlantone	1786	4.76
Neophytadiene	1840	2.94
Perhydrofarnesyl acetone	1847	2.6
Monoterpene hydrocarbons		41.75
Oxygenated monoterpenes		10.38
Sesquiterpene hydrocarbons		6.46
Oxygenated sesquiterpenes		33.73
Total		**92.32**

RI* = Retention indices as determined on HP-5MS column

HPLC-UV quantitative analysis

We analyzed for the first time the polyphenols from *T.minuta* in Iran. Table 3 shows the standard chromatogram values of 9 individual phenolic substances

in the aerial parts of the plant, have been carried out by HPLC-UV. It is noteworthy that the separation of all examined compounds was carried out in 50 min. Nine phenolic compounds were analyzed and eight compounds were determined: 4-hydroxy benzoic acid, caffeic acid, syringic, vanillic acid, *p*-coumaric acid, ferulic acid, caffeic acid and rutin (flavonoid glycosides). By examining the HPLC profiles we observe that sinapic acid (5.86±0.1 mg/g) and 4-hydroxy benzoic acid (0.79±0.07 mg/g) are predominant in volatile oil and methanolic extract, respectively. Also gallic acid is not in the samples. However, the pattern of polyphenols indicated that the plant contains sinapic acid derivatives rather than hydroxybenzoic acid derivatives. Our results was supported by several studies in the literature reported that leaves of *T.minuta* exhibits high levels of hydroxycinnamic acid and quercetin derivatives (32±2 and 10±1 mg/g dw, respectively).[28] In fact, phenolic acids have gained considerable attention because of their potential protective role against oxidative damage diseases.[21]

Table 2. Amount of various fatty acids in *T.minuta* oil

No	Fatty acid	Acronym	Concentration (%)
1	Capric acid	C10:0	24.15 ± 0.5
2	Lauric acid	C12:0	16.58 ± 0.7
3	Myristic acid	C14:0	11.02 ± 0.4
4	Palmitic acid	C16:0	30.74 ± 0.4
5	Palmitoleic acid	C16:1	1.19 ± 0.3
6	Stearic acid	C18:0	0.24 ± 0.05
7	Oleic acid	C18:1	0.01 ± 0.03
8	**Linoleic acid**	C18:2	5.75 ± 0.5
9	**Linolenic acid**	C18:3	1.86 ± 0.1
10	Arachidic acid	C20:0	5.3 ± 0.5
11	Behenic acid	C22:0	1.32 ± 0.2
12	Erucic acid	C22:1	1.82 ± 0.2
	TSFA (Total saturated fatty acids)		89.35
	TUFA (Total un saturated fatty acids)		10.65
	TUFA/TSFA		0.1

Each value is the mean ± SD of three independent measurements

Determination of total polyphenols and flavonoid contents

The Folin–Ciocalteu reagent is widely used for the colorimetric in vitro assay of polyphenolic antioxidants. Plant phenolics constitute a large group of secondary metabolites which act as primary antioxidants.[29] As shown in Table 4, total phenolic contents in the oil of *T.minuta* was 153.27±0.9 mg GAE/g dry plant sample. Lower total phenolic contents were found in the methanol extract of the plant (34.17±0.6 mg GAE/g dry extract). In the past years a study performed by Ranilla et al. on selected leaves showed 67±7 0.6 mg GAE/g of phenolic compounds in the dry weight of the extracts (methanolic) of *Tagetes minuta*.[28] Our results seem to be consistent with other research which found *Tagetes minuta* is rich of phenolic acids and can be considered as a invaluable source of natural antioxidants.

In terms of TFC, the oil of *T. minuta* (63.79±0.1 mg/g, $p < 0.05$) was richer in flavonoids, than the extract (14.86±0.4 mg/g, $p < 0.05$) (Table 4). Previously, Kaisoon et al. discovered that the flowers of this genus had 68.9 mg/g of flavonoid content.[30] Flavonoids are a large family of plant polyphenolics that act as free-radical scavengers and the biological function is related to their chemical structure (hydroxyl groups).[31]

Antioxidant activity

The DPPH method is an simple, rapid, valid accurate and sensitive approach to evaluate the antioxidant activity of a special composition or plant extracts.[32] Especially, EO of *T.minuta* (DPPH=66.23±0.92%, IC_{50}=29.31±0.8 µg/ml) has more antioxidant potential than its methanolic extracts (DPPH=36.21±1.44%, IC_{50}=48.67±0.8 µg/ml) (Table 4). This antioxidant activity is in line with those of previous studies with I_{C50} between 35-344 µg/ml.[19] Thus, the study suggests that these fractions (The methanol extract and the volatile oil) are good sources of antioxidant compounds. However, the extraction techniques and time of extraction can highly affect the results of DPPH assay.[33]

Table 3. Content of phenolic compounds in essential oil (**A**) and methanolic extract (**B**) of *T.minuta*

No	Phenolic compound	Calibration curve*	R^2	Plant material (mg/g DW)	
				A	B
1	Rutin	Y=2e+06x-1e+06	0.998	-	0.36 ± 0.02
2	Galic acid	Y=2E+06x-2E+06	0.997	-	-
3	Caffeic acid	Y=1E+06x-2E+06	0.988	2.82 ± 0.06 [a]	0.75 ± 0.06 [b]
4	4- Hydroxy benzoic acid	Y=838158x-1E+06	0.998	2.96 ± 0.08 [a]	0.79 ± 0.07 [a]
5	Vanillic acid	Y=3E+06x-29609	0.999	0.27 ± 0.05 [a]	0.05 ± 0.01 [a]
6	P-coumaric acid	Y=82.887x-59041	0.998	1.58 ± 0.02 [a]	0.65 ± 0.1 [a]
7	Syringic acid	Y=13571x-3682.9	0.985	4.62 ± 0.1 [a]	0.18 ± 0.03 [b]
8	Ferulic acid	Y=165138x-136553	0.988	2.63 ± 0.05 [a]	0.74 ± 0.09 [b]
9	Sinapic acid	Y=20727x-9590	0.997	5.86 ± 0.1 [a]	0.56 ± 0.1 [b]

* Linear calibration curves for the HPLC-UV analysis of the phenolic compounds. Each value is presented as the mean ± SD (n=3). Mean values in the same row followed by a different letter (a,b) are significantly different (p <0.05)

Table 4. The content of total polyphenols, flavonoids and antioxidant capacity parameters in the plant

Samples	TPC (mg GAE/g)	TFC (mg QUE/g)	DPPH (%)	IC_{50} (µg/mL)
EO	153.27 ± 0.9 [a]	63.79 ± 0.1 [a]	66.23 ± 0.92 [b]	29.31 ± 0.8 [b]
Extract	34.17 ± 0.6 [b]	14.86 ± 0.4 [b]	36.21 ± 1.44 [c]	48.67 ± 0.8 [a]
Gallic acid	-	-	93.12 ± 0.4 [a]	0.15 ± 0.01 [c]

Each value is the mean ± SD of three independent measurements. Mean values in the same column followed by a different letter (a-c) are significantly different (p <0.05). GAE: Gallic acid equivalents; QUE: Quercetin equivalents

Conclusion

The present study demonstrates that the volatile oil of *Tagetes minuta* is rich in monoterpenes with two major components dihydrotagetone and spathulenol. The oil tested shows significant quantitative and qualitative variations when compared with previous reports from Iran and abroad. The differences could be possibly due to genetic variation and environmental factors. This research also revealed that the aerial parts of this aromatic plant are various sources of oily components, especially the essential ones, as well as of good natural sources of unsaturated fatty acids (such as linoleic acid). On the other hand, it was found that the native *Tagetes* oil is a non negligible source of phenolic compounds.

Therefore, in addition to traditional uses this medicinal Plant can also be grown and utilized in Pharmaceutical and food industries.

Acknowledgments

The authors would like to express their gratitude to Scientific Research Projects Coordination Unit of Urmia University for financial support (Project Number: 996/2015/D30).

Conflict of Interest

The authors declare no conflict of interest.

References

1. Naqinzhad A, Saeidi Mehrvarz SH. Some new records for Iran and flora Iranica area collected from Boujagh National Park, N. Iran. *Iran J Bot* 2007;13(2):112-9.

2. Hadjiakhoondi A, Vatandoost H, Khanavi M, Abaeeb MR, Karami M. Biochemical investigation of different extracts and larvicidal activity of *Tagetes minuta* L. on Anopheles Stephensi Larvae. *Iran J Pharm Sci* 2005;1(2):81-4.

3. Shahzadi I, Hassan A, Khan UW, Shah MM. Evaluating biological activities of the seed extracts from *Tagetes minuta* L. found in Northern Pakistan. *J Med Plants Res* 2010;4(20):2108-12.

4. Shahzadi I, Shah MM. Acylated flavonol glycosides from *Tagetes minuta* with antibacterial activity. *Front Pharmacol* 2015;6:195. doi: 10.3389/fphar.2015.00195

5. Buchbauer G. The detailed analysis of essential oils leads to the understanding of their properties. *Perfumer Flavorist* 2000;25(2):64-7.

6. Farshbaf-Moghaddam M, Omidbeigi R, Sefidkon F. Chemical composition of essential oil *Tagetes minuta* from Iran. *Iran J Pharm Res* 2004;3:83-4.

7. Meshkatalsadat MH, Safaei-ghomi J, Moharramipour S, Nasseri M. Chemical characterization of volatile components of *Tagetis minuta* L. cultivated in south west of Iran by nanoscaleinjection. *Dig J Nanomater Biostruct* 2010;5(1):101-6.

8. Moradalizadeh M, Mehrabpanah M, Salajeghe M, Nayebli M. Chemical constituents of the essential oils from the leaves, flowers and seeds of *TAGETES MINUTA* L. by GC/MS. *Int J Adv Biol Biom Res* 2013;1(9):1124-8.

9. EL-Deeb KS, Abbas FA, Fishawy A, Mossa SJ. Chemical composition of the essential oil of *Tagetes minuta* L. growing in Saudi Arabia. *Saudi Pharm J* 2004;12:51-3.

10. Senatore F, Napolitano F, Mohamed MAH, Harris PJC, Mnkeni PNS, Henderson J. Antibacterial activity of *Tagetes minuta* L. (Asteraceae) essential oil with different chemical composition. *Flavour Fragr J* 2004;19(6):574-8. doi: 10.1002/ffj.1358

11. Chamorro ER, Ballerini G, Sequeira AF, Velasco GA, Zalazar MF. Chemical composition of essential oil from *Tagetes minuta* L. leaves and flowers. *J Argent Chem Soc* 2008;96(1-2):80-6.

12. Gil A, Ghersa CM, Perelman S. Root thiophenes in *Tagetes minuta* L. accessions from Argentina: genetic and environmental contribution to changes in concentration and composition. *Biochem Syst Ecol* 2002;30(1):1-13. doi: 10.1016/S0305-1978(01)00058-8

13. Moghaddam M, Omidbiagi R. Chemical composition of the essential oil of *Tagetes minuta* L. *J Essent Oil Res* 2007;19(1):3-4. doi: 10.1080/10412905.2007.9699213

14. Rahimi-Nasrabadi M, Nazarian S, Farahani H, Fallah-Koohbijari GR, Ahmadi F, Batooli H. Chemical composition, antioxidant, and antibacterial

activities of the essential oil and methanol extracts of *Eucalyptus largiflorens* F. muell. *Int J Food Prop* 2013;16(2):369-81. doi: 10.1080/10942912.2010.551310

15. Fasina OO, Hallman H, Craig-Schmidt M, Clements C. Predicting temperature-dependence viscosity of vegetable Oils from fatty acid composition. *J Am Oil Chem Soc* 2006;83(10):899-903. doi: 10.1007/s11746-006-5044-8

16. Nikolas BK, Theophanis K. Calculation of iodine value from measurements of fatty acid methyl esters of some oils: comparison with the relevant American oil chemists society method. *J Am Oil Chem Soc* 2000;77(12):1235-8.

17. Ahmad M, Sabir AW, Waheed I, Kamalud Din, Bhatty MK. *Tagetes minuta* L.Syn.T. glandulifera fatty acid composition of the seed oil. *Pak J Sci Ind Res* 1987;30(2):700-1.

18. Petcu E, Arsintescu A, Stanciu D. The effect of drought stress on fatty acid composition in some Romanian sunflower hybrids. *Rom Agric Res* 2001;12:39-43.

19. Parejo I, Bastida J, Viladomat F, Codina C. Acylated quercetagetin glycosides with antioxidant activity from *Tagetes maxima*. *Phytochemistry* 2005;66(19):2356-62. doi: 10.1016/j.phytochem.2005.07.004

20. Taheri-Shirazi M, Gholami H, Kavoosi G, Rowshan V, Tafsiry A. Chemical composition, antioxidant, antimicrobial and cytotoxic activities of *Tagetes minuta* and *Ocimum basilicum* essential oils. *Food Sci Nutr* 2014;2(2):146-55. doi: 10.1002/fsn3.85

21. Pandey KB, Rizvi SI. Plant polyphenols as dietary antioxidants in human health and disease. *Oxid Med Cell Longev* 2009;2(5):270-8. doi: 10.4161/oxim.2.5.9498

22. Adams RP. Identification of essential oil components by gas chromatography-mass spectrometry. USA: Allured Publishing Corporation; 2007.

23. Akbari V, Jamei R, Heidari R, Jahanban-Sfahlan A. Antiradical activity of different parts of Walnut (Juglans regia L.) fruit as a function of genotype. *Food Chem* 2012;135(4):2404-10. doi: 10.1016/j.foodchem.2012.07.030

24. Kahkonen MP, Hopia AI, Vuorela HJ, Rauha JP, Pihlaja K, Kujala TS, et al. Antioxidant activity of plant extracts containing phenolic compounds. *J Agric Food Chem* 1999;47(10):3954-62. doi: 10.1021/jf990146l

25. Shin Y, Liu RH, Nock JF, Holliday D, Watkins CB. Temperature and relative humidity effects on quality, total ascorbic acid, phenolics and flavonoid concentrations, and antioxidant activity of strawberry. *Postharvest Biol Technol* 2007;45(3):349-57. doi: 10.1016/j.postharvbio.2007.03.007

26. Hatano T, Kagawa H, Yasuhara T, Okuda T. Two new flavonoids and other constituents in licorice root: their relative astringency and radical scavenging

effects. *Chem Pharm Bull (Tokyo)* 1998;36(6):2090-97. doi: 10.1248/cpb.36.2090

27. William EC. Importance of n−3 fatty acids in health and disease. *Am J Clin Nutr* 2000;71(1):171S-5S. doi: 10.1093/ajcn/71.1.171S

28. Ranilla LG, Kwon YI, Apostolidis E, Shetty K. Phenolic compounds, antioxidant activity and in vitro inhibitory potential against key enzymes relevant for hyperglycemia and hypertension of commonly used medicinal plants, herbs and spices in Latin America. *Bioresour Technol* 2010;101(12):4676-89. doi: 10.1016/j.biortech.2010.01.093

29. Muchuweti M, Nyamukonda L, Chagonda LS, Ndhlala AR, Mupure C, Benhura M. Total phenolic content and antioxidant activity in selected medicinal plants of Zimbabwe. *Int J Food Sci Technol* 2006;42(6):33-8. doi: 10.1111/j.1365-2621.2006.01258.x

30. Kaisoon O, Siriamornpuna S, Weerapreeyakul N, Meeso N. Phenolic compounds and antioxidant activities of edible flowers from Thailand. *J funct Foods* 2011;3(2):88-99. doi: 10.1016/j.jff.2011.03.002

31. Naczk M, Shahidi F. Phenolics in cereals, fruits and vegetables: occurrence, extraction and analysis. *J Pharm Biomed Anal* 2006;41(5):1523-42. doi: 10.1016/j.jpba.2006.04.002

32. Koleva II, Van Beek TA, Linssen JP, de Groot A, Evstatieva LN. Screening of plant extracts for antioxidant activity: a comparative study on three testing methods. *Phytochem Anal* 2002;13(1):8-17. doi: 10.1002/pca.611

33. Polatoglua K, Karakoc OC, Goren N. Phytotoxic, DPPH scavenging, insecticidal activities and essential oil composition of *Achillea vermicularis*, *A. teretifolia* and proposed chemotypes of *A. biebersteinii* (Asteraceae). *Ind Crops Prod* 2013;51:35-45. doi: 10.1016/j.indcrop.2013.08.052

23

A Review of Herbal Therapy in Multiple Sclerosis

Sina Mojaverrostami[1]* , Maryam Nazm Bojnordi[2,3], Maryam Ghasemi-Kasman[4] , Mohammad Ali Ebrahimzadeh[5] , Hatef Ghasemi Hamidabadi[2,6]

[1] Young Researchers and Elite Club, Behshahr Branch, Islamic Azad University, Behshahr, Iran.
[2] Department of Anatomy & Cell Biology, Faculty of Medicine, Mazandaran University of Medical Sciences, Sari, Iran.
[3] Cellular and Molecular Research Center, Department of Anatomy & Cell Biology, Faculty of Medicine, Mazandaran University of Medical Sciences, Sari, Iran.
[4] Cellular and Molecular Biology Research Center, Health Research Institute, Babol University of Medical Sciences, Babol, Iran.
[5] Pharmaceutical Sciences Research Center, School of Pharmacy, Mazandaran University of Medical Sciences, Sari, Iran.
[6] Immunogenetic Research Center, Department of Anatomy & Cell Biology, Faculty of Medicine, Mazandaran University of Medical Sciences, Sari, Iran.

Article info

Keywords:
· Multiple sclerosis
· Inflammation
· Demyelination
· Remyelination
· Herbal therapy

Abstract
Multiple sclerosis is a complex autoimmune disorder which characterized by demyelination and axonal loss in the central nervous system (CNS). Several evidences indicate that some new drugs and stem cell therapy have opened a new horizon for multiple sclerosis treatment, but current therapies are partially effective or not safe in the long term. Recently, herbal therapies represent a promising therapeutic approach for multiple sclerosis disease. Here, we consider the potential benefits of some herbal compounds on different aspects of multiple sclerosis disease. The medicinal plants and their derivatives; *Ginkgo biloba, Zingiber officinale, Curcuma longa, Hypericum perforatum, Valeriana officinalis, Vaccinium macrocarpon, Nigella sativa, Piper methysticum, Crocus sativus, Panax ginseng, Boswellia papyrifera, Vitis vinifera, Gastrodia elata, Camellia sinensis, Oenothera biennis, MS14* and *Cannabis sativa* have been informed to have several therapeutic effects in MS patients.

Introduction

Multiple sclerosis (MS) is an autoimmune disease that mostly occurs in young adulthood.[1] The etiology of MS disease is still not well understood, but both genetic and environmental factors were found to have important roles in MS disease initiation or progression.[2] In MS disease, inflammatory cells demolish myelin sheath in the CNS which weakens action potential conduction.[3] Two cardinal properties of MS are acute inflammation that associated with demyelination and another one is axonal loss.[4] After injury, oligodendrocyte precursor cells (OPCs) which are residing at parenchyma continuously produce myelinating oligodendrocytes.[3-5] In addition, regarding to the ability of neural stem cells for differentiation to OPCs, these stem cells are considered as an important source for remyelination.[6-8] These endogenous stem cells proliferate, migrate and differentiate to OPCs after brain injuries. However, endogenous OPCs can produce myelin and improve some aspects of the MS disease, but endogenous repair may fail in long term.[7,9] Therefore, several studies have focused on different approaches (including targeting specific signaling pathways, stem cell therapy, suppressing the inflammation process and reprogramming of glial cells to OPCs ...) that improve myelination.[10] Despite the potential benefits of stem cell therapy in the improvement of myelin repair,[11] its clinical application has been hampered because of the possibility of teratoma formation, cell rejection and ethical problems.[12,13] Therefore, there is still a need for developing new drugs which have no or less considerable side effects.

The pathophysiology of MS is not well elucidated, which makes its' treatment strategy very difficult and perplexing.[14] At the present time, most of the strategies in MS treatment are focused on preventing of inflammation in the CNS.[15] Interferon beta (IFN-beta) was firstly confirmed as an effective drug for treatment of MS in 1993.[16] Afterward, different drugs were introduced for curing MS such as glatiramer acetate, natalizumab, alemtuzumab and fingolimod.[14] All of these mentioned drugs were partially effective and their remarkable adverse effects makes them unsuitable for prolonged use.[17] For example, several studies indicated the adverse effects of IFN-beta consumption including, stroke, headache, migraine and depression.[17] Until now, no absolute treatment has been found for MS, therefore,

---

*Corresponding author: Sina Mojaverrostami, Email: sinamojaver@gmail.com

trying to find a completely effective and safe treatment is still ongoing.

Use of complementary and alternative medicine (CAM), in particular herbal remedies have noticeably risen in MS patients over the last decades.[18,19] Herbal therapy is known as a helpful strategy for curing the different disorders from ancient to the present time.[20] Previous studies reported that medicinal plants have several therapeutic effects in different disorders such as cancers, diabetes and neurodegenerative diseases.[21,22] Recently, a growing number of findings have indicated that some herbal compounds improve myelin repair and lead to suppression of inflammation.[23,24] Also, there are many studies that reported the anti-inflammatory and antioxidant effects of medicinal plants, as well as other helpful properties which make them as a natural, safe and reliable remedy for treatment of neurodegenerative diseases.[25,26] Perivious studies have indicated that MS patients are interested in using herbal medicines to control their disease symptoms.[26] For example in China, Chinese herbal medicine (CHM) is widely used by MS patients for ameloriating the severity of disease.[27] The beneficial effects of CHM in MS disease is occured by reduction of the severity of MS disease; including antioxidative properties, anti-apoptotic effects, anti-inflammatory properties and promoting the differentiation of local stem cells to myelin producing cells.[28] MS patients usually use CAM, and medicinal plants as a member of this family plays a crucial role to cure MS and its' associated symptoms.[29] Different herbal medicines are recommended for MS patients, but the understanding of their efficacy is not well described. In this review; we will discuss some of herbal compounds beneficial effects on MS disease (Table 1 and Table 2). We conducted a search for all English language articles in Google Scholar, Science Direct, Scopus, PubMed and Medline for medicinal plants, that have been used for their therapeutic potentials in MS disease, studies which their publication dates from January 1960 to April 2018 were used.

Table1. Summary of herbal medicines used in the treatment of Multiple sclerosis

Plant	Author (Country)	Design of study	Dosage	Number	Duration of study	Effects	Ref
Ginkgo biloba	Johnson et al (USA)	Clinical trial-Double-blind, placeo-controlled	240 mg/day of ginkgo extract	22 MS patients	4 weeks	Treatment with ginkgo extract relieved fatigue with no adverse effect in MS patients	34
	Lovera et al (USA)	Clinical trial-Double-blind, placeo-controlled	240 mg/day of ginkgo extract	38 MS patients	12 weeks	Improvement of the cognitive performance were reported in treated group	37
	Brochet et al (France)	Clinical trial-Double-blind, placeo-controlled	240 and 360 mg/day of ginkgolide B	104 MS patients	1 week	ginkgolide B was not an effective treatment for exacerbations of MS	180
Zingiber officinale	Jafarzadeh et al (Iran)	EAE model of MS in mice	200 and 300 mg/kg ginger extract	24	4 weeks	Ginger extract ameliorated EAE severity and modulated the expression of IL-27, IL-33	43
Curcuma longa	Xie et al (Japan)	EAE model of MS in rats	100 and200 mg/kg curcumin extract	21	2 weeks	Curcumin decreased the inflammation and the severity of EAE	53
	Natarajan and Bright (USA)	EAE model of MS in SJL/J mice	50 and 100 µg curcumin in 25 µl DMSO / day	-	4 weeks	Curcumin decreased CNS inflammation and demyelination also,decreased the severity of EAE	54
	Mohajeri et al (Iran)	EAE model of MS in rats	12.5 mg/kg of curcumin	20	17 days	Treatment with polymerized nano-curcumin decreased the severity of EAE and increased the remyelination	23
Oenothera biennis	Firouzi et al (Iran)	Double blind, randomized clinical trial	18–21 g/day Evening primrose oil and *C. sativa* oils	100 MS patients	24 weeks	Treatment with co-supplemented *C. sativa* and *evening primrose* oils decreased the clinical score in MS patients	158
	Horrobin (Canada)	Double blind, randomized clinical trial	-	14 MS patients	24 weeks	Treatment with colchicine and evening primrose oil improved manual dexterity test and clinical score in MS patients	159
Hypericum perforatum	Naziroglu et al (Turkey)	In-vitro study on neutrophils of MS patients	20 µM/ml *H. perforatum* for 2 hours	9 MS patients	-	Treatment with *H. perforatum* indicated the protective effects on oxidative stress in MS patients	69
Vaccinium macrocarpon	Gallien et al (France)	Double blind, clinical trial, placebo-controlled	36 mg/day Cranberry extract(proanthocyanidins)	171 MS patients	1 year	Treatment with cranberry extract versus placebo did not prevent UTI occurrence in MS patients	81
Nigella sativa	Fahmy et al (Egypt)	EAE model of MS in rats	2.8 g/kg *Nigella sativa* extract	22	4 weeks	*N. sativa* ameliorated the clinical signs of EAE, suppressed inflammation and enhanced remyelination in the CNS	85
	Noor et al (Egypt)	EAE model of MS in rats	2.8 g/kg *Nigella sativa* extract	22	4 weeks	*N. sativa* suppressed inflammation in EAE rats. Also, *N sativa* enhanced remyelination in the cerebellum and reduced the expression of TGF β1	87

Plant	Author (Country)	Design of study	Dosage	Number	Duration of study	Effects	Ref
Crocus sativus	Ghaffari et al (Iran)	EAE model of MS in rats	Intrahippocampal (5and 10 µg/rat) injection of the saffron	35	3 days	Local injection of saffron extract modulated the oxidative stress markers (reduced the activity of GPx and SOD enzymes), through scavenging of ROS	103
	Ghazavi et al (Iran)	EAE model of MS in C57bl/6 mice	100 µL saffron extract	20	3 weeks	Treatment with saffron decreased inflammation in the spinal cord and decreased the severity of EAE	102
Panax ginseng	Hwang et al (Korea)	EAE model of MS in C57bl/6 mice	200 µg of an acidic polysaccharide of *Panax ginseng*	-	33 days	Acidic polysaccharide of *Panax ginseng* decreased the infiltration of inflammatory cells in the CNS, also suppressed EAE score by inhibiting the proliferation of T cells and the production of inflammatory cytokines	113
	Etemadifar et al (Iran)	Randomized Double-blind, placeo-controlled	250 mg ginseng tablets	52 MS patients	12 weeks	Ginseng treatment had no adverse effect on MS patients as well as reduced fatigue and had a positive effect on quality of life	114
Boswellia papyrifera	Sedighi et al (Iran)	Randomized, double-blinded, placebo-controlled study	600 mg of *B. papyrifera*	80 MS patients	8 weeks	*B. papyrifera* improved the visuospatial memory of MS patients	124
Vitis vinifera	Sato et al (USA)	EAE model of MS in C57bl/6 mice	20 mg/kg per day	-	8 weeks	Resveratrol treatment worsened the demyelination and inflammation without neuroprotective effects in the CNS	129
	Kelly et al (USA)	EAE model of MS in C57bl/6 mice	100 and 250 mg/kg Sigma resveratrol	-	4 weeks	Resveratrol delayed the onset of EAE and had a significant neuroprotective effect as well as prevents neuronal loss	130
	Shindler et al (USA)	EAE model of MS in SJL/J mice	500 and 1000 mg/kg resveratrol	62	4 weeks	Resveratrol treatment prevented neuronal loss during optic neuritis and reduced neurological dysfunction during EAE	131
Camellia sinensis	Mahler et al (Germany)	Randomized, double-blinded, placebo-controlled study	600 mg/d EGCG	18 MS patients	12 weeks	Treatment with EGCG improved muscle metabolism during moderate exercise in MS patients	155
MS14	Tafreshi et al (Iran)	EAE model of MS in C57bl/6 mice	MS14 containing 30% of the diet	14	20 days	*Treatment with MS14 ameliorated the clinical signs of EAE and reduced neuropathological changes*	163
	Kalan et al (Iran)	EAE model of MS in C57bl/6 mice	MS14 containing 30% of the diet	25	35 days	MS14 decreased EAE symptoms and lymphocyte infiltration into the CNS	164
	Kalan et al (Iran)	EAE model of MS in C57bl/6 mice	MS14 containing 30% of the diet	25	35 days	Treatment with MS14 reduced clinical signs of EAE, demyelination and IL-6 production	165
Cannabis sativa	Zajicek et al (UK)	Randomized, placebo-controlled trial	Capsules containing 2.5 mg of THC and 1.25 mg of cannabidiol	630 MS patients	15 weeks	cannabinoids improved patients' mobility and improved in spasticity	173
	Zajicek et al (UK)	Double blind, placebo controlled, phase III study	Capsules containing cannabidiol 0.8–1.8 mg and 2.5 mg THC	279 MS patients	12 weeks	Treatment with cannabinoids improved the relief from muscle stiffness in MS patients	172
	Wade et al (UK)	Double-blind, randomized, placebo-controlled study	120 mg cannabidiol and 120 mg THC	160 MS patients	10 weeks	Treatment with cannabinoids improved patient's spasticity, without any adverse effects	174
	Greenberg et al (USA)	Double-blind, randomized, placebo-controlled study	Smoking one marijuana cigarette containing 1.54% THC	10 MS patients	3 days	Smoking marijuana improved eyes-open and eyes-closed tests, and noise variance values	178
	Brady et al (USA)	Open-label, pilot study	2.5 mg of THC and 2.5 mg CBD per spray	10 MS patients	8 weeks	Cannabinoids decreased urinary urgency, number and volume of incontinence episodes, frequency and nocturia in MS patients. Also, spasticity and quality of sleep improved significantly in the treated group	179

Table 2. Use of herbal medicines in Multiple sclerosis, according to the symptomatic problems

Usage	Plant	References
Antidepressant	Hypericum perforatum Crocus sativus	69,101
Sleeping problem	Piper methysticum Valeriana officinalis	73,93
Improvement in cognitive impairment	Ginkgo biloba Boswellia papyrifera	36,124
Urinary system dysfunction	Vaccinium macrocarpon Cannabis sativa	79,179
Fatigue	Ginkgo biloba Panax ginseng	114,34
Anti-inflammatory and neuroprotective	Ginkgo biloba Zingiber officinale Curcuma longa Oenothera biennis Nigella sativa Crocus sativus Panax ginseng Boswellia papyrifera Vitis vinifera Gastrodia elata Camellia sinensis Cannabis sativa MS14	33,34,87,101,113,124,130,14 0,134,159,164,167

Ginkgo biloba

Ginkgo biloba L. (well-known as ginkgo), is one of the oldest living tree species from the family Ginkgoaceae. Ginkgo is native to Korea and China, but now it can be found all over the world.[30] Ginkgo refers to an extract of the leaves of the G. biloba trees, which traditionally used as a remedy to improve the mental alertness and memory.[31] The current reputation of G. biloba can be attributed to a pioneeering research that informed G. biloba is an effective cure for cognitive issues.[32]

Studies have shown that anti-inflammatory and inhibiting the platelet-activating factor (PAF) properties of ginkgo extract (EGB761) are effective on MS disease.[33,34] Ginkgolides is the major component of G. biloba, its effect on the PAF activity represents the possible therapeutic role of this plant on MS.[34] PAF's role in inflammation process is obviously introduced, so ginkgo can inhibit this process.[35] In addition, ginkgo reverses cognitive impairment and reduces fatigue in MS patients.[36,37] G. biloba is generally safe with no side or adverse effects[38] but in some few cases, dizziness, headaches and ocular bleeding associated with its usage.[30] Consumption of G. biloba is almost safe and has obvious therapeutic effects for MS patients; improving functional status (fatigue) of people with MS and neuroprotective activities are the valuable medical properties of G. biloba.

Zingiber officinale

Zingiber officinale Roscoe (Ginger), is an aromatic plant in the family Zingiberaceae. Z. officinale is native to India and commonly grown in Asia, tropical Africa and Latin America.[38] Ginger root is routinely used as an aromatic spice and a traditional drug.[39] Recent studies acknowledged the anti-cancer,[40] antioxidant[41] and anti-inflammatory activities of ginger.[42]

Anti-inflammatory capacity of ginger is the reason of its consumption by MS patients.[43] Gingerols and its dehydrated derivatives (shogaols), are the major components of the ginger that exhibit anti-inflammatory effects.[44] The anti-inflammatory effects of 6-shogaol were reported by inhibiting the expression of inducible nitric oxide synthase (iNOS) and cyclooxygenase- 2 (COX-2) in macrophages, as well as preventing dopamine reduction and reducing apoptose rate in CNS.[45] 10-gingerol is another important component of ginger which attributited with anti-inflammatory effect in fresh ginger.[46] 10-gingerols inhibits LPS-induced NO and production of pro-inflammatory cytokines by inhibiting the NF-jB activation.[46] Positive effects of ginger and its' active compounds (6-shogaol and 10-gingerol) were approved in animal models of MS, by exerting anti-inflammatory and neuroprotective effects, but still clinical studies on MS patients are needed to confirm these results.

Curcuma longa

Curcuma longa L. is a tropical plant, native to southern and southeastern tropical Asia.[47] C. longa is belonging to the ginger family, Zingiberaceae. A yellow coloring-matter obtained from the roots of C. longa, is named curcumin.[47] Curcumin is widely used as a dietary spice and pigment. Curcumin is commonly consumed as an Asian folk remedy for treating biliary disorders, anorexia, cough, sinusitis and sore throat.[48] Studies indicated that curcumin exerts a wide range of biological activities, including anti-inflammatory,[49] antitumor[50] and antioxidants effects.[51]

Anti-inflammatory effect of curcumin has been obviously examined in different studies.[44,52] Curcumin does its anti-inflammatory role in two major ways: (1) inhibition of pro-inflammatory cytokines and (2) inhibition of Th17 differentiation and its related pathways.[52] Curcumin ameloriated the severity of experimental autoimmune encephalomyelitis (EAE), as a animal model of MS disease, also reduced the infiltration of inflammatory cells to the CNS.[52] Curcumin modulates inflammatory process by decreasing the expression of the different pro-inflammatory and inflammatory cytokines.[44,53] In one study, polymerized form of nano-curcumin was used for treating EAE model of MS, which demonstrated anti-inflammatory and antioxidative effects as well as increasing remyelination and decreasing EAE score.[23] Furthermore, curcumin can decrease the secerity of MS disease by blocking IL-12 signaling pathway in T cells.[54] Side effects of curcumin is associated with high dose consumption which causes nausea and diarrhea.[55] Although, therapeutic effects of curcumin were demonstrated in different studies but human studies are certainly needed to confirm the recommendation of curcumin in MS patients.

Hypericum perforatum

Hypericum perforatum L. better known as St John's Wort is a flowering plant from the family *Hypericaceae*. *H. perforatum* is a native plant in Europe and Asia but today has worldwide spread.[30] From the ancient time, *H. perforatum* was popular plant because it had a wide range of therapeutic effects for different diseases such as anxiety, depression and menstrual disorders.[56] Currently, *H. perforatum* is used for treating the inflammation-related disorders,[57] cancers[58] and neurodegenerative diseases.[59]

The usage of *H. perforatum* in MS disease is related to its antidepressant effects.[60,61] Hypericin is the main antidepressant component of *H. perforatum* which stimulates capillary blood flow in brain.[62] Studies have showed that Hypericin strongly inhibits the MAO enzymes and has a strong affinity for Sigma receptors which regulate dopamine level.[63] Recent studies have shown that hypericin acts as an antagonist for adenosine, benzodiazepine and GABA receptors.[64] Many studies emphasis on another constituent, Hyperforin, for the therapeutic effects of this plant. It has been reported that Hyperforin has antidepressant effects as a result of inhibiting the uptake of dopamine, serotonin, noradrenaline, GABA, and L-glutamate.[65,66] There are some clinical studies which have shown the effectiveness of *H. perforatum* on depression conditions.[60,67,68] *H. perforatum* can be recommended to MS patients due to its antidepressant, antioxidative and anti-inflammatory effects.[69]

Valeriana officinalis

Valeriana officinalis L. (Valerian) is native to Europe, North America and parts of Asia.[68] Valerian is a plant in the family of *Caprifoliaceae*, the root and rhizome of this herb are used for different medicinal purposes.[68] In ancient Greek, valerian had various medicinal applications, for example, for digestive problems, epilepsy and urinary tract infections.[70] In addition, valerian was introduced as a treatment for sleeping problems and insomnia.[71]

Sleep disturbance is the most important cause of fatigue in MS patients.[72] Clinical trials demonstrated that major component of *V. officinalis* root extract, valerenic acid, is effective in treatment of mild-to-moderate sleeping disorders.[73] Like benzodiazepines which are GABA-analogs, valerenic acid has particular affinity for the $GABA_A$ receptor.[30] Limited adverse effects such as stomachache and allergic reaction have been observed in patients under treatment of valerenic acids.[30,74] Consumption of *V. officinalis* can be suggested to MS patients due to the ameliorating effects on sleeping problems and fatigue status.

Vaccinium macrocarpon

Vaccinium macrocarpon (Cranberry, Large Cranberry), is a North American species of cranberry in *Ericaceae* family. Cranberry juice is obtained from the *V. macrocarpon* fruit.[75] Cranberry has been traditionally used for treatment of bladder and kidney disorders by Native Americans.[75,76]

MS patients are susceptible to the urinary tract colonizations (UTC) and urinary tract infections (UTIs), as a result of the bladder dysfunction in MS disease.[77] Studies have shown that cranberry juice or its produced-capsules is a beneficial remedy for treatment of UTIs.[78] It has been reported that cranberry can inhibit *Escherischia coli* adherence to the urethra.[79] Cranberry has two substantial compounds, fructose and proanthocyanidin, that stick to the fimbriae of *E. coli* and effectively hindering the bacteria's ability to attach to the urethra.[79] There are a few clinical studies that examined the preventive effects of cranberry on UTIs in MS patients.[80] However, in different studies cranberry was found to be effective against urinary tract infections, but in one clinical trial of MS patients, it not showed acceptable prevention from urinary tract infections.[81]

Nigella sativa

Nigella sativa L. usually known as black seed is widely used as a medicinal plant belongs to the family *Ranunculaceae*. Black seed is native to Southern Europe, Southwest Asia and North Africa.[82] Seeds and oil of *N. sativa* has a long historical and religious background for treatment of various illnesses such as headache, back pain and gastrointestinal problems.[83,84] Several studies have shown that black seed has diverse therapeutic effects, including anticancer, analgesic, antimicrobial, anti-inflammatory, renal protective and antioxidant properties.[84,85] Thymoquinone is the active compound of *N. sativa* seeds.[86]

There are several evidences that indicated the anti-inflammatory capacity of black seed oil.[85,87] In vitro studies demonstrated the inhibitory effects of *N. sativa* oil and its active compound, thymoquinone, on the production of inflammatory mediators {such as IL-1b, IL-6, TNF-a, IFN-c and PGE2}.[88,89] In addition, Black seed oil inhibited COX and 5-LO pathways of arachidonate metabolism.[89,90] Thymoquinone also potently inhibiting the non-enzymatic peroxidation in brain phospholipid liposomes.[84] The therapeutic effects of *N. sativa* in animal models of MS were reported. *N. sativa* enhanced remyelination in CNS, reduced inflammation processes and suppressed the expression of TGF β1 in EAE models of MS disease.[87]

Piper methysticum

Piper methysticum (kava kava) is a psychoactive herb in the family *Piperaceace*, which has been used in the Pacific Islands for hundreds of years. The root of this plant is well-known for its sedative and anesthetic properties.[80] Kava traditionally used for producing a comforting and relaxing drink.[80,91]

Combination of kava and valerian seems to be more effective for treatment of stress-induced insomnia than either herb alone.[92] The active compound of kava is cavalactones, which interacts with $GABA_A$ receptors and decreases anxiety and sleeping problems.[93,94] Kava also can potentiate the sedating effects of the drugs that usually used in MS disease such as Lioresal (Baclofen).[95] Extensive use of kava may lead to hepatotoxicity, hepatic necrosis and cholestasis hepatitis.[96] It can be concluded that kava alone or in combination with other herbal medicines is a promising candidate for treating anxiety disorders of MS patients.

Crocus sativus

Crocus sativus L. (Saffron) is a flowering plant in the family *Iridaceae*. Saffron stigma has been widely used as a medicinal plant for healing the different disorders.[97] Saffron has been commonly used as an herbal drug for its sedative, stimulant and anticatarrhal properities.[97,98] Several studies suggested that saffron can be effective in treatment of hypertension and memory impairments. Additionally, saffron has been demonstrated anti-inflammatory and antitussive effects.[99] Crocetin and crocin are the two main active compounds of saffron stigma, which have a wide range of therapeutic activitis.[100] Antidepressant and anti-neuroinflammatory effects of saffron are evidently effective in MS disease.[101-103] Crocin exerts its anti-inflammatory effects via inhibiting syncytin-1 and nitric oxide (NO)-induced astrocyte and oligodendrocyte cytotoxicity, also decreases neurological injuries in experimental autoimmune encephalomyelitis (EAE).[104,105] Syncytin-1 is highly expresses in microglia, astrocytes and glial cell of MS lesions.[106] Studies have shown that crocin has antidepressant effects in mild to moderate depression.[99] Excessive consumption of saffron induces dizziness, nausea, vomiting and diarrhea.[107] Depression is a common condition in MS disease which adversely affect health status. According to this point, antidepressant activity of saffron can be highly helpful in depressive disorders of MS patients.

Panax ginseng

Panax ginseng also known as Asian ginseng is a traditional herbal medicine in Asia for thousands of years, which belongs to the *Araliaceae* family.[108] Ginseng root is traditionally used in powdered form to regenerate the body and mind, increase physical strength and prevent aging.[109] The main active compound of *P. ginseng* is ginsenosides, that exhibits anti-inflammatory, antioxidant, and anti-apoptotic properties.[110,111] In addition, *P. ginseng* is one of the most useful medicinal plants for curing different neuroinflammatory diseases such as Parkinson's disease, Alzheimer's disease, Huntington's disease and Multiple sclerosis.[112] Some evidences have indicated that ginseng can decrease the inflammation and fatigue, which may be useful in MS patients.[113,114] Ginseng reduced the severity of EAE by inhibiting the proliferation of T cells, inhibiting the production of the inflammatory cytokines (FN-γ, IL-1β and IL-17) and depleting of CD25+ cells.[113] In clinical studies ginseng led to fatigue improvement and had a positive effect on quality of life.[114] Excessive intake of ginseng can lead to several adverse effects including hypertension, insomnia, rashes and diarrhea.[115] We can deduce that ginseng is an effective remedy for curing MS-related fatigue and enhancing quality of life in these patients.

Boswellia papyrifera

Boswellia papyrifera belongs to the *Burseraceae* family.[116] Gum production through resin of *B. papyrifera*, has high economic value.[117] The resin of *B. papyrifera* has been traditionally used in treatment of ulcers, chronic inflammation and for memory support.[118] The main active compound of *B. papyrifera* resin is boswellic acids.[119] Several studies have indicated the different therapeutic effects of boswellic acids such as anti-inflammatory, antitumor and antioxidant effects.[120,121] Cognitive impairment is a common clinical symptom in MS patients, with incidence rates up to 70%.[122] Cognitive deficits in MS patients affect various aspects including attention, information processing efficiency, processing speed, long term memory and visual learning.[123] Anti-inflammatory and neuroprotective properties of *B. papyrifera*, reversed the cognitive impairments in MS patients.[124] In one clinical trial, patients with MS which received *B. papyrifera*, had a significant visuospatial memory improvement compared to the control group.[124] Administration of *B. papyrifera* enhances cognitive impairment in MS patients, but still there is a need for large scale trials to completely clarify the therapeutic effects of *B. papyrifera* in MS patients.

Vitis vinifera

Vitis vinifera L. (common grape vine) is one of the most important fruit crops in the world from the family *Vitaceae*. V. vinifera is cultivated in the most countries of Europe, Northern Africa and Western Asia.[125] The leaves and seeds of this plant have various medicinal properties.

Resveratrol (*trans*-3, 4, 5-trihydroxystilbene) is a phenolic compound that produced in the grapes in response to injuries of fungal pathogens.[126] Resveratrol has been reported to have several pharmaceutical effects such as anti-inflammatory, anticancer, antioxidant and antiviral properties.[127,128]

Both neuroprotective and anti-inflammatory effects of resveratrol were informed in several researches.[129-131] Resveratrol exhibits neuroprotective effects by inhibiting the microglia activation and decreasing the pro-inflammatory factors production through the MAPKs, phosphoinositide3-kinase (PI3-K)/Akt, glycogen synthase kinase-3β (GSK-3β) and NADPH oxidase signaling pathway.[127,132,133] Resveratrol can cross the blood–brain barrier (BBB), therefore it can be an ideal candidate for treating neuroinflammatory and neurodegenerative diseases.[129,134] Excessive intake of common grape causes gastrointestinal side effects including nausea, abdominal pain, flatulence and diarrhea.[135] Neuroprotective effects of *V. vinifera* were demonstrated in different neurodegenerative diseases, but more specific studies on MS disease are needed to determine it's therapeutic role in MS.

Gastrodia elata

Gastrodia elata Blume (tianma) is a saprophytic herb from the family *Orchidaceae*. *G. elata* is a traditional Chinese plant, native to the oriental countries.[136] Tianma is the dried rhizome of the *G. elata* which were used as a traditional herbal medicine for a variety of conditions such as headaches, vertigo and hypertension.[137] In addition, tianma is commonly used for the treatment of neurodegenerative disorders and memory improvement.[138,139]

Due to neuroprotective and anti-neuroinflammatory effects of *G. elata,* it can be considered as a promising candidate for MS therapy. *G. elata* reduces oxygen free radicals and protects against neuronal damage.[137,140,141] *G. elata* indicated anxiolytic-like properties via the GABA-ergic nervous system.[142] It has been reported that *G. elata* has protective effects against global ischemia, nitric oxide synthase activity and apoptosis.[143] Gastrodin is the main active component of the tianma which mediates its neuroprotective effects.[144] Vanillin and Benzyl alcohol are the other active compouds of *G. elata* that have anti-inflammatory effects by inhibiting the generation of reactive oxygen species (ROS) and inhibiting the activities of cyclooxygenase- (COX-) 1 and COX-2.[145] *G. elata* plays an important protective role in the neurorestorative processes, therefore it can be a helpful remedy for MS patients. however, future animal models and clinical studies of MS disease are needed to clarify the possible therapeutic effects of this plant on MS patients.

Camellia sinensis

Camellia sinensis L. is well known as green tea, one of the oldest beverages in the world from the *Theaceae* family.[146,147] Dried leaves of *C. sinensis* are used in green tea production.[147] Green tea is used for several different purposes including weight loss, cardiovascular disorders, inflammation and neuroprotective effects.[148]

Green tea exhibits anti-inflammatory and neuroprotective properties.[149,150] Epigallocatechin-3-gallate (EGCG) is one of the most important active compounds of green tea which is attributed to anti-inflammatory and neuroprotective properties of this plant.[134] EGCG is a polyphenol compound that inhibits the production of inflammatory mediators such as TNF-α, IL-1β and IL-6 and improvs the neuroprotection in nervous system.[151,152] In other studies, EGCG inhibited LPS-induced microglial activation and protected against inflammation-mediated dopaminergic neuronal injury.[153] Regular and habitual consumption of green tea is safe, but, consuming high doses causes liver toxicity.[154] Green tea has anti-inflammatory effects which can protect CNS from neurodegenerative diseases such as MS. Also, green tea regulates energy expenditure in the body which may relief MS-related fatigue.[155]

Oenothera biennis

Oenothera biennis L. (Evening primrose) is a species in the family of *Onagraceae*. Evening primrose oil is produced from the seeds of *O. biennis* which has numerous pharmacological effects.[156] The traditional consumptions of this plant was for the treatment of swelling in the body, then were used for other problems such as skin disorders, gastro-intestinal disorders and asthma.[157] Two parts of the plant; flowers and seeds, are used for extracting the oils.

The application of Evening primrose oil in treatment of MS is related to its anti-inflammatory and immune-modulating effects.[158,159] These beneficial effects largely related to the evening primrose oil abundant supply of polyunsaturated fatty acids (PUFA) content.[159] Gamma-linolenic acid is a precursor of prostaglandin and it is responsible for anti-inflammatory effects of evening primrose oil.[158] In clinical trials, Evening primrose oil led to significant performance improvement in the manual dexterity test.[159] In another clinical study gamma-linolenic acid rich oil had an obvious effect in relapsing-remitting MS, which meaningfully decreased the relapse rate and the progression of disease.[160] However, more clinical trials are needed to prove the therapeutic effects of Evening primrose oil in MS patients.

MS14 (*Penaeus latisculatus, Apium graveolens and Hypericum perforatum*)

MS14 is an Iranian natural herbal-marine drug, which has obvious therapeutic effects on MS patients.[161,162] MS14 consists of 90% *Penaeus latisculatus*, 5% *Apium graveolens* and 5% *Hypericum perforatum*.[163] In both animal models and human clinical trials, MS14 was effective in treatment of MS.[162,164] Antioxidant and anti-inflammatory effects, are the two features of MS14 that halt the progression of MS disease.[161] MS14 showed some benefits on quality of life and improvement of patients' mobility (lower limb).[162] The neuroprotective and anti-inflammatory properties of MS14 were reported by suppressing the proliferation responses of T cells and decreasing the expression levels of IL-6, IL-5, IL-10, TNF-α and IL-1β. Furthermore, MS14 inhibited the inflammatory cell infiltration into the CNS and up-regulated LCN2 in all stages of EAE.[164,165] Oral consumption of MS14 was reported properly safe without any adverse effects.[162] MS14 is an herbal-marine drug that has beneficial effects in MS disease and other neroudegenerative disorders, but still more studies are needed to find various mechanisms and pathways that MS14 shows it's neuroprotective effects.

Cannabis sativa

Cannabis sativa L. (Bang, Marijuana, and Hachis) is a flowering plant in the genus *Cannabis* from the *Cannabaceae* family. *C. sativa* is native to Western and Central Asia, but extensively cultivated in Asia and Europe.[166] *C. sativa* has traditionally been used for healing the different diorders such as allergies, inflammation and sexually transmitted diseases.[167] Seeds, leaves and flowers of *C. sativa* was reported to have various therapeutic and medicinal values. There are numerous studies that indicated the pharmacological usage of *C. sativa,* including analgesic effect, anticancer activity, anti-inflammatory activity, central nervous system depressant activity and immunomodulatory effect.[166]

C. sativa is the most important and the most common plant which is using for treating of MS. There are numerous studies that indicated cannabinoids consumption reduced muscle stiffness, bladder disturbance, spasms, neuropathic pain and sleep disorders in MS patients.[168,169] The major compound of *C. sativa* is Δ-9tetrahydrocannabinol (THC).[170] THC binds to cannabinoid receptors (CBR) in the CNS and acts as a partial agonist to CB1 and CB2 receptors.[171] THC was shown to have anti-inflammatory and neuroprotective properties.[167] Some studies have shown the applications of cannabinoids for improvments of spasticity in MS, consumption of cannabinoids led to significant improvement in patient-reported spasticity.[172-174] Also, the combination of THC and cannabidiol (CBD) was more effective for treatment of moderate to severe refractory spasticity in MS patients.[175] Cannabinoids and their synthetic drugs indicated attractive anti-inflammatory effects in animal models of MS.[176] Synthetic cannabinoids can reduce inflammation by suppressing the TNF-α production in the brain. Also, Synthetic cannabinoids can improve motor function by preventing the infiltration of immune cells into the CNS, and can decrease the pro-inflammatory cytokines secretion such as IFN-μ, IL-17, IL-6, IL-1β and TNF-α.[167] Sativex is a combination of the two derived cannabinoids of the *C. sativa*; THC and CBD, which has been formulated for oromucosal mouth spray to relief neuropathic pain, spasticity, sleeping difficulties, bladder disturbance and other symptoms associated with MS.[177] Orally administration of THC can decrease the intensity of several signs and symptoms of MS such as, decreasing spasticity, rigidity, tremor, as well as improving walking ability, performance of handwriting and bladder control.[169] Smoking marijuana in patients with MS demonstrated to have some advantageous effects, including healing the spasticity, pain, tremor and emotional dysfunction.[178] In one clinical trial, cannabinoids decreased the urinary symptoms, urinary incontinence, frequency of urination and nocturia in treated group.[179] There are some adverse effects associated with *C. sativa* such as the risks of cancer, cardiovascular disease, nausea, vomiting and impaired driving.[61]

Conclusion

Medicinal plants have opened a new horizon in curing neurodegenerative disorders such as Parkinson's disease, AD and MS. literature data review indicated that herbal medicines could be effective in the treatment of MS disease and its' related symptoms, by reducing the demyelination, improving remyelination and suppressing the inflammation in the CNS. On the basis of the above mentioned review, it can be concluded that the anti-inflammatory effect is the main reason of medicinal plants therapeutic effects in MS disease, through which medicinal plants ameliorate the severity of disease and reduce neuropathological changes. Anti-inflammatory effects of medicinal plants usually occur through inhibiting the inflammatory cell infiltration into the CNS, decreasing the production of pro-inflammatory and inflammatory cytokines. Further studies are needed to disclose the exact mechanisms of action, through which medicinal plants exhibit their anti-inflammatory and neuroprotective effects. Given that most studies of herbal therapy effects in MS have been done on animal models, still there is a great need for approving these studies by clinical trials to recommend these mentioned plants for MS patients. In addition to neuroprotective effect, medicinal plants have other beneficial effects for MS patients, such as sedation, improving sleep quality, anti-depressant effects, relief muscle stiffness and reducing bladder disturbance.

Conflicts of Interest

All authors declare no conflicts of interest.

References

1. Camina-Tato M, Fernandez M, Morcillo-Suarez C, Navarro A, Julia E, Edo MC, et al. Genetic association of CASP8 polymorphisms with primary progressive multiple sclerosis. *J Neuroimmunol* 2010;222(1-2):70-5. doi: 10.1016/j.jneuroim.2010.03.003

2. Hasan KM, Walimuni IS, Abid H, Datta S, Wolinsky JS, Narayana PA. Human brain atlas-based multimodal MRI analysis of volumetry,

diffusimetry, relaxometry and lesion distribution in multiple sclerosis patients and healthy adult controls: Implications for understanding the pathogenesis of multiple sclerosis and consolidation of quantitative MRI results in MS. *J Neurol Sci* 2012;313(1-2):99-109. doi: 10.1016/j.jns.2011.09.015

3. Franklin RJ, Ffrench-Constant C. Remyelination in the CNS: From biology to therapy. *Nat Rev Neurosci* 2008;9(11):839-55. doi: 10.1038/nrn2480

4. Fancy SP, Kotter MR, Harrington EP, Huang JK, Zhao C, Rowitch DH, et al. Overcoming remyelination failure in multiple sclerosis and other myelin disorders. *Exp Neurol* 2010;225(1):18-23. doi: 10.1016/j.expneurol.2009.12.020

5. Franklin RJ, Kotter MR. The biology of CNS remyelination: The key to therapeutic advances. *J Neurol* 2008;255 Suppl 1:19-25. doi: 10.1007/s00415-008-1004-6

6. Fancy SP, Zhao C, Franklin RJ. Increased expression of Nkx2.2 and Olig2 identifies reactive oligodendrocyte progenitor cells responding to demyelination in the adult CNS. *Mol Cell Neurosci* 2004;27(3):247-54. doi: 10.1016/j.mcn.2004.06.015

7. Gensert JM, Goldman JE. Endogenous progenitors remyelinate demyelinated axons in the adult CNS. *Neuron* 1997;19(1):197-203. doi: 10.1016/S0896-6273(00)80359-1

8. Nazm Bojnordi M, Ghasemi HH, Akbari E. Remyelination after lysophosphatidyl choline-induced demyelination is stimulated by bone marrow stromal cell-derived oligoprogenitor cell transplantation. *Cells Tissues Organs* 2014;200(5):300-6. doi: 10.1159/000437350

9. Bjartmar C, Trapp BD. Axonal and neuronal degeneration in multiple sclerosis: Mechanisms and functional consequences. *Curr Opin Neurol* 2001;14(3):271-8. doi: 10.1097/00019052-200106000-00003

10. Nazm Bojnordi M, Movahedin M, Tiraihi T, Javan M, Ghasemi Hamidabadi H. Oligoprogenitor cells derived from spermatogonia stem cells improve remyelination in demyelination model. *Mol Biotechnol* 2014;56(5):387-93. doi: 10.1007/s12033-013-9722-0

11. Pourabdolhossein F, Hamidabadi HG, Bojnordi MN, Mojaverrostami S. Stem cell therapy: A promising therapeutic approach for multiple sclerosis. In: Zagon IS, McLaughlin PJ, editors. Multiple sclerosis: Perspectives in treatment and pathogenesis. Brisbane (AU): Codon Publications; 2017. P. 85-108.

12. Herberts CA, Kwa MS, Hermsen HP. Risk factors in the development of stem cell therapy. *J Transl Med* 2011;9(1):29. doi: 10.1186/1479-5876-9-29

13. Sanganalmath SK, Bolli R. Cell therapy for heart failure: A comprehensive overview of experimental and clinical studies, current challenges, and future directions. *Circ Res* 2013;113(6):810-34. doi: 10.1161/CIRCRESAHA.113.300219

14. Kasarełło K, Cudnoch-Jędrzejewska A, Członkowski A, Mirowska-Guzel D. Mechanism of action of three newly registered drugs for multiple sclerosis treatment. *Pharmacol Rep* 2017;69(4):702-8. doi: 10.1016/j.pharep.2017.02.017

15. Katsavos S, Anagnostouli M. Biomarkers in multiple sclerosis: An up-to-date overview. *Mult Scler Int* 2013;2013:340508. doi: 10.1155/2013/340508

16. Salvetti M, Landsman D, Schwarz-Lam P, Comi G, Thompson AJ, Fox RJ. Progressive MS: From pathophysiology to drug discovery. *Mult Scler* 2015;21(11):1376-84. doi: 10.1177/1352458515603802

17. de Jong HJI, Kingwell E, Shirani A, Cohen Tervaert JW, Hupperts R, Zhao Y, et al. Evaluating the safety of β-interferons in MS: A series of nested case-control studies. *Neurology* 2017;88(24):2310-20. doi: 10.1212/WNL.0000000000004037

18. Kim S, Chang L, Weinstock-Guttman B, Gandhi S, Jakimovski D, Carl E, et al. Complementary and alternative medicine usage by multiple sclerosis patients: Results from a prospective clinical study. *J Altern Complement Med* 2018;24(6):596-602. doi: 10.1089/acm.2017.0268

19. Dayapoglu N, Tan M. Use of complementary and alternative medicine among people with multiple sclerosis in eastern turkey. *Neurology Asia* 2016;21(1):63-71

20. Mikaili P, Mojaverrostami S, Moloudizargari M, Aghajanshakeri S. Pharmacological and therapeutic effects of mentha longifolia L. And its main constituent, menthol. *Anc Sci Life* 2013;33(2):131-8. doi: 10.4103/0257-7941.139059

21. Agyare C, Spiegler V, Asase A, Scholz M, Hempel G, Hensel A. An ethnopharmacological survey of medicinal plants traditionally used for cancer treatment in the Ashanti region, ghana. *J Ethnopharmacol* 2018;212:137-52. doi: 10.1016/j.jep.2017.10.019

22. Dehghan-Shahreza F, Beladi-Mousavi SS, Rafieian-Kopaei M. Medicinal plants and diabetic kidney disease; an updated review on the recent findings. *Immunopathol Persa* 2016;2(1):e04.

23. Mohajeri M, Sadeghizadeh M, Najafi F, Javan M. Polymerized nano-curcumin attenuates neurological symptoms in eae model of multiple sclerosis through down regulation of inflammatory and oxidative processes and enhancing neuroprotection and myelin repair. *Neuropharmacology* 2015;99:156-67. doi: 10.1016/j.neuropharm.2015.07.013

24. Piao Y, Liang X. Chinese medicine in diabetic peripheral neuropathy: Experimental research on nerve repair and regeneration. *Evid Based Complement Alternat Med* 2012;2012:191632. doi: 10.1155/2012/191632

25. Kaplan M, Mutlu EA, Benson M, Fields JZ, Banan A, Keshavarzian A. Use of herbal preparations in the

treatment of oxidant-mediated inflammatory disorders. *Complement Ther Med* 2007;15(3):207-16. doi: 10.1016/j.ctim.2006.06.005

26. Olsen SA. A review of complementary and alternative medicine (CAM) by people with multiple sclerosis. *Occup Ther Int* 2009;16(1):57-70. doi: 10.1002/oti.266

27. Miller RE. An investigation into the management of the spasticity experienced by some patients with multiple sclerosis using acupuncture based on traditional chinese medicine. *Complement Ther Med* 1996;4(1):58-62. doi: 10.1016/S0965-2299(96)80058-6

28. Song L, Zhou QH, Wang HL, Liao FJ, Hua L, Zhang HF, et al. Chinese herbal medicine adjunct therapy in patients with acute relapse of multiple sclerosis: A systematic review and meta-analysis. *Complement Ther Med* 2017;31:71-81. doi: 10.1016/j.ctim.2017.02.004

29. Claflin SB, van der Mei IAF, Taylor BV. Complementary and alternative treatments of multiple sclerosis: A review of the evidence from 2001 to 2016. *J Neurol Neurosurg Psychiatry* 2018;89(1):34-41. doi: 10.1136/jnnp-2016-314490

30. Beaubrun G, Gray GE. A review of herbal medicines for psychiatric disorders. *Psychiatr Serv* 2000;51(9):1130-4. doi: 10.1176/appi.ps.51.9.1130

31. Wesnes KA, Ward T, McGinty A, Petrini O. The memory enhancing effects of a ginkgo biloba/panax ginseng combination in healthy middle-aged volunteers. *Psychopharmacology (Berl)* 2000;152(4):353-61. doi: 10.1007/s002130000533

32. Le Bars PL, Katz MM, Berman N, Itil TM, Freedman AM, Schatzberg AF. A placebo-controlled, double-blind, randomized trial of an extract of ginkgo biloba for dementia. *JAMA* 1997;278(16):1327-32. doi: 10.1001/jama.1997.03550160047037

33. Venkatesan R, Ji E, Kim SY. Phytochemicals that regulate neurodegenerative disease by targeting neurotrophins: A comprehensive review. *Biomed Res Int* 2015;2015:814068. doi: 10.1155/2015/814068

34. Johnson SK, Diamond BJ, Rausch S, Kaufman M, Shiflett SC, Graves L. The effect of Ginkgo biloba on functional measures in multiple sclerosis: A pilot randomized controlled trial. *Explore (NY)* 2006;2(1):19-24. doi: 10.1016/j.explore.2005.10.007

35. Braquet P, Esanu A, Buisine E, Hosford D, Broquet C, Koltai M. Recent progress in ginkgolide research. *Med Res Rev* 1991;11(3):295-355. doi: 10.1002/med.2610110303

36. Yadav V, Bever C Jr, Bowen J, Bowling A, Weinstock-Guttman B, Cameron M, et al. Summary of evidence-based guideline: Complementary and alternative medicine in multiple sclerosis: report of the guideline development subcommittee of the American Academy Of Neurology. *Neurology* 2014;82(12):1083-92. doi: 10.1212/WNL.0000000000000250

37. Lovera J, Bagert B, Smoot K, Morris CD, Frank R, Bogardus K, et al. Ginkgo biloba for the improvement of cognitive performance in multiple sclerosis: A randomized, placebo-controlled trial. *Mult Scler* 2007;13(3):376-85. doi: 10.1177/1352458506071213

38. Haniadka R, Rajeev AG, Palatty PL, Arora R, Baliga MS. Zingiber officinale (ginger) as an anti-emetic in cancer chemotherapy: A review. *J Altern Complement Med* 2012;18(5):440-4. doi: 10.1089/acm.2010.0737

39. Palatty PL, Haniadka R, Valder B, Arora R, Baliga MS. Ginger in the prevention of nausea and vomiting: A review. *Crit Rev Food Sci Nutr* 2013;53(7):659-69. doi: 10.1080/10408398.2011.553751

40. Surh YJ. Anti-tumor promoting potential of selected spice ingredients with antioxidative and anti-inflammatory activities: A short review. *Food Chem Toxicol* 2002;40(8):1091-7. doi: 10.1016/S0278-6915(02)00037-6

41. Eguchi A, Murakami A, Ohigashi H. Novel bioassay system for evaluating anti-oxidative activities of food items: Use of basolateral media from differentiated Caco-2 cells. *Free Radic Res* 2005;39(12):1367-75. doi: 10.1080/10715760500045624

42. Haniadka R, Saldanha E, Sunita V, Palatty PL, Fayad R, Baliga MS. A review of the gastroprotective effects of ginger (Zingiber officinale Roscoe). *Food Funct* 2013;4(6):845-55. doi: 10.1039/c3fo30337c

43. Jafarzadeh A, Mohammadi-Kordkhayli M, Ahangar-Parvin R, Azizi V, Khoramdel-Azad H, Shamsizadeh A, et al. Ginger extracts influence the expression of IL-27 and IL-33 in the central nervous system in experimental autoimmune encephalomyelitis and ameliorates the clinical symptoms of disease. *J Neuroimmunol* 2014;276(1-2):80-8. doi: 10.1016/j.jneuroim.2014.08.614

44. Ha SK, Moon E, Ju MS, Kim DH, Ryu JH, Oh MS, et al. 6-Shogaol, a ginger product, modulates neuroinflammation: A new approach to neuroprotection. *Neuropharmacology* 2012;63(2):211-23. doi: 10.1016/j.neuropharm.2012.03.016

45. Ali BH, Blunden G, Tanira MO, Nemmar A. Some phytochemical, pharmacological and toxicological properties of ginger (Zingiber officinale Roscoe): A review of recent research. *Food Chem Toxicol* 2008;46(2):409-20. doi: 10.1016/j.fct.2007.09.085

46. Ho SC, Chang KS, Lin CC. Anti-neuroinflammatory capacity of fresh ginger is attributed mainly to 10-gingerol. *Food Chem* 2013;141(3):3183-91. doi: 10.1016/j.foodchem.2013.06.010

47. Amirghofran Z. Herbal medicines for immunosuppression. *Iran J Allergy Asthma Immunol* 2012;11(2):111-9.

48. Srimal R, Dhawan B. Pharmacology of diferuloyl methane (curcumin), a non-steroidal anti-

inflammatory agent. *J Pharm Pharmacol* 1973;25(6):447-52. doi: 10.1111/j.2042-7158.1973.tb09131.x

49. Huang HC, Jan TR, Yeh SF. Inhibitory effect of curcumin, an anti-inflammatory agent, on vascular smooth muscle cell proliferation. *Eur J Pharmacol* 1992;221(2-3):381-4. doi: 10.1016/0014-2999(92)90727-L

50. Aggarwal BB, Kumar A, Bharti AC. Anticancer potential of curcumin: Preclinical and clinical studies. *Anticancer res* 2003;23(1A):363-98.

51. Naidu KA, Thippeswamy NB. Inhibition of human low density lipoprotein oxidation by active principles from spices. *Mol Cell Biochem* 2002;229(1-2):19-23.

52. Xie L, Li XK, Takahara S. Curcumin has bright prospects for the treatment of multiple sclerosis. *Int Immunopharmacol* 2011;11(3):323-30. doi: 10.1016/j.intimp.2010.08.013

53. Xie L, Li XK, Funeshima-Fuji N, Kimura H, Matsumoto Y, Isaka Y, et al. Amelioration of experimental autoimmune encephalomyelitis by curcumin treatment through inhibition of IL-17 production. *Int Immunopharmacol* 2009;9(5):575-81. doi: 10.1016/j.intimp.2009.01.025

54. Natarajan C, Bright JJ. Curcumin Inhibits Experimental Allergic Encephalomyelitis by Blocking IL-12 Signaling Through Janus Kinase-STAT Pathway in T Lymphocytes. *J Immunol* 2002;168(12):6506-13. doi: 10.4049/jimmunol.168.12.6506

55. Chainani-Wu N. Safety and anti-inflammatory activity of curcumin: A component of tumeric (Curcuma longa). *J Altern Complement Med* 2003;9(1):161-8. doi: 10.1089/107555303321223035

56. Henderson L, Yue QY, Bergquist C, Gerden B, Arlett P. St John's wort (Hypericum perforatum): Drug interactions and clinical outcomes. *Br J Clin Pharmacol* 2002;54(4):349-56. doi: 10.1046/j.1365-2125.2002.01683.x

57. Dost T, Ozkayran H, Gokalp F, Yenisey C, Birincioglu M. The effect of Hypericum perforatum (St. John's Wort) on experimental colitis in rat. *Dig Dis Sci* 2009;54(6):1214-21. doi: 10.1007/s10620-008-0477-6

58. Schempp CM, Kirkin V, Simon-Haarhaus B, Kersten A, Kiss J, Termeer CC, et al. Inhibition of tumour cell growth by hyperforin, a novel anticancer drug from St. John's wort that acts by induction of apoptosis. *Oncogene* 2002;21(8):1242-50. doi: 10.1038/sj.onc.1205190

59. Lu YH, Du CB, Liu JW, Hong W, Wei DZ. Neuroprotective effects of Hypericum perforatum on trauma induced by hydrogen peroxide in PC12 cells. *Am J Chin Med* 2004;32(3):397-405. doi: 10.1142/S0192415X04002053

60. Werneke U, Horn O, Taylor DM. How effective is St. John's wort? The evidence revisited. *J Clin Psychiatry* 2004;65(5):611-7. doi: 10.4088/jcp.v65n0504

61. Bowling AC. Complementary and alternative medicine in multiple sclerosis. *Continuum (Minneap Minn)* 2010;16(5 Multiple Sclerosis):78-89. doi: 10.1212/01.CON.0000389935.84660.a5

62. DerMarderosian A, Beutler JA. The Review of Natural Products. St Louis, MO: Facts and Comparisons; 2002.

63. Suzuki O, Katsumata Y, Oya M, Bladt S, Wagner H. Inhibition of monoamine oxidase by hypercin. *Planta Med* 1984;50(3):272-4. doi: 10.1055/s-2007-969700

64. Chavez ML, Chavez PI. Saint John's wort. *Hosp Pharm* 1997;32:1621-32.

65. Cervo L, Rozio M, Ekalle-Soppo CB, Guiso G, Morazzoni P, Caccia S. Role of hyperforin in the antidepressant-like activity of hypericum perforatum extracts. *Psychopharmacology (Berl)* 2002;164(4):423-8. doi: 10.1007/s00213-002-1229-5

66. Zanoli P. Role of hyperforin in the pharmacological activities of St. John's wort. *CNS Drug Rev* 2004;10(3):203-18. doi: 10.1111/j.1527-3458.2004.tb00022.x

67. Linde K, Ramirez G, Mulrow CD, Pauls A, Weidenhammer W, Melchart D. St John's wort for depression--an overview and meta-analysis of randomised clinical trials. *BMJ* 1996;313(7052):253-8. doi: 10.1136/bmj.313.7052.253

68. LaFrance WC Jr, Lauterbach EC, Coffey CE, Salloway SP, Kaufer DI, Reeve A, et al. The use of herbal alternative medicines in neuropsychiatry. A report of the ANPA committee on research. *J Neuropsychiatry Clin Neurosci* 2000;12(2):177-92. doi: 10.1176/jnp.12.2.177

69. Naziroglu M, Kutluhan S, Övey İS, Aykur M, Yurekli VA. Modulation of oxidative stress, apoptosis, and calcium entry in leukocytes of patients with multiple sclerosis by hypericum perforatum. *Nutr Neurosci* 2014;17(5):214-21. doi: 10.1179/1476830513Y.0000000083

70. Brown DJ. Herbal prescriptions for better health: Your everyday guide to prevention, treatment, and care. Rocklin, CA: Prima Publishing; 1996.

71. Hsu PP. Natural medicines comprehensive database. *J Med Libr Assoc* 2002;90(1):114.

72. Fleming WE, Pollak CP. Sleep disorders in multiple sclerosis. *Semin Neurol* 2005;25(1):64-8. doi: 10.1055/s-2005-867075

73. Barton DL, Atherton PJ, Bauer BA, Moore DF Jr, Mattar BI, LaVasseur BI, et al. The use of Valeriana officinalis (Valerian) in improving sleep in patients who are undergoing treatment for cancer: a phase III randomized, placebo-controlled, double-blind study (NCCTG Trial, N01C5). *J Support Oncol* 2011;9(1):24-31. doi: 10.1016/j.suponc.2010.12.008

74. Willey LB, Mady SP, Cobaugh DJ, Wax PM. Valerian overdose: A case report. *Vet Hum Toxicol* 1995;37(4):364-5.

75. Dugoua JJ, Seely D, Perri D, Mills E, Koren G. Safety and efficacy of cranberry (vaccinium macrocarpon) during pregnancy and lactation. *Can J Clin Pharmacol* 2008;15(1):e80-6

76. Lynch DM. Cranberry for prevention of urinary tract infections. *Am Fam Physician* 2004;70(11):2175-7.

77. Betts CD, D'Mellow MT, Fowler CJ. Urinary symptoms and the neurological features of bladder dysfunction in multiple sclerosis. *J Neurol Neurosurg Psychiatry* 1993;56(3):245-50. doi: 10.1136/jnnp.56.3.245

78. Guay DR. Cranberry and urinary tract infections. *Drugs* 2009;69(7):775-807. doi: 10.2165/00003495-200969070-00002

79. Liu Y, Black MA, Caron L, Camesano TA. Role of cranberry juice on molecular-scale surface characteristics and adhesion behavior of escherichia coli. *Biotechnol Bioeng* 2006;93(2):297-305. doi: 10.1002/bit.20675

80. Schultz A. Efficacy of cranberry juice and ascorbic acid in acidifying the urine in multiple sclerosis subjects. *J Community Health Nurs* 1984;1(3):159-69. doi: 10.1207/s15327655jchn0103_5

81. Gallien P, Amarenco G, Benoit N, Bonniaud V, Donzé C, Kerdraon J, et al. Cranberry versus placebo in the prevention of urinary infections in multiple sclerosis: A multicenter, randomized, placebo-controlled, double-blind trial. *Mult Scler* 2014;20(9):1252-9. doi: 10.1177/1352458513517592

82. Khare CP. Encyclopedia of indian medicinal plants. New York: Springes-Verlag; 2004.

83. El-Dakhakhny M. Studies on the Egyptian Nigella sativa L. IV. Some pharmacological properties of the seeds' active principle in comparison to its dihydro compound and its polymer. *Arzneimittelforschung* 1965;15(10):1227-9.

84. Salem ML. Immunomodulatory and therapeutic properties of the Nigella sativa L. Seed. *Int Immunopharmacol* 2005;5(13-14):1749-70. doi: 10.1016/j.intimp.2005.06.008

85. Fahmy HM, Noor NA, Mohammed FF, Elsayed AA, Radwan NM. Nigella sativa as an anti-inflammatory and promising remyelinating agent in the cortex and hippocampus of experimental autoimmune encephalomyelitis-induced rats. *J Basic Appl Zool* 2014;67(5):182-95. doi: 10.1016/j.jobaz.2014.08.005

86. Ghosheh OA, Houdi AA, Crooks PA. High performance liquid chromatographic analysis of the pharmacologically active quinones and related compounds in the oil of the black seed (Nigella sativa L.). *J Pharm Biomed Anal* 1999;19(5):757-62. doi: 10.1016/S0731-7085(98)00300-8

87. Noor NA, Fahmy HM, Mohammed FF, Elsayed AA, Radwan NM. Nigella sativa amliorates inflammation and demyelination in the experimental autoimmune encephalomyelitis-induced Wistar rats. *Int J Clin Exp Pathol* 2015;8(6):6269-86.

88. Mansour M, Tornhamre S. Inhibition of 5-lipoxygenase and leukotriene C4 synthase in human blood cells by thymoquinone. *J Enzyme Inhib Med Chem* 2004;19(5):431-6. doi: 10.1080/14756360400002072

89. Houghton PJ, Zarka R, de las Heras B, Hoult JR. Fixed oil of Nigella sativa and derived thymoquinone inhibit eicosanoid generation in leukocytes and membrane lipid peroxidation. *Planta Med* 1995;61(1):33-6. doi: 10.1055/s-2006-957994

90. El-Dakhakhny M, Madi NJ, Lembert N, Ammon HP. Nigella sativa oil, nigellone and derived thymoquinone inhibit synthesis of 5-lipoxygenase products in polymorphonuclear leukocytes from rats. *J Ethnopharmacol* 2002;81(2):161-4. doi: 10.1016/S0378-8741(02)00051-X

91. Williamson EM. Synergy and other interactions in phytomedicines. *Phytomedicine* 2001;8(5):401-9. doi: 10.1078/0944-7113-00060

92. Wheatley D. Stress-induced insomnia treated with kava and valerian: Singly and in combination. *Hum Psychopharmacol* 2001;16(4):353-6. doi: 10.1002/hup.299

93. Jussofie A, Schmiz A, Hiemke C. Kavapyrone enriched extract from *Piper methysticum* as modulator of the GABA binding site in different regions of rat brain. *Psychopharmacology* 1994;116(4):469-74. doi: 10.1007/BF02247480

94. Davies LP, Drew CA, Duffield P, Johnston GA, Jamieson DD. Kava pyrones and resin: Studies on $GABA_A$, $GABA_B$ and benzodiazepine binding sites in rodent brain. *Pharmacol Toxicol* 1992;71(2):120-6. doi: 10.1111/j.1600-0773.1992.tb00530.x

95. Bowling AC. Complementary and alternative medicine and multiple sclerosis. Demos Medical Publishing; 2006.

96. Volz HP, Kieser M. Kava-kava extract WS 1490 versus placebo in anxiety disorders--A randomized placebo-controlled 25-week outpatient trial. *Pharmacopsychiatry* 1997;30(1):1-5. doi: 10.1055/s-2007-979474

97. Rios JL, Recio MC, Giner RM, Manez S. An update review of saffron and its active constituents. *Phytother Res* 1998;10(3):189-93.

98. Hosseinzadeh H, Younesi HM. Petal and stigma extracts of crocus sativus L. Have antinociceptive and anti-inflammatory effects in mice. *BMC Pharmacol* 2002;2:7. doi: 10.1186/1472-6882-4-12

99. Khazdair MR, Boskabady MH, Hosseini M, Rezaee R, Tsatsakis AM. The effects of crocus sativus (saffron) and its constituents on nervous system: A review. *Avicenna J Phytomed* 2015;5(5):376-91.

100. Abdullaev Jafarova F, Caballero-Ortega H, Riveron-Negrete L, Pereda-Miranda R, Rivera-Luna R, Manuel Hernandez J, et al. In vitro evaluation of

the chemopreventive potential of saffron. *Rev Invest Clin* 2002;54(5):430-6.

101. Akhondzadeh S, Fallah-Pour H, Afkham K, Jamshidi AH, Khalighi-Cigaroudi F. Comparison of Crocus sativus L. and imipramine in the treatment of mild to moderate depression: a pilot double-blind randomized trial [ISRCTN45683816]. *BMC Complement Altern Med* 2004;4(1):12. doi: 10.1186/1472-6882-4-12

102. Ghazavi A, Mosayebi G, Salehi H, Abtahi H. Effect of Ethanol Extract of Saffron (Crocus sativus L.) on the Inhibition of Experimental Autoimmune Encephalomyelitis in C57bl/6 Mice. *Pak J Biol Sci* 2009;12(9):690-5. doi: 10.3923/pjbs.2009.690.695

103. Ghaffari S, Hatami H, Dehghan G. The effect of ethanolic extract of saffron (Crocus sativus L.) on oxidative stress markers in the hippocampus of experimental models of MS. *Med J Tabriz Univ Med Sci Health Serv* 2015;37(1):40-9.

104. Christensen T. Association of human endogenous retroviruses with multiple sclerosis and possible interactions with herpes viruses. *Rev Med Virol* 2005;15(3):179-211. doi: 10.1002/rmv.465

105. Antony JM, Van Marle G, Opii W, Butterfield DA, Mallet F, Yong VW, et al. Human endogenous retrovirus glycoprotein-mediated induction of redox reactants causes oligodendrocyte death and demyelination. *Nat Neurosci* 2004;7(10):1088-95. doi: 10.1038/nn1319

106. Barnett MH, Prineas JW. Relapsing and remitting multiple sclerosis: Pathology of the newly forming lesion. *Ann Neurol* 2004;55(4):458-68. doi: 10.1002/ana.20016

107. Schmidt M, Betti G, Hensel A. Saffron in phytotherapy: Pharmacology and clinical uses. *Wien Med Wochenschr* 2007;157(13-14):315-9. doi: 10.1007/s10354-007-0428-4

108. Baker JT, Borris RP, Carté B, Cordell GA, Soejarto DD, Cragg GM, et al. Natural product drug discovery and development: New perspectives on international collaboration. *J Nat Prod* 1995;58(9):1325-57. doi: 10.1021/np50123a003

109. Choi KT. Botanical characteristics, pharmacological effects and medicinal components of Korean Panax ginseng C A Meyer. *Acta Pharmacol Sin* 2008;29(9):1109-18. doi: 10.1111/j.1745-7254.2008.00869.x

110. Kim MH, Lee YC, Choi SY, Cho CW, Rho J, Lee KW. The changes of ginsenoside patterns in red ginseng processed by organic Acid impregnation pretreatment. *J Ginseng Res* 2011;35(4):497-503. doi: 10.5142/jgr.2011.35.4.497

111. Yuan CS, Wang CZ, Wicks SM, Qi LW. Chemical and pharmacological studies of saponins with a focus on american ginseng. *J Ginseng Res* 2010;34(3):160-7. doi: 10.5142/jgr.2010.34.3.160

112. Cho IH. Effects of panax ginseng in neurodegenerative diseases. *J Ginseng Res* 2012;36(4):342-53. doi: 10.5142/jgr.2012.36.4.342

113. Hwang I, Ahn G, Park E, Ha D, Song JY, Jee Y. An acidic polysaccharide of panax ginseng ameliorates experimental autoimmune encephalomyelitis and induces regulatory T cells. *Immunol Lett* 2011;138(2):169-78. doi: 10.1016/j.imlet.2011.04.005

114. Etemadifar M, Sayahi F, Abtahi SH, Shemshaki H, Dorooshi GA, Goodarzi M, et al. Ginseng in the treatment of fatigue in multiple sclerosis: A randomized, placebo-controlled, double-blind pilot study. *Int J Neurosci* 2013;123(7):480-6. doi: 10.3109/00207454.2013.764499

115. Siegel RK. Ginseng abuse syndrome. Problems with the panacea. *JAMA* 1979;241(15):1614-5. doi: 10.1001/jama.1979.03290410046024

116. Mertens M, Buettner A, Kirchhoff E. The volatile constituents of frankincense - a review. *Flavour Fragrance J* 2009;24(6):279-300. doi: 10.1002/ffj.1942

117. Tadesse W, Desalegn G, Alia R. Natural gum and resin bearing species of Ethiopia and their potential applications. *Invest Agrar Sist Recur For* 2007;16(3):211-21. doi: 10.5424/srf/2007163-01010

118. Mahmoudi A, Hosseini-Sharifabad A, Monsef-Esfahani HR, Yazdinejad AR, Khanavi M, Roghani A, et al. Evaluation of systemic administration of Boswellia papyrifera extracts on spatial memory retention in male rats. *J Nat Med* 2011;65(3-4):519-25. doi: 10.1007/s11418-011-0533-y

119. Banno N, Akihisa T, Yasukawa K, Tokuda H, Tabata K, Nakamura Y, et al. Anti-inflammatory activities of the triterpene acids from the resin of Boswellia carteri. *J Ethnopharmacol* 2006;107(2):249-53. doi: 10.1016/j.jep.2006.03.006

120. Ammon HP. Modulation of the immune system by Boswellia serrata extracts and boswellic acids. *Phytomedicine* 2010;17(11):862-7. doi: 10.1016/j.phymed.2010.03.003

121. Omura Y, Horiuchi N, Jones MK, Lu DP, Shimotsuura Y, Duvvi H, et al. Temporary anti-cancer & anti-pain effects of mechanical stimulation of any one of 3 front teeth (1st incisor, 2nd incisor, & canine) of right & left side of upper & lower jaws and their possible mechanism, & relatively long term disappearance of pain & cancer parameters by one optimal dose of DHEA, Astragalus, Boswellia Serrata, often with press needle stimulation of True ST. 36. *Acupunct Electrother Res* 2009;34(3-4):175-203. doi: 10.3727/036012909803860997

122. Langdon DW. Cognition in multiple sclerosis. *Curr Opin Neurol* 2011;24(3):244-9. doi: 10.1097/WCO.0b013e328346a43b

123. Langdon DW, Amato MP, Boringa J, Brochet B, Foley F, Fredrikson S, et al. Recommendations for a brief international cognitive assessment for multiple sclerosis (BICAMS). *Mult Scler* 2012;18(6):891-8. doi: 10.1177/1352458511431076

124. Sedighi B, Pardakhty A, Kamali H, Shafiee K, Hasani BN. Effect of Boswellia papyrifera on

cognitive impairment in multiple sclerosis. *Iran J Neurol* 2014;13(3):149-53.

125. Chiou A, Karathanos VT, Mylona A, Salta FN, Preventi F, Andrikopoulos NK. Currants (Vitis vinifera L.) content of simple phenolics and antioxidant activity. *Food Chem* 2007;102(2):516-22. doi: 10.1016/j.foodchem.2006.06.009

126. Frémont L. Biological effects of resveratrol. *Life Sci* 2000;66(8):663-73. doi: 10.1016/S0024-3205(99)00410-5

127. Das S, Das DK. Anti-inflammatory responses of resveratrol. *Inflamm Allergy Drug Targets* 2007;6(3):168-73. doi: 10.2174/187152807781696464

128. de la Lastra CA, Villegas I. Resveratrol as an antioxidant and pro-oxidant agent: Mechanisms and clinical implications. *Biochem Soc Trans* 2007;35(Pt 5):1156-60. doi: 10.1042/BST0351156

129. Sato F, Martinez NE, Shahid M, Rose JW, Carlson NG, Tsunoda I. Resveratrol exacerbates both autoimmune and viral models of multiple sclerosis. *Am J Pathol* 2013;183(5):1390-6. doi: 10.1016/j.ajpath.2013.07.006

130. Fonseca-Kelly Z, Nassrallah M, Uribe J, Khan RS, Dine K, Dutt M, et al. Resveratrol neuroprotection in a chronic mouse model of multiple sclerosis. *Front Neurol* 2012;3:84. doi: 10.3389/fneur.2012.00084

131. Shindler KS, Ventura E, Dutt M, Elliott P, Fitzgerald DC, Rostami A. Oral resveratrol reduces neuronal damage in a model of multiple sclerosis. *J Neuroophthalmol* 2010;30(4):328-39. doi: 10.1097/WNO.0b013e3181f7f833

132. Bi XL, Yang JY, Dong YX, Wang JM, Cui YH, Ikeshima T, et al. Resveratrol inhibits nitric oxide and TNF-α production by lipopolysaccharide-activated microglia. *Int Immunopharmacol* 2005;5(1):185-93. doi: 10.1016/j.intimp.2004.08.008

133. Meng XL, Yang JY, Chen GL, Wang LH, Zhang LJ, Wang S, et al. Effects of resveratrol and its derivatives on lipopolysaccharide-induced microglial activation and their structure-activity relationships. *Chem Biol Interact* 2008;174(1):51-9. doi: 10.1016/j.cbi.2008.04.015

134. Choi DK, Koppula S, Suk K. Inhibitors of microglial neurotoxicity: Focus on natural products. *Molecules* 2011;16(2):1021-43. doi: 10.3390/molecules16021021

135. Patel KR, Scott E, Brown VA, Gescher AJ, Steward WP, Brown K. Clinical trials of resveratrol. *Ann N Y Acad Sci* 2011;1215(1):161-9. doi: 10.1111/j.1749-6632.2010.05853.x

136. Ahn EK, Jeon HJ, Lim EJ, Jung HJ, Park EH. Anti-inflammatory and anti-angiogenic activities of Gastrodia elata blume. *J Ethnopharmacol* 2007;110(3):476-82. doi: 10.1016/j.jep.2006.10.006

137. Tsai CF, Huang CL, Lin YL, Lee YC, Yang YC, Huang NK. The neuroprotective effects of an extract of Gastrodia elata. *J Ethnopharmacol* 2011;138(1):119-25. doi: 10.1016/j.jep.2011.08.064

138. Yu SJ, Kim JR, Lee CK, Han JE, Lee JH, Kim HS, et al. Gastrodia elata blume and an active component, p-hydroxybenzyl alcohol reduce focal ischemic brain injury through antioxidant related gene expressions. *Biol Pharm Bull* 2005;28(6):1016-20 doi: 10.1248/bpb.28.1016

139. Van Kampen J, Robertson H, Hagg T, Drobitch R. Neuroprotective actions of the ginseng extract G115 in two rodent models of Parkinson's disease. *Exp Neurol* 2003;184(1):521-9. doi: 10.1016/j.expneurol.2003.08.002

140. Manavalan A, Ramachandran U, Sundaramurthi H, Mishra M, Sze SK, Hu JM, et al. Gastrodia elata Blume (tianma) mobilizes neuro-protective capacities. *Int J Biochem Mol Biol* 2012;3(2):219-41.

141. Kim BW, Koppula S, Kim JW, Lim HW, Hwang JW, Kim IS, et al. Modulation of LPS-stimulated neuroinflammation in BV-2 microglia by Gastrodia elata: 4-hydroxybenzyl alcohol is the bioactive candidate. *J Ethnopharmacol* 2012;139(2):549-57. doi: 10.1016/j.jep.2011.11.048

142. Jung JW, Yoon BH, Oh HR, Ahn JH, Kim SY, Park SY, et al. Anxiolytic-like effects of Gastrodia elata and its phenolic constituents in mice. *Biol Pharm Bull* 2006;29(2):261-5. doi: 10.1248/bpb.29.261

143. Hsieh CL, Chen CL, Tang NY, Chuang CM, Hsieh CT, Chiang SY, et al. Gastrodia elata BL mediates the suppression of nNOS and microglia activation to protect against neuronal damage in kainic acid-treated rats. *Am J Chin Med* 2005;33(4):599-611. doi: 10.1142/S0192415X0500320X

144. Wu HQ, Xie L, Jin XN, Ge Q, Jin H, Liu GQ. The effect of vanillin on the fully amygdala-kindled seizures in the rat. *Yao Xue Xue Bao* 1989;24(7):482-6.

145. Lee JY, Jang YW, Kang HS, Moon H, Sim SS, Kim CJ. Anti-inflammatory action of phenolic compounds from *Gastrodia elata* root. *Arch Pharm Res* 2006;29(10):849-58. doi: 10.1007/BF02973905

146. Gramza-Michalowska A, Regula J. Use of tea extracts (Camelia sinensis) in jelly candies as polyphenols sources in human diet. *Asia Pac J Clin Nutr* 2007;16(Suppl 1):43-6.

147. Graham HN. Green tea composition, consumption, and polyphenol chemistry. *Prev Med* 1992;21(3):334-50. doi: 10.1016/0091-7435(92)90041-F

148. Chacko SM, Thambi PT, Kuttan R, Nishigaki I. Beneficial effects of green tea: A literature review. *Chin Med* 2010;5:13. doi: 10.1186/1749-8546-5-13

149. Yang F, de Villiers WJ, McClain CJ, Varilek GW. Green tea polyphenols block endotoxin-induced tumor necrosis factor-production and lethality in a murine model. *J Nutr* 1998;128(12):2334-40. doi: 10.1093/jn/128.12.2334

150. Koh SH, Lee SM, Kim HY, Lee KY, Lee YJ, Kim HT, et al. The effect of epigallocatechin gallate on suppressing disease progression of ALS model mice. *Neurosci Lett* 2006;395(2):103-7. doi: 10.1016/j.neulet.2005.10.056

151. Neyestani TR, Gharavi A, Kalayi A. Selective effects of tea extract and its phenolic compounds on human peripheral blood mononuclear cell cytokine secretions. *Int J Food Sci Nutr* 2009;60(Suppl 1):79-88. doi: 10.1080/09637480802158184

152. Mandel SA, Avramovich-Tirosh Y, Reznichenko L, Zheng H, Weinreb O, Amit T, et al. Multifunctional activities of green tea catechins in neuroprotection. Modulation of cell survival genes, iron-dependent oxidative stress and PKC signaling pathway. *Neurosignals* 2005;14(1-2):46-60. doi: 10.1159/000085385

153. Li R, Huang YG, Fang D, Le WD. (-)-Epigallocatechin gallate inhibits lipopolysaccharide-induced microglial activation and protects against inflammation-mediated dopaminergic neuronal injury. *J Neurosci Res* 2004;78(5):723-31. doi: 10.1002/jnr.20315

154. Molinari M, Watt KD, Kruszyna T, Nelson R, Walsh M, Huang WY, et al. Acute liver failure induced by green tea extracts: Case report and review of the literature. *Liver Transpl* 2006;12(12):1892-5. doi: 10.1002/lt.21021

155. Mähler A, Steiniger J, Bock M, Klug L, Parreidt N, Lorenz M, et al. Metabolic response to epigallocatechin-3-gallate in relapsing-remitting multiple sclerosis: A randomized clinical trial. *Am J Clin Nutr* 2015;101(3):487-95. doi: 10.3945/ajcn.113.075309

156. Balch SA, McKenney CB, Auld DL. Evaluation of gamma-linolenic acid composition of evening primrose (Oenothera) species native to Texas. *HortScience* 2003;38(4):595-8.

157. Horrobin DF. Nutritional and medical importance of gamma-linolenic acid. *Prog Lipid Res* 1992;31(2):163-94. doi: 10.1016/0163-7827(92)90008-7

158. Rezapour-Firouzi S, Arefhosseini SR, Mehdi F, Mehrangiz EM, Baradaran B, Sadeghihokmabad E, et al. Immunomodulatory and therapeutic effects of Hot-nature diet and co-supplemented hemp seed, evening primrose oils intervention in multiple sclerosis patients. *Complement Ther Med* 2013;21(5):473-80. doi: 10.1016/j.ctim.2013.06.006

159. Horrobin DF. Multiple sclerosis: The rational basis for treatment with colchicine and evening primrose oil. *Med Hypotheses* 1979;5(3):365-78. doi: 10.1016/0306-9877(79)90018-5

160. Harbige LS, Sharief MK. Polyunsaturated fatty acids in the pathogenesis and treatment of multiple sclerosis. *Br J Nutr* 2007;98(S1):S46-53. doi: 10.1017/S0007114507833010

161. Ahmadi A, Habibi G, Farrokhnia M. MS14, an iranian herbal-marine compound for the treatment of multiple sclerosis. *Chin J Integr Med* 2010;16(3):270-1. doi: 10.1007/s11655-010-0270-1

162. Naseri M, Ahmadi A, Gharegozli K, Nabavi M, Faghihzadeh S, Ashtarian N, et al. A double blind, placebo-controlled, crossover study on the effect of MS14, an herbal-marine drug, on quality of life in patients with multiple sclerosis. *J Med Plant Res* 2009;3(4):271-5.

163. Tafreshi AP, Ahmadi A, Ghaffarpur M, Mostafavi H, Rezaeizadeh H, Minaie B, et al. An Iranian herbal-marine medicine, MS14, ameliorates experimental allergic encephalomyelitis. *Phytother Res* 2008;22(8):1083-6. doi: 10.1002/ptr.2459

164. Ebrahimi-Kalan A, Soleimani Rad J, Kafami L, Mohammadnejad D, Habibi Roudkenar M, Khaki AA, et al. MS14 down-regulates lipocalin2 expression in spinal cord tissue in an animal model of multiple sclerosis in female C57BL/6. *Iran Biomed J* 2014;18(4):196-202.

165. Ebrahimi Kalan A, Soleimani Rad J, Kafami L, Mohamadnezhad D, Khaki AA, Mohammadi Roushandeh A. MS14, a marine herbal medicine, an immunosuppressive drug in experimental autoimmune encephalomyelitis. *Iran Red Crescent Med J* 2014;16(7):e16956. doi: 10.5812/ircmj.16956

166. Kuddus M, Ginawi IAM, Al-Hazimi A. Cannabis sativa: An ancient wild edible plant of India. *Emir J Food Agric* 2013;25(10):736-45. doi: 10.9755/ejfa.v25i10.16400

167. Saito VM, Rezende RM, Teixeira AL. Cannabinoid modulation of neuroinflammatory disorders. *Curr Neuropharmacol* 2012;10(2):159-66. doi: 10.2174/157015912800604515

168. Zajicek J, Fox P, Sanders H, Wright D, Vickery J, Nunn A, et al. Cannabinoids for treatment of spasticity and other symptoms related to multiple sclerosis (CAMS study): Multicentre randomised placebo-controlled trial. *Lancet* 2003;362(9395):1517-26. doi: 10.1016/S0140-6736(03)14738-1

169. Pertwee RG. Cannabinoids and multiple sclerosis. *Pharmacol Ther* 2002;95(2):165-74. doi: 10.1016/S0163-7258(02)00255-3

170. Borgelt LM, Franson KL, Nussbaum AM, Wang GS. The pharmacologic and clinical effects of medical cannabis. *Pharmacotherapy* 2013;33(2):195-209. doi: 10.1002/phar.1187

171. Zajicek JP, Apostu VI. Role of cannabinoids in multiple sclerosis. *CNS Drugs* 2011;25(3):187-201. doi: 10.2165/11539000-000000000-00000

172. Zajicek JP, Sanders HP, Wright DE, Vickery PJ, Ingram WM, Reilly SM, et al. Cannabinoids in multiple sclerosis (CAMS) study: Safety and efficacy data for 12 months follow up. *J Neurol Neurosurg Psychiatry* 2005;76(12):1664-9. doi: 10.1136/jnnp.2005.070136

173. Zajicek J, Reif M, Schnelle M. Cannabis extract in the treatment of muscle stiffness and other

symptoms in multiple sclerosis-Results of the MUSEC study. 25th Congress of the European Committee for Treatment and Research in Multiple Sclerosis. 2009.

174. Wade DT, Makela P, Robson P, House H, Bateman C. Do cannabis-based medicinal extracts have general or specific effects on symptoms in multiple sclerosis? A double-blind, randomized, placebo-controlled study on 160 patients. *Mult Scler* 2004;10(4):434-41. doi: 10.1191/1352458504ms1082oa

175. Grotenhermen F, Müller-Vahl K. The therapeutic potential of cannabis and cannabinoids. *Dtsch Arztebl Int* 2012;109(29-30):495-501. doi: 10.3238/arztebl.2012.0495

176. Wirguin I, Mechoulam R, Breuer A, Schezen E, Weidenfeld J, Brenner T. Suppression of experimetal autoimmune encephalomyelitis by cannabinoids. *Immunopharmacology* 1994;28(3):209-14. doi: 10.1016/0162-3109(94)90056-6

177. Kmietowicz Z. Cannabis based drug is licensed for spasticity in patients with MS. *BMJ* 2010;340:c3363. doi: 10.1136/bmj.c3363

178. Greenberg HS, Werness SA, Pugh JE, Andrus RO, Anderson DJ, Domino EF. Short-term effects of smoking marijuana on balance in patients with multiple sclerosis and normal volunteers. *Clin Pharmacol Ther* 1994;55(3):324-8. doi: 10.1038/clpt.1994.33

179. Brady CM, DasGupta R, Dalton C, Wiseman OJ, Berkley KJ, Fowler CJ. An open-label pilot study of cannabis-based extracts for bladder dysfunction in advanced multiple sclerosis. *Mult Scler* 2004;10(4):425-33. doi: 10.1191/1352458504ms1063oa

24

Effect of *Cucurbita Maxima* on Control of Blood Glucose in Diabetic Critically Ill Patients

Ata Mahmoodpoor[1], Mahsa Medghalchi[2], Hossein Nazemiyeh[3,4], Parina Asgharian[5,4], Kamran Shadvar[6], Hadi Hamishehkar[7]*

[1] Department of Anesthesiology, Tabriz University of Medical Sciences, Tabriz, Iran.
[2] Iranian Evidence Based Medicine Center of Excellence, Tabriz University of Medical Sciences, Tabriz, Iran.
[3] Research Center for Pharmaceutical Nanotechnology, Tabriz University of Medical Sciences, Tabriz, Iran.
[4] Department of Pharmacognosy, Faculty of Pharmacy, Tabriz University of Medical Sciences, Tabriz, Iran.
[5] Student Research Committee, Tabriz University of Medical Sciences, Tabriz, Iran.
[6] Cardiovascular Research Center, Tabriz University of Medical Sciences, Tabriz, Iran.
7 Drug Applied Research Center, Tabriz University of Medical Sciences, Tabriz, Iran.

Article info

Keywords:
· Cucurbita maxima
· Blood glucose
· Hyperglycemia
· Critical illness
· Intensive care unit

Abstract

Purpose: Cucurbita maxima Duchense (*C. maxima*) has been widely used in China and Mexico as a hypoglycemic plant for controlling blood glucose in diabetic patients. Furthermore, in northwest of Iran, this plant is used traditionally for controlling of diabetes. We examined the effect of *C. maxima* pulp besides insulin on control of hyperglycemia in diabetic patients admitted to Intensive care unit (ICU).

Methods: Twenty critically ill patients who were admitted to the ICU were enrolled in this study. 5g lyophilized powder of *C. maxima* was administrated every 12 hours for 3 days. Moreover, blood glucose level and insulin dose were measured every 1-4 hours during 3 days before administration and 3days at the time of *C. maxima* administration.

Results: The average of glucose level in 3 days before *C. maxima* administration was 214.9 ± 55.7 mg/dl, while in 3 days during *C. maxima* administration it was decreased to 178.4 ± 36.1 mg/dl (P<0.001). Additionally, the average insulin dose during 3 days before intervention was 48.05 ± 36.5 IU and during the 3 days of *C. maxima* administration was decreased to 39.5 ± 27.8 IU (P=0.06).

Conclusion: It seems that *C. maxima* may decrease high blood glucose level fast and effective in diabetic critically ill patients.

Introduction

Hyperglycemia frequently occurs after injury or critical illness in diabetic patients. Prevalence of Insulin resistance in the most of critically ill patients causes impairment in the blood glucose control.[1] Stress mediators like stress hormones, cytokines and the central nervous system are involved in carbohydrate metabolism particularly in the liver and skeletal muscle.[2] Systemic catecholamine release, cytokine release following systemic inflammation and direct systemic stimulation can all result in hepatic glycogenolysis and finally hyperglycemia.[3] In septic patients, pathological activation of the innate immune system can induce insulin resistance and hyperglycemia.[4] As a result, development of hyperglycemia and insulin resistance is more common in patients admitted to Intensive Care Unit (ICU). Hyperglycemia has been identified as an independent risk factor for undesirable outcomes in critically ill patients and it can cause complications including severe infections, polyneuropathy, multiple organ failure and furthermore death.[5,6]

In intensive care setting, using of oral anti-diabetic medications from Biguanide and Thiazolidinedione family is limited. In addition, Metformin is contraindicated in patients with sepsis, metabolic acidosis, renal failure, and unstable hemodynamic because lactic acidosis may be developed as a fatal consequent.[7] Peripheral edema is common with Pioglitazone particularly in patients suffering from congestive heart failure.[8] These complications are common among patients admitted to ICU. Hence, introducing a drug augmenting insulin sensitivity and better control of blood glucose in such patients seems to be valuable. In this regard, using herbal products is increasing.[9,10] *Cucurbita maxima* Duchense (*C. maxima*) (English name: Winter squash) has been known as a medical plant; it belongs to the family of Cucurbitaceae.[11,12] *C. maxima* is a dicotyledonous seed vegetable. It has flexible succulent stem with trifoliate, alternate and also leafstalk leaves.[11,13,14] The biological active components of *C. maxima* fruit include polysaccharides, para aminobenzoic acid, fixed oils,

---

*Corresponding author: Hadi Hamishehkar, Email: hamishehkar@tbzmed.ac.ir,

proteins and peptides[13,15] sterol, flavonoids[16] tannins, phenolics and saponins.[17] In addition, pectin, as a water-soluble fiber is a common and main compound of pumpkin plants.[18] Several pharmacological activities such as anti-oxidant, anti-diabetic properties,[19,20] anti-hyperlipidemic, hepatoprotective[21] and anti- cancer,[22] have been reported by different species of these plants. The active hypoglycemic components of *C. maxima* have been found in the fruit pulp[13] and seeds[11] which defined to be beneficial for the diabetic rats and also human who are type2 diabetic patients. Among 200 Chinese medical plants which have known as anti-diabetic plants, *C. maxima* and *C. moschata* have been frequently used.[23] Moreover, its use for diabetes was reported from Mexico[16] Since there is no information regarding the effect of *C. maxima* on blood glucose control levels in patients admitted to ICU, the objective of this preliminary study was to examine the effect of *C. maxima* pulp besides insulin on glucose level in diabetic patients admitted to ICU.

Materials and Methods
Preparation of winter squash powder
The fruits of *C. maxima* were collected from East Azarbaijan province (Iran) during November 2013. After matching with available references by professional herbalis, round Pepo fruit and developed tendril had been considered for *C.maxima* with voucher number as CV. Buttercup squash TBZ-fph 1713. and also, retained in the herbarium of the Faculty of Pharmacy, Tabriz University of Medical Sciences, Iran. The fruits were thoroughly washed with potable water and cleanser then, were sliced in little pieces to be processed in an electric domestic extractor. After obtaining the juice, the volume reduced in rotary evaporator in 37°C. After that, the juice was powdered using freeze dryer, and stored at 4°C for 4 months.

Participants
This was an uncontrolled before-after clinical trial has been performed at two ICUs of two hospitals affiliated to Tabriz University of Medical Sciences. This study included the patients were admitted to ICUs between the first of January 2014 to May 2016. Patients aged 18 years or older and also, were diabetic with lack of appropriate response to insulin therapy (their blood glucose levels were higher than 160 mg/dl in spite of insulin therapy used on sliding scale in therapy for 24h), have been entered into the study.[24] 12 patients had diabetes type 1 and 8 patients had type 2 diabetes received insulin in their Medicinal diet. We excluded patients with no evidence of diabetes from diabetic patients with controlled blood glucose levels using insulin therapy. The study protocol was approved by the ethic committee of the Tabriz University of medical science and was recorded in the International Clinical Trials Registry Platform (ICTRP) with identifier IRCT201311118307N2.

Study Protocol

In the study of Acosta-Patin˜o and colleagues[25] who performed on type 2 diabetes, the dose of *Cucurbita ficifolia* was 4 ml/kg of fruit juice. Accordingly, and considering the average weight of 70 kg for patients, after drying 280 ml of juice in oven, the amount of dry matter remained was 9 grams. Therefore, in this study, the dose of *Cucurbita maxima* was assumed to be 10 grams per day in two divided doses. This dose is close to that of the plant used in traditional medicine (one glass of *C. maxima* fruit juice every day)

The patients received 5 g of the *C. maxima* powder every 12 hours for 3 days. Blood levels of glucose and the dose of insulin were measured every 1-4 hours depending on severity of hyperglycemia. The data were collected during 3 days before and within 3 days of *C. maxima* administration.

For all patients, Acute Physiology and Chronic Health Evaluation (APACHE II) and Sequential Organ Failure Assessment score (SOFA) were calculated daily to determine the severity of primary disease and organ failure, respectively.

Statistical Analysis
We are planning a study of a continuous response variable from matched pairs of study subjects. Prior data from a pilot study with 6 patients have indicated that the difference in the response of matched pairs is normally distributed with standard deviation of 29.5. The difference in the mean response of matched pairs was 30, and then the sample size calculated to be 12 pairs of subjects to be able to reject the null hypothesis that this response difference is zero with probability (power =0.9). The Type I error probability associated with the test of null hypothesis is 0.05. For increasing the power of study, we included 20 patients in our study. Paired-samples t-test was used to compare mean blood glucose level 3 days before administration of *C. maxima* with 3 days of *C. maxima* administration and repeated measures analysis of variance was used to detect significant changes in the blood glucose and prescribed insulin for patients during sequential measured times. Greenhouse-Geisser test was used when Mauchly's test of sphericity was significant to test the significant changes of blood glucose and insulin within group. A two-sided P value less than 0.05 was considered significant. All statistical analyses were performed with the SPSS software (Statistical Package for the Social Sciences, version 16.0, SPSS Inc, Chicago, Ill, USA).

Results
A total of 20 patients, 11 males and 9 females, aged 45-82 years, enrolled in the study with a follow-up period of 6 days. Table 1 shows the characteristics and disease severity for enrolled patients. The medications that patients received during the study and affecting blood glucose were listed in the Table 1. Eight patients received beta blocker and fluoroquinolones, 5 patients beta blocker, 4 patients fluoroquinolones, 2 patients corticosteroids and one patient received beta blocker and corticosteroids

Table 1. Severity of disease and characteristics of patients*

Age, years (min-max)	65.4 ± 10.9 (45-79)
Sex, Male no (%)	11 (55%)
SOFA (admission)	5.1 ± 2.1
SOFA (mean of 3 days before *C. maxima* Administration)	4.9 ± 1.6
SOFA (mean of 3 days of *C. maxima* Administration)	5.08 ± 2.24
APACHE II (admission)	18.8 ± 6.9
APACHE II (mean of 3 days before *C. maxima* Administration)	18.4 ± 6.5
APACHE II (mean of 3 days of *C. maxima* Administration)	18.5 ± 7.8
GCS (admission)	10.2 ± 3.3
HA1c	9.35 ± 2.5
Drugs, number of patients	
Beta Blocker	14
Corticosteroids	3
Fluoroquinolones	12

*Values are shown as the percentage (number) or mean ± standard deviation; SOFA: Sequential Organ Failure Assessment score; APACHE II: Acute Physiology and Chronic Health Evaluation; *C. maxima*: Cucurbita maxima; GCS: Glasgow Coma Scale

There were no significant changes in the average of APACHE II and SOFA scores following the administration of *C. maxima*. (P>0.05).
The effect of *C. maxima* on blood glucose levels and infused insulin dose is shown in Table 2.

Table 2. Blood glucose levels and insulin dose in diabetic patients admitted in ICU before and after the oral administration of *C. maxima* powder

Day	BS (mg/dL)	Ins.Dose (unit)
Before *C. maxima* administration		
-3	209.2 ± 41.3	36.7 ± 31.1
-2	218.2 ± 66.2	49.4 ±37.8
-1	217.4 ± 59.1	58.01 ± 38.8
Mean	214.9 ± 55.7	48.05 ± 36.5
After *C. maxima* administration		
1	182.6 ± 33.1	43.6 ± 31.8
2	175.1 ± 28.1	40.3 ± 26.9
3	177.4 ± 46.3	34.9 ± 25.1
Mean	178.4 ± 36.1	39.5 ± 27.8
MD (95% CI), Pv*	(22.5 – 50.6), <0.001	(-5.2 – 17.2), 0.28

BS: blood sugar, Ins: insulin, MD: Mean Difference, CI: Confidence Interval, *C. maxima*: Cucurbita maxima
*Results based on Paired T test comparing mean blood glucose level before and after *C. maxima* administration

The average glucose level in 3 days before *C. maxima* administration was 214.9 ± 55.7 mg/dl and in 3 days after that blood glucose level decreased to 178.4 ± 36.1 mg/dl. The amount of decrease was significant compared with the pre- *C. maxima* administration level (P<0.001). In addition, repeated measurements analysis for blood glucose levels during the study days showed significant decrease (P= 0.002) (Figure1). Pairwise Comparisons

among average glucose level in 3 days before *C. maxima* administration and blood glucose level in each 3 days after *C. maxima* administration showed statistically significant differences (p<0.05).

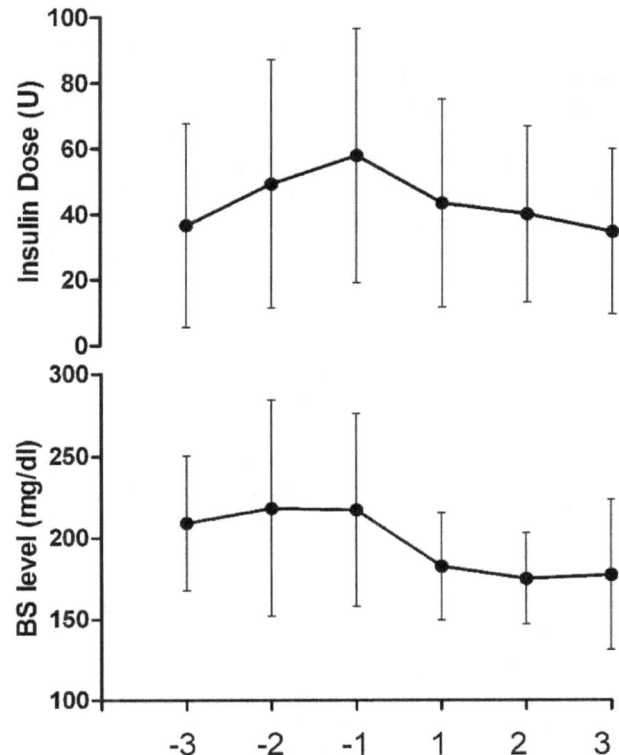

Figure 1. BS; Blood Sugar. Changes in consumed insulin dose and blood glucose levels during 6 days of study. -3 to -1 implies 3 days before intervention and 1 to 3 show 3 days during *C. maxima* powder prescription for patients.

The average dose of infused insulin during 6 days has been summarized in Table 2. In first 3 days, the average insulin dose was 48.05 ± 36.5 IU and during the last 3 days, it decreased to 39.5 ± 27.8 IU (P=0.06). There were not any significant differences among the average dose of infused insulin during 3 days before *C. maxima* administration and the average insulin doses in each 3 days after *C. maxima* administration (p>0.05).

Discussion
Results of the present study indicated that administration of 5g *C. maxima* powder twice daily for 3days in diabetic patients admitted to ICU significantly reduced blood glucose level as compared to that in 3days before *C. maxima* administration. In addition, this plant was able to decrease insulin dose, though it was insignificant. Our results were in line with Asghary et al,[26] they showed that, treating diabetic rats by other species of *Cucurbita* fruit powder (*C. pepo*) reduced blood glucose level significantly and increase the blood insulin level. The results of that study demonstrated blood glucose decreasing effect of Pumpkin was as well as glibenclamide. Furthermore, other study,[11] has demonstrated the effect of different extracts of *C. maxima*

seeds on decreasing the level of blood glucose concentration in streptozotocin induced diabetic rats.

Previous studies have indicated that Protein-bound polysaccharides (PBPs) found in other species of *Cucurbita* have anti-diabetic properties. Li et al[27] carried out examination to evaluate the effect of orally administered different doses of PBPs of pumpkin on diabetic rats. In mentioned study, PBPs indicated hypoglycemic activity, even stronger than that observed with 20 mg/kg of glibenclamide. Based on the results of that study, it can be suggested that different doses of PBPs may have hypoglycemic effect. The phytochemical investigation indicated the different extracts of *C. maxima* contain carbohydrates, flavanoids, tannins, phenolics, pectines and saponins.[17] Pumpkin polysaccharides could increase anti-oxidant capacity by elevating glutathione peroxidase and superoxide dismutase activity and also, decreasing the malonaldehyde in mice serum.[28] On the other hand, flavonoides (like quercetine) and saponines[26-30] have antioxidant activities which play a main role in anti-diabetic effect of pumpkin especially in critically ill patients who oxidative stress may cause insulin resistance and diabetes. Additionally, it has shown that[31] pumpkin's polysaccharides and pectines increase the serum insulin levels and reduce blood glucose.

In a clinical study,[25] ten Type 2 diabetic patients with moderate hyperglycemia received 4 ml/kg row extract of *C. ficifolia* fruit pulp. The average blood glucose level was 217.2 ± 30.4 mg/dl at baseline. 5 h after the *C. ficifolia* administration, blood glucose reached 150.8 ± 31.3 mg/dl. Hence, the results demonstrated a hypoglycemic effect by *C. ficifolia* in type 2 diabetic patients with moderate hyperglycemia.

In intensive care setting, safe and fast acting anti-diabetic agents are urgently needed to improve insulin resistance and decrease the blood glucose. The results of this preliminary study indicated that hypoglycemic effect of *C. maxima* is obvious from the first day of administration and it continued during last 3 days. However, the APACHE II and SOFA scores did not reduce in last 3 days, showing independency of the reduced blood glucose level, from improvement of illness severity in patients. In this study, none of the studied patients experienced undesirable side effects from the *C. maxima*. So, this plant seems an appropriate therapeutic to use in ICU. Further studies are needed to explore active ingredients as well as potential mechanisms of *C. maxima* responsible for its hypoglycemic effect and the mechanisms involved. Long-term larger studies are also strongly needed to confirm its hypoglycemic effects in diabetic patients admitted to ICU.

Limitations of the study
1. The sample size calculated to be 10 pairs of subjects but we included 20 patients in our study to increase the power of study, as regards 20 patients are not enough to support clinical usage of C. maxima, we need more subjects in future studies.

2. This study was a pre-post study but of increasing the power of study we need a control group in future studies.
3. We have not checked the adverse effects of C. maxima powder in patients. Also we suggest this study to take place in patients with renal failure, liver failure and patients with active infections.
4. Stability and uniformity tests of the obtained C. maxima powder did not performed in this study.
5. Complementary analysis such as bioassay guided isolated of from anti-diabetic compounds have not been performed. Based on our results, it is suggested for to considering in future projects to evaluate pure compounds anti-diabetic effects.

Acknowledgments
We are grateful to Shahrokh Teshnehdel and ICU staffs of Imam Reza and Shohada hospitals for their cooperation in this investigation. Applied Research Center of Tabriz University of Medical Science is greatly appreciated for supporting the study.

Conflict of Interest
The authors declared no potential conflicts of interest with respect to the research, authorship, and/or publication of this article.

References
1. Mahmoodpoor A, Hamishehkar H, Shadvar K, Beigmohammadi M, Iranpour A, Sanaie S. Relationship between glycated hemoglobin, intensive care unit admission blood sugar and glucose control with icu mortality in critically ill patients. *Indian J Crit Care Med* 2016;20(2):67-71. doi: 10.4103/0972-5229.175938
2. Van Cromphaut SJ. Hyperglycaemia as part of the stress response: The underlying mechanisms. *Best Pract Res Clin Anaesthesiol* 2009;23(4):375-86.
3. Frayn KN. Hormonal control of metabolism in trauma and sepsis. *Clin Endocrinol (Oxf)* 1986;24(5):577-99.
4. Samuel VT, Shulman GI. Mechanisms for insulin resistance: Common threads and missing links. *Cell* 2012;148(5):852-71. doi: 10.1016/j.cell.2012.02.017
5. Li L, Messina JL. Acute insulin resistance following injury. *Trends Endocrinol Metab* 2009;20(9):429-35. doi: 10.1016/j.tem.2009.06.004
6. Mahmoodpoor A, Hamishehkar H, Beigmohammadi M, Sanaie S, Shadvar K, Soleimanpour H, et al. Predisposing factors for hypoglycemia and its relation with mortality in critically ill patients undergoing insulin therapy in an intensive care unit. *Anesth Pain Med* 2016;6(1):e33849. doi: 10.5812/aapm.33849
7. McCulloch DK. Metformin in the treatment of adults with type 2 diabetes mellitus. In: UpToDate, Post TW

(Ed), UpToDate, Waltham, MA. (Accessed on Apr 2018) https://www.uptodate.com

8. Yki-Järvinen H. Thiazolidinediones. *N Engl J Med* 2004;351(11):1106-18. doi: 10.1056/NEJMra041001

9. Mohamad Shahi M, Haidari F, Shiri MR. Comparison of effect of resveratrol and vanadium on diabetes related dyslipidemia and hyperglycemia in streptozotocin induced diabetic rats. *Adv Pharm Bull* 2011;1(2):81-6. doi: 10.5681/apb.2011.012

10. Sunarwidhi AL, Sudarsono S, Nugroho AE. Hypoglycemic effect of combination of azadirachta indica a. Juss. And gynura procumbens (lour.) merr. Ethanolic extracts standardized by rutin and quercetin in alloxan-induced hyperglycemic rats. *Adv Pharm Bull* 2014;4(Suppl 2):613-8. doi: 10.5681/apb.2014.090

11. Sharma A, Sharma AK, Chand T, Khardiya M, Yadav KC. Antidiabetic and antihyperlipidemic activity of Cucurbita maxima Duchense (pumpkin) seeds on streptozotocin induced diabetic rats. *J Pharmacogn Phytochem* 2013;1(6):108-16.

12. Saganuwan AS. Tropical plants with antihypertensive, antiasthmatic, and antidiabeteic value. *J Herbs Spices Med Plants* 2009;15(1):24–44. doi:10.1080/10496470902787477

13. Adams GG, Imran S, Wang S, Mohammad A, Kok S, Gray DA, et al. The hypoglycaemic effect of pumpkins as anti-diabetic and functional medicines. *Food Res Int* 2011;44(4):862-67. doi:10.1016/j.foodres.2011.03.016

14. Lazos ES. Nutritional, fatty acid, and oil characteristics of pumpkin and melon seeds. *J Food Sci* 1986;51(5):1382–3. doi: 10.1111/j.1365-2621.1986.tb13133.x

15. Buchbauer G, Boucek B, Nikiforov A. On the aroma of Austrian pumpkin seed oil: correlation of analytical data with olfactoric characteristics. *Ernahrung/Nutrition* 1998; 22(6):246–9.

16. Andrade-Cetto A, Heinrich M. Mexican plants with hypoglycaemic effect used in the treatment of diabetes. *J Ethnopharmacol* 2005;99(3):325-48. doi: 10.1016/j.jep.2005.04.019

17. Marles RJ, Farnsworth NR. Antidiabetic plants and their active constituents. *Phytomedicine* 1995;2(2):137-89. doi: 10.1016/s0944-7113(11)80059-0

18. Fissore EN, Matkovic L, Wider E, Rojas AM, Gerschenson LN. Rheological properties of pectin-enriched products isolated from butternut (Cucurbita moschata Duch ex Poiret). *LWT-Food Sci Technol* 2009;42(8):1413-21. doi:10.1016/j.lwt.2009.03.003

19. Caili F, Huan S, Quanhong L. A review on pharmacological activities and utilization technologies of pumpkin. *Plant Foods Hum Nutr* 2006;61(2):73-80. doi: 10.1007/s11130-006-0016-6

20. Xia T, Wang Q. Antihyperglycemic effect of cucurbita ficifolia fruit extract in streptozotocin-induced diabetic rats. *Fitoterapia* 2006;77(7-8):530-3. doi: 10.1016/j.fitote.2006.06.008

21. Makni M, Fetoui H, Gargouri NK, Garoui el M, Jaber H, Makni J, et al. Hypolipidemic and hepatoprotective effects of flax and pumpkin seed mixture rich in omega-3 and omega-6 fatty acids in hypercholesterolemic rats. *Food Chem Toxicol* 2008;46(12):3714-20. doi: 10.1016/j.fct.2008.09.057

22. Pan H, Qiu X, Li H, Jin J, Yu C, Zhao J. Effect of pumpkin extracts on tumor growth inhibition in S180-bearing mice. *Pract Prev Med* 2005;12:745-7.

23. Jia W, Gao W, Tang L. Antidiabetic herbal drugs officially approved in china. *Phytother Res* 2003;17(10):1127-34. doi: 10.1002/ptr.1398

24. Stapleton RD, Heyland DK, Glycemic control and intensive insulin therapy in critical illness. In: UpToDate, Post TW (Ed), UpToDate, Waltham, MA. (Accessed on December 2017) https://www.uptodate.com

25. Acosta-Patino JL, Jimenez-Balderas E, Juarez-Oropeza MA, Diaz-Zagoya JC. Hypoglycemic action of cucurbita ficifolia on type 2 diabetic patients with moderately high blood glucose levels. *J Ethnopharmacol* 2001;77(1):99-101.

26. Asgary S, Moshtaghian SJ, Setorki M, Kazemi S, Rafieian-kopaei M, Azadeh A, et al. Hypoglycaemic and hypolipidemic effects of pumpkin (Cucurbita pepo L.) on alloxan-induced diabetic rats. *Afr J Pharm Pharmaco* 2011;5(23):2620-6. doi: 10.5897/AJPP11.635

27. Quanhong L, Caili F, Yukui R, Guanghui H, Tongyi C. Effects of protein-bound polysaccharide isolated from pumpkin on insulin in diabetic rats. *Plant Foods Hum Nutr* 2005;60(1):13-6.

28. Xu GH. A study of the possible antitumour effect and immunom petence of pumpkin polysaccharide. *J Wuhan Prof Med Coll* 2000;28(4):1-4.

29. Rauter AP, Martins A, Borges C, Mota-Filipe H, Pinto R, Sepodes B, et al. Antihyperglycaemic and protective effects of flavonoids on streptozotocin-induced diabetic rats. *Phytother Res* 2010;24 Suppl 2:S133-8. doi: 10.1002/ptr.3017

30. Abdel-Hassan IA, Abdel-Barry JA, Tariq Mohammeda S. The hypoglycaemic and antihyperglycaemic effect of citrullus colocynthis fruit aqueous extract in normal and alloxan diabetic rabbits. *J Ethnopharmacol* 2000;71(1-2):325-30.

31. Mukherjee PK, Maiti K, Mukherjee K, Houghton PJ. Leads from indian medicinal plants with hypoglycemic potentials. *J Ethnopharmacol* 2006;106(1):1-28. doi: 10.1016/j.jep.2006.03.021

25

Physiological and Biochemical Effects of *Echium Amoenum* Extract on Mn^{2+}-Imposed Parkinson Like Disorder in Rats

Leila Sadeghi[1]* , **Farzeen Tanwir**[2] , **Vahid Yousefi Babadi**[3]

[1] *Department of Animal Biology, Faculty of Natural Sciences, University of Tabriz, Tabriz, Iran.*
[2] *Matrix Dynamics Group, University of Toronto, Canada.*
[3] *Department of Physiology, Payam Noor University of Iran, Iran.*

Article info

Keywords:
· Catecholamine
· Cognitive disorder
· Depression like behavior
· Hippocampus
· Manganism
· Mitochondria dysfunction

Abstract

Purpose: Manganism is a cognitive disorder take places in peoples are exposed to environmental manganese pollution. Overexposure to manganese ion (Mn^{2+}) mainly influences central nervous system and causes symptoms that increase possibility of hippocampal damages.

Methods: In this study rats were administrated by two different doses of MnCl$_2$ and behavioral and physiological consequences were evaluated. We also investigated effects of *E. Amoenum* on Mn^{2+}-imposed toxicity by behavioral, biochemical, immunoblotting and histological studies on hippocampus tissue.

Results: Results showed metal overexposure increases oxidative stress mainly by lipid peroxidation and reactive oxygen species overproduction. Histological studies and caspase 3 analyses by immunoblotting revealed Mn^{2+} induced apoptosis from mitochondrial-dependent pathway in the presence of low metal dose. This study provides evidence that oral administration of *E. amoenum* extract inhibited manganese neurotoxicity by oxidative stress attenuation and apoptosis reduction that lead to improved depression like behavior. Plant extract also increased catecholamine content in Mn^{2+} treated hippocampus.

Conclusion: As molecular and pathophysiological effects of *E. amoenum*, it could be considered as a pre-treatment for Parkinson and Parkinson like disorders in high-risk people.

Introduction

Manganese (Mn) plays key role in mammalian brain development and function as a trace element.[1] Mn^{2+} is cofactor of important enzymes such as glutamine synthetase, pyruvate decarboxylase, serine/threonine protein phosphatase I, Mn-superoxide dismutase and arginase, which are required for neurotransmitter synthesis, metabolism and antioxidant defense system.[2] It is also the fourth most widely used heavy metal in the industry such as textile bleaching, leather tanning and iron, steel, potassium permanganate, hydroquinone, glass and ceramics production.[2,3] By considering high application of Mn^{2+} in today's life, exposing to this poisonous metal is predictable especially in miners and factory workers.[4] Previous studies confirmed Mn^{2+} overdose causes Parkinson like disorder known as manganism that accompanied by tremors, odd movements, mask like face, and body stiffness that first observed in miners.[3] The risk of Mn^{2+} exposure is not limited to miners or welders. The environmental accessibility and high Mn^{2+} concentration in water or food represent a source of contamination for the general population.[4] As previous study, systemic injected Mn^{2+} mainly accumulated in central nervous system (CNS) and damaged it.[5] Our prior results also showed acute dose of Mn^{2+} causes reduction of catecholamine level in the brain tissue by unknown mechanism.[6] The main theories for damaging mechanisms of heavy metals are mitochondrial dysfunction and oxidative stress.[7] Plants, especially *Echium amoenum*, are important source of antioxidants and cell protectants can be used for CNS toxicity.[8] *E. amoenum* Fisch, a common traditional herbal medicine, is widely used as an effective treatment for tranquillizer, diaphoretic, cough, sore throat and pneumonia.[8,9] Dried violet-blue petals of *E. amoenum* have been recently recognized as an important source of phenolic compounds like rosmarinic acid, cyaniding and delphinidin that could be extracted by water solvents.[10] By considering molecular composition, it is believed that this plant has antibacterial, antioxidant, analgesic, anxiolytic, antidepressant and immunomodulatory properties.[10-13] It has been shown that *E. amoenum* aqueous extract is effective treatment for obsessive-compulsive disorder and pancreatitis.[14,15] Neuroprotective effects of cyanidin 3-glucoside, the most common anthocyanin in petals of this plant, have been investigated previously and results showed it can inhibit inflammation by blocking the c-Jun and NF-κB factors translocation into the nucleus.[16] Therefor its possible *E. amoenum* aqueous extract prevents toxic effects induced by heavy metals such as Mn^{2+} in CNS.

*Corresponding author: Leila Sadeghi, Email: l.sadeghi@tabrizu.ac.ir

The main goal of this study is evaluation of the $MnCl_2$ toxicity in the rat hippocampus by biochemical analysis, behavioral assessment and histological studies. Hippocampus tissue plays an important role in hippocampal-dependent learning and memory, depressive-like behaviors and cognitive disorders similar to manganism, therefore we investigated Mn^{2+} toxicity in hippocampus tissue.[17,18] Two different doses of metal were used to dose dependent assessment of physiological and biochemical parameters. This study also estimated *E. amoenum* aqueous extract improving effects on the neurotoxicity imposed by high dose of $MnCl_2$.

Materials and Methods

2,7 dichlorofluoresc indiacetate (DCFHDA), thiobarbituric acid, and *5,5'-Dithiobis* (2-nitrobenzoic acid) riboflavin and nitro blue tetrazolium were purchased from Sigma Chemical Company. All other solvents and chemicals were of the highest grade-commercially available.

Experimental design and plant extraction

In vivo study was conducted on experimental animals and using adult male Wistar rats weighing 250-300 g obtained from the animal house of martyr portal. Animals with average age of 4.5-6 months were selected. Testing was carried out at temperature of 20-25 centigrade degree and that day duration was 12 hours and dark period was 12 hours. Municipal tap water was used as drinking water and animal feed as nutrition (compressed feed). We have 4 experimental groups in this study and 8 rats in each group. The first group was daily injected by physiological saline (0.9 % NaCl) for 15 days, the second group was daily injected by 10 mg/kg $MnCl_2$ in saline as vehicle during 15 days, third group was injected daily by 15 mg/kg $MnCl_2$ in saline for 15 days and fourth group was administrated by 15 mg/kg $MnCl_2$ + 5 mg/kg *E. amoenum* extract for same time duration. $MnCl_2$ and extract doses determined according to previous study[19] and some experiments (data not shown). Although there are many methods for plant extract preparing, but few scientific reports are available in the literature on lyophilized extracts of fresh violet petals of *E. amoenum*, as this type of extraction causes better antioxidant and cell protective potential in rats.[20] Sample was collected after approval of agricultural experts. The fresh violet petals of *E. amoenum* were thoroughly washed with tap water and its juice was obtained using a blender. After obtaining the juice, it was lyophilized to get the dry powder using freeze dryer. We used 5 mg/kg of plant extract in saline for orally administration of rats before 15 mg/kg $MnCl_2$ intraperitoneally injection.

Behavioral assessment

Forced swimming test (FST)

As previous standard protocol,[21] rats were placed in a transparent plexiglass cylinder (20 cm diameter and 50 cm height) filled with warm water (25 °C and 30 cm depth). The classical procedure uses a two-day protocol.

The first day of habituation, the rats were forced to swim for 15 min; 24 h after, on the test day three categories of behavioral activity (climbing, swimming and immobility) were recorded during the 5 min test period. Immobilization time considered as time between introduction of a rat into the pool and making only those movements necessary to keep its head above water without struggling. Immediately after each experience rats were dried and kept warm before returning to their home cage.

Sucrose preference test (SPT)

SPT estimates hedonia (pleasure-seeking) or its deficient (anhedonia) by monitoring preference of rats to sucrose water.[22] Rats were placed in individual cages with food and water. At first, rats were adapted to having two water bottles in the cage lid for 72 hours and their position was randomly changed as many times as possible to avoid a place preference. The bottles were fitted with ball-bearing sipper tubes to prevent fluid leak. After this acclimation, rats had the free choice of either bottle for water drinking. Then one of the bottles filled with 1% sucrose solution during 48 hours test. Water and sucrose solution intake was measured daily. The locations of two bottles were switched daily to reduce side bias. Sucrose preference was calculated as follows: 100 * [sucrose consumption (g)/(sucrose consumption (g) + water intake (g))] and averaged over the 2 days of testing.

Reactive oxygen species (ROS) measurement

ROS generation was measured according to the methods of Keston and Brandt[23] and Lebel et al.[24] with some modifications. The method used to measure the oxidative conversion of DCFH-DA to dichlorofluorescin (DCFH) as a fluorescent compound. Hippocampus homogenates were diluted 1:10 in buffer to obtain a concentration of 5 mg tissue/ml. Then the homogenates were pipetted into 24-well plates (0.45 ml/ well) and allowed to warm to room temperature for 5 min. At that time, 5 μl of DCFH-DA (10 μM final concentration) was added to each well and the plates preincubated for 15 min at room temperature to allow the DCFH-DA to be incorporated into any membrane-bound vesicles and the diacetate group cleaved by esterases. After the preincubation, 50 μl of the appropriate concentration of Fe^{2+} was added to the wells. After 30 min, DCFH-DA converted into non-fluorescent DCFH, which reacts with ROS to form the fluorescent product DCF. DCF fluorescence was determined at 485 nm excitation and 530 nm emission using a (Perkin Elmer luminescence spectrometer LS 55) fluorescence spectrophotometer. The slit width was 5 nm for both excitation and emission. Background fluorescence (conversion of DCFH to DCF in the absence of homogenate) was corrected by the inclusion of parallel blanks. ROS content was expressed as DCF fluorescence/mg protein/min in comparison with control. Protein concentration in homogenates was determined using Bradford method[25] and did not differ between groups.

Lipid peroxidation (LPO) measurement

Hippocampus tissue samples were used for measurement of lipid peroxidation as a marker of oxidative stress.[26] Tissue was separated after anesthesia and homogenized with ice cold buffer containing 0.15 M KCl to obtain 1:10 (w/v) homogenates. Aliquots of homogenate (1 ml) were incubated at 37°C for 3 h in a shaker. Then, 1ml of 10% aqueous trichloroacetic acid (TCA) was added and mixed. The mixture was then centrifuged at 800 g for 10 min. Then, supernatant (1 ml) was mixed with 1ml of 0.67% thiobarbituric acid and placed in a boiling water bath for 10 min. The mixture was cooled and diluted with 1ml distilled water. The absorbance of the solution was then read using spectrophotometer at 532 nm. In this process malondialdehyde (MDA) as a final product of lipid peroxidation reacts with tiobarbitouric acid (TBA) (this reaction completes in 100°C) and releases TBARS that absorbs 532 nm light.[27] Results were expressed as percent of MDA production compared to the control.

Antioxidant enzymes assay

Superoxide dismutase (SOD)

SOD activity was measured spectrophotometrically according to the riboflavin/nitro blue tetrazolium (NBT/RF) assay method.[28] This indirect method involves the inhibition of NBT reduction. In the NBT/RF method, SOD competes with NBT for O_2^- generated by the RF under illumination. The 1.5 ml reaction mixture (50 mM KH_2PO_4, pH 7.8, 0.1 mM EDTA), 2 mM riboflavin and 57 µM NBT) were used. Since generation of O_2^- radicals in the NBT/RF assay is driven by light, samples were subsequently illuminated from above for 15 min by 4 fluorescence tubes (40 W, 30 cm distance) giving 199 µmol photons m^2 s^{-1}. Afterwards, absorbance was measured at 560 nm. Fifty percent inhibition was calculated by regression using the linear part of a natural semi-log curve after which the specific activity was calculated. One unit of SOD activity was defined as the amount of enzyme that inhibits 50% of NBT photochemical reduction.

Catalase (CAT)

Catalase activity was measured following the method of Aebi with minor modifications.[29] The principle of this method was based on the hydrolyzation of H_2O_2 and decreased absorbance at 240 nm. The conversion of H_2O_2 into water and 1/2 oxygen per minute at 25 °C and phosphate buffer (pH 7) was considered to be the enzyme reaction velocity.

Catecholamine measurement

24 hours after last treatment rats were anesthetized with ketamine/xylazine and hippocampus was separated from sculpture. Fresh tissue or tissue that had been frozen in liquid nitrogen and stored at −80 °C were homogenized in cold 0.05 N HClO₄ containing dihydroxybenzylamine

as internal standard. The supernatant after 15 min centrifugation at 12000 g was processed according to Felice et al., except that 0.1 N HClO₄ was used to elute the amines from the alumina.[30] Catecholamine converts to fluorescent substance in alkaline environment and in the presence of ascorbic acid and iodine as a strong oxidant.[30] Fluorescence studies were carried out on a Perkin Elmer luminescence spectrometer LS 55. The excitation wavelength was set at 405 nm and the emission spectra were recorded in 515 nm. Excitation and emission slit were both set at 5 nm.

Western blotting analysis

Caspase 3 and caspase 9 have important role in mitochondria dependent and independent apoptosis pathway respectively so were selected to be quantified via western blot by using specific antibodies (rat specific anti-Caspase-3 and anti-Caspase-9 antibodies purchased from Abcam company). Western blotting was carried out according to our previous study,[31] after SDS-PAGE, the proteins were transferred onto PVDF membrane actively at 140 V for 1.5-2 h in the transfer buffer. After completion of the transfer and blocking, membrane was probed with the primary and secondary specific antibodies and was washed four times in TBST (50 mM Tris, pH 7.5, 150 mM NaCl, 0.05 % Tween 20) between incubations. Bands containing specific proteins were visualized using an ECL detection system according to the manual. Anti β-actin (1:1,000) (Cell Signaling Technology) was used as a housekeeping control. The density was calculated through ImageJ 1.46r; Java 1.6.0_20 software for each band.

Statistical evaluation

All values were expressed as the mean ± standard error of mean (S.E.M). Data was analyzed using one-way ANOVA followed by the post-hoc Duncan multiple range test for analysis of biochemical data using SPSS version 11. Differences were considered significant at $p < 0.05$.

Results and Discussion

Extensive application of the Mn^{2+} in industry and its pollution in the environment, expose human and animal to the manganese neurotoxicity.[4] This study examines toxic effects of $MnCl_2$ on Wistar rats as a suitable model. Therefore we administrated rats by 10 and 15 mg/kg $MnCl_2$ intraperitoneally and assessed behavioral parameters of depression such as body weight dynamic, sucrose preference and immobilizing time in forced swimming test. We also measured ROS, LPO and oxidative stress barriers such as catalase and SOD for examine the role of Mn^{2+} in oxidative damages in rat brain. Catecholamine as an important neurotransmitter in health and normal application of brain was measured. $MnCl_2$ role in cell death was estimated by measuring of the apoptosis involved proteins and tissue sections analysis. We also assessed *Echium amoenum* extract effects on Mn^{2+}-induced neurotoxicity as an important traditional medicine grows in northern part of Iran.[9,10] This plant has been recognized as an important source of phenolic compounds like rosmarinic acid, cyanidin and delphinidin which potentially have chemoprotective effects against toxic metals that are increasing in life today.[4,13] By considering chemical nature of antioxidants and biocompatibility, saline was used in extraction process. Manganese toxicity upon overexposure (manganism) was reported to be accompanied by Parkinson and depression like behavior assigns in miners and welders.[2,4] By considering cognitive disorder as main problem in patients suffer from manganism, its predictable hippocampus is one of the affected tissues in CNS that has not been studied previously.[17,18]

Behavioral assessment

Body weight

Body weight dynamics is a sensitive indicator for chemical toxicants.[32] Previous studies have shown that administration of toxic nanoparticles such as AgNPs and ZnNPs significantly decreased body weight growth rate in rats.[32,33] Therefore to investigate whether exposure to $MnCl_2$ could be considered as a global health issue, we monitored the mortality rate, food consumption, water intake, and body weight dynamic of experimental groups during study. Results showed water/food and survival of rats were not changed significantly in treated rats during experiment. But body weight progressive curve was affected by both doses of $MnCl_2$ and metal treated animals showed a slow increase in body weight. The rats were injected by $MnCl_2$ revealed growing body weight with a mean ± S.E.M. of 304.7 ± 15.2 g in 10 mg/kg Mn^{2+}-treated rats, 297.2 ± 10.4 in 15 mg/kg Mn^{2+}-treated rats and 323.4 ± 12.9 g in control after 15 days. As Figure 1, slop of the body growing curve is dose dependent and has an inverse relationship with Mn^{2+} dose. Interestingly E. amoenum extract improved Mn^{2+} effect, as Figure 1 showed. Body weight of rats that received plant extract in addition to high dose of Mn^{2+}, increases near to the control, 320 ± 13.1 g at the end of experiment.

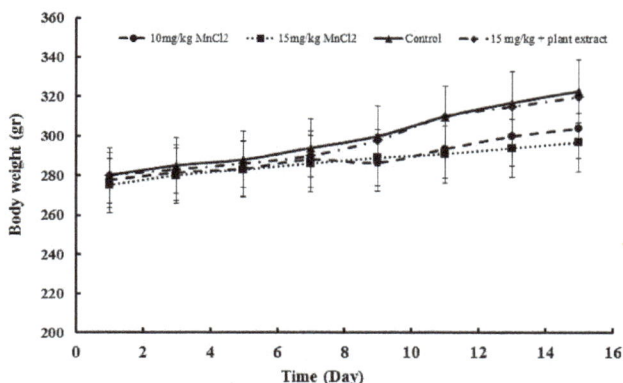

Figure 1. Body weight dynamic during the experimental period. Results showed weight loss in manganese treated rats that improved by oral administration of E. amoenum extract. Each data indicates the mean ± S.E.M.

Forced swimming test (FST)

FST was done to assess depressive-like behavior[21] as a result of $MnCl_2$ injection. Recorded immobility time for 10 mg/kg $MnCl_2$ treated rats is 80.54 ± 4.65 sec, for 15 mg/kg is 101.34 ± 6.43 sec and in control is 15.20 ± 3.23 sec. Therefore Mn^{2+} treatment significantly increased immobility time compared to the control that refer to depression in Mn^{2+} treated rats dose dependently. Figure 2 revealed daily treatment of rats that received 15 mg/kg Mn^{2+} with plant extract reduced immobilization time significantly from 80.54 ± 4.65 sec to 20.22 ± 3.43 sec that approved aqueous extract of E. amoenum relieved depression like behaviors signs. Plant extract slightly increased immobility time in control rats but it's not significant (P<0.05).

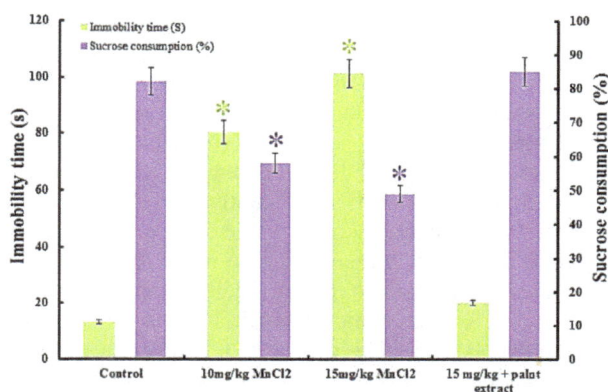

Figure 2. Depression like behavior test. Increased immobilization time and decreased sucrose preference confirmed depression like behavior in rats that received manganese dose dependently. Results showed E. amoenum extract compensates metal toxic effects. Each value indicates the mean ± S.E.M. Asterisk symbols showed significant changes by P<0.05.

Sucrose preference test (SPT)

Sucrose preference test is one of the most commonly used assays for depression in rodents,[22] so we used this test to anhedonia evaluation in Mn^{2+} or/and plant extract treated rats and control. Results showed sucrose consumption decreased significantly in Mn^{2+} received rats dose dependently (Figure 2). Sucrose intake in rats received 10 mg/kg is 58.02 ± 5.13 %, in rats administrated with 15 mg/kg is 49.32 ± 4.29 % and in control rats is 82.16 ± 8.56 %. Decreased sucrose preference refers to depression like behavior in rats as a result of Mn^{2+} injection especially in rats that received high dose. Figure 2 also showed decreased sucrose consumption was improved by plant extract in rats that received high dose of metal (85.45 ± 4.76 %). Control rats which received an equal dose of plant extract don't show significant differences in sucrose intake (data not shown).

Oxidative stress in hippocampus tissue

Noticed depression like behavior and previous studies approved one of the important targets for metals toxicity is CNS.[5-7] To investigate whether the administration of toxic doses of Mn^{2+} creates oxidative stress in hippocampus tissue, we studied ROS content and oxidative barrier enzymes activity in four experimental groups.

ROS measurement

ROS are chemically reactive molecules mainly contain super oxide, peroxide and hydroxyl groups that basically are produced by mitochondria during normal metabolism in low concentration but acute stress increases it by causing mitochondrial dysfunction.[34] Therefore, ROS measurement will give a useful report from oxidative state of the hippocampus tissue related to experimental groups. Figure 3 revealed Mn^{2+} induced high DCF fluorescence intensity that refers to ROS overproduction in hippocampus tissue. 10 mg/kg $MnCl_2$ administration raised ROS level more than 2.5 folds and by increasing metal dose to 15 mg/kg, ROS elevated to more than 3 folds rather than control. Therefore $MnCl_2$ administration causes harsh oxidative stress in hippocampus tissue by overproduction of ROS molecules (Figure 3). Previous studies showed heavy metals damaged mitochondria and interrupted respiratory chain that lead to reactive molecules production.[35] ROS content of $MnCl_2$ treated hippocampus decreased significantly by plant extract. The antioxidant capacity of phenolic compounds in plant extract is attributed to their ability in metal ions and ROS molecules chelating, so protect cell compounds from oxidation.[31] Apoptosis and necrosis in living system are main outcomes of ROS overproduction.[36] Plant effects on ROS level of control rats are not significant that approved *E. amoenum* possibly doesn't affect healthy function of mitochondrial.

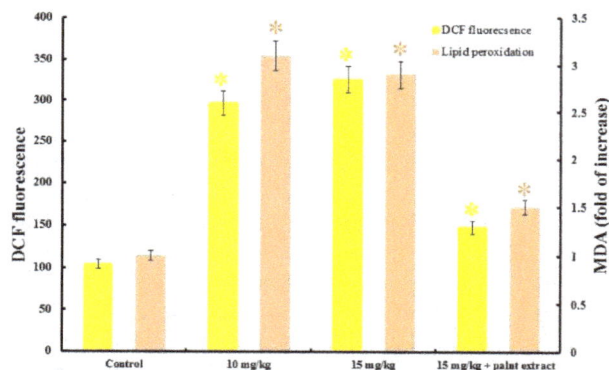

Figure 3. Oxidative stress investigation. Rising of the DCF fluorescence in hippocampus related to metal treated rats refer to ROS overproduction. Increased ROS molecules causes lipid peroxidation that showed by high malondialdehyde content. Interestingly increased oxidative stress attenuated by *E. amoenum* extract. Each data indicates the mean ± S.E.M. Asterisk symbols showed significant changes by P<0.05.

Lipid peroxidation (LPO) evaluation

LPO is the most popular indicator of oxidative stress can be used as a marker of cell membrane injuries also.[26,37] Overproduced reactive molecules attack to the cell membrane lipids and damage it by lipid peroxidation.[38] Malondialdehyde (MDA) is the most known secondary products of lipid peroxidation could be evaluated by thiobarbituric acid method.[27] The rats which received

both doses of metal showed increased MDA about 3 folds than control, that were initially caused by increased free radicals (Figure 3). As Figure 3, plant extract treatment reduces MDA level (about 2 folds) in hippocampus tissue of rats that received 15 mg/kg $MnCl_2$. Therefore MDA level increased in the presence of $MnCl_2$ dose dependently that refers to elevated lipid peroxidation as a result of metal toxicity (Figure 3). Plant extract contains antioxidant molecules that diminished ROS level and consequently reduced MDA in metal treated rats.

SOD and catalase activity measurement

Hippocampus tissue samples were used for measurement of superoxide dismutase (SOD) and catalase (CAT) activities as the most popular antioxidants barrier in biological systems. Since the Mn^{2+} treated rats produce an oxidative stress which could be exhausted by the antioxidative ability of SOD and CAT.[39] Therefore, we estimated both enzyme activities in four experimental groups. Activities of both enzymes were increased in rats who received 10 and 15 mg/kg $MnCl_2$ (Figure 4). SOD and CAT activity that induced by Mn^{2+}, were reduced by plant extract near to the control. As Figure 4, 15 mg/kg $MnCl_2$ causes activation of SOD to 7.8 unit and catalase to 1.35 mmol/min but plant extract decreased it to 2.3 unit and 0.56 mmol/min respectively, while activity of enzymes in control rats are 2.1 unit and 0.52 mmol/min for SOD and catalase respectively. Difference between control group, rats that received 15 mg/kg $MnCl_2$ + plant extract and normal rats that received plant extract are not significant (P<0.05). By considering ROS overproduction in Mn^{2+} administrated rats, increased activity of the SOD and catalase (Figure 3) refers to an adaptation of hippocampus cells to neutralize the extra produced oxidant compounds.[40] The increased SOD activity possibly resulted from SOD overexpression that is regulated by Mn^{2+} as essential cofactor of this enzyme.[2]

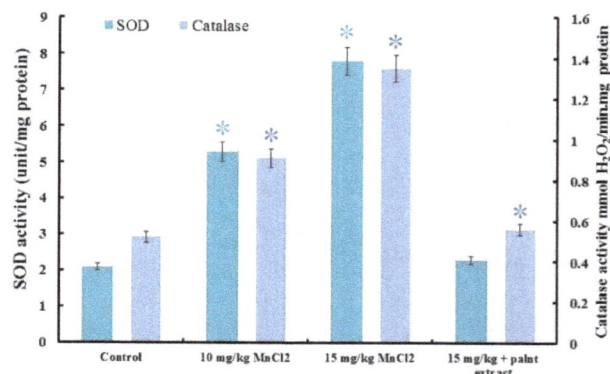

Figure 4. Antioxidant enzyme assessment. Oxidative stress imposed by manganese toxicity causes improving of the superoxide dismutase and catalase enzymes activity in hippocampus tissue as an adaptation to toxic stress. Antioxidant enzymes activity decreased in rats that received plant extract. Each value indicates the mean ± S.E.M. Asterisk symbols showed significant changes by P<0.05.

Catecholamine content of hippocampus tissue

Catecholamines, including dopamine and norepinephrine, are most the important neurotransmitters that mediate a variety of functions in CNS, such as motor control, cognition, emotion, memory processing, and endocrine modulation.[41] Dysfunctions in catecholamine neurotransmission are related to some neuropsychiatric disorders specially Parkinson disease and epilepsy.[31] Similar neuropsychiatric signs in Parkinson disease and manganism possibly are caused by equal molecular events.[2] Therefore catecholamine content of hippocampus tissue was compared between experimental groups as follow: 10 mg/kg MnCl₂, 142.43 ± 12.52 ng/mg protein; 15 mg/kg MnCl₂, 91.45 ± 4.52 ng/mg protein; 15 mg/kg MnCl₂ + plant extract, 250.45 ± 12.34 ng/mg protein and control rats, 210.32 ± 10.23 ng/mg protein. Decreased catecholamine may be caused by increased dopaminergic cell death in the presence of metal ions.[7] Diminished catecholamine was returned near to (even more than) the control by plant extraction treatment, while these kinds of neurotransmitters have dual action (Neurotoxic and neuroprotective) and according to previous experiments, high doses of catecholamine induces apoptosis in the neurons.[42] Control rats that received plant extract showed increase in catecholamine content (224.41 ± 14.29 ng/mg protein) but it's not significant and does not accompanied with abnormal neurobehaviours. Relieving effects of *E. amoenum* in molecular level especially catecholamine rising, finally lead to improved depression like behavior in rats treated by toxic doses of metal as discussed above.

Caspase 9 and caspase 3 analysis

Raised oxidative stress and reduced catecholamine possibly cause cell death in metal treated hippocampus. Catecholamine level of brain is important in healthy function and survival of neurons and decreased catecholamine lead to neurodegeneration in some neurological disease.[42] ROS overproduction was caused by mitochondrial dysfunction or/and inefficient antioxidant barrier that lead to mitochondrial-dependent and –independent apoptosis with different molecular mechanisms.[43] Caspase 9 involves in mitochondrial-independent and caspase 3 participates in mitochondrial-dependent apoptosis.[44,45] Our experiments revealed in rats that received 10 mg/kg MnCl₂ only caspase 9 increased significantly but in rats treated by 15 mg/kg MnCl₂ both of the caspase 3 and caspase 9 increased in hippocampus (Figure 5). These results confirmed more sensitivity of the mitochondria against metal toxicity. Manganese overexposing well documented to result in a disrupted Fe²⁺ homeostasis that lead to mitochondrial dysfunction.[44] As Figure 5, increased expression of the caspase 3 and 9 that induced by 15 mg/kg of metal was improved by oral administration of plant extract.

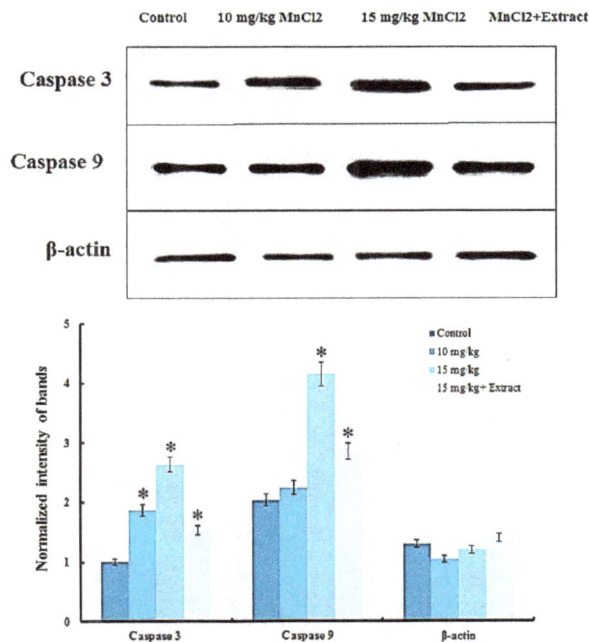

Figure 5. Immunoblotting studies. Up-regulation of caspase 3 and 9 during manganese intoxication refers to increased apoptosis in metal received rats. *E. amoenum* extraction significantly decreased neurodegeneration in hippocampus tissue. The intensity of bands was quantified by ImageJ software. The data were expressed as mean ± S.E.M of three independent experiments. Asterisk (*) was used to denote statistical significance (P<0.05).

Histological studies

The biological significance and toxicological importance of any changes which are found between tissue section in control and experimental groups have been considered as biochemical results confirmation. Therefore after the end of experimental time course, rats were anesthetized and brain tissue separated from scalp. Tissue samples were treated by formalin for fixation and stained by hematoxilin-eosin method and then studied by light microscope.[46] Results showed presence of necrotic and apoptotic cells in tissues were administrated by 10 and 15 mg/kg MnCl₂ (Figure 6). Early apoptotic nuclei have a condensed appearance that frequently seen in MnCl₂ administrated tissue especially in 15 mg/kg MnCl₂ received rats. Increased apoptosis in the metal treated rats accompanied by decreased level of the catecholamine may be due to catecholamine positive role in cell survival or catecholamine producing cell death in Mn²⁺ neurotoxicity. Histology results also were confirmed by elevated level of caspase 3 and 9 in intoxicated rats. As Figure 6, amounts of condensed apoptotic and deformed necrotic cells reduced in tissues related to rats received plant extract+15 mg/kg MnCl₂ that accompanied by decreased caspases and improved behavioral abnormalities also.

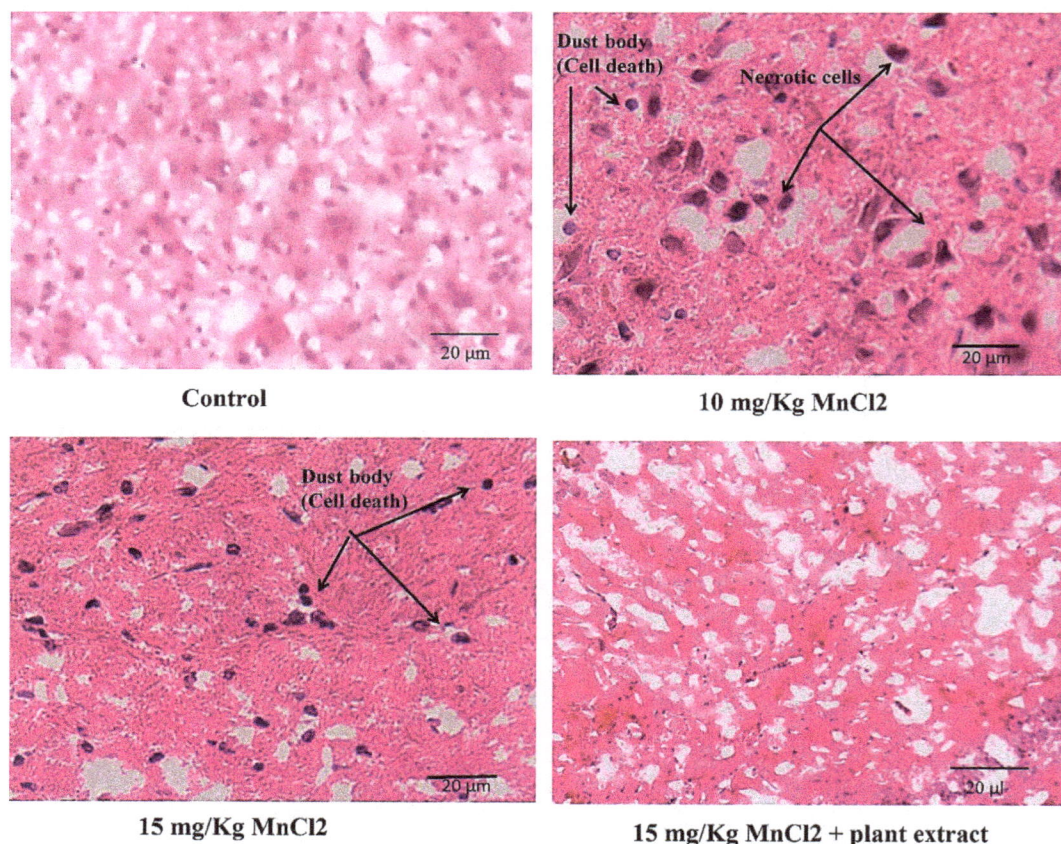

Figure 6. Histological studies. Hematoxylin/eosin staining of hippocampus sections revealed presence of the apoptotic and necrotic cells in MnCl₂ treated rat hippocampus rather than control. Result showed oral administration of *E. amoenum* extraction significantly decreased apoptotic and necrotic cells in hippocampus.

Conclusion

Pathophysiological signs of manganism in human and animal models suggest hippocampus as a possible affected tissue. Our biochemical results approved hash oxidative damages in the presence of MnCl₂ doses that attenuated by plant extract. Increased expression of the caspase 9 in low dose of Mn²⁺ revealed, metal toxicity causes mitochondrial dysfunction at first and then induces oxidative damages that lead to mitochondrial independent apoptosis in the presence of high metal dose (caspase 3 upregulation). Despite the prevalent use of *E. amoenum* as an antidepressant, there are no pharmacological data to support such effects. Our molecular and biochemical studies confirmed *E. amoenum* extract inhibited apoptosis from both described pathways possibly by ROS molecules scavenging, mitochondrial dysfunction improving and metal ions trapping. All of the identified beneficial effects or possibly uncharacterized mechanisms lead to decreased depressive behaviors. Investigated therapeutic effects of *E. amoenum* on Mn²⁺ neurotoxicity revealed this plant could be considered in antidepressant drug design and as supplement against all of the metals toxicity or oxidative damages. By considering physiological and molecular

similarities between manganism and Parkinson disease and also *E. amoenum* role in catecholamine overproduction, this plant could be used as natural co-treatment in associated diseases.

Conflict of Interest

All of the Authors have no conflict of interest to declare.

References

1. O'Neal SL, Zheng W. Manganese Toxicity Upon Overexposure: a Decade in Review. *Curr Environ Health Rep* 2015;2(3):315-28. doi: 10.1007/s40572-015-0056-x

2. Kwakye GF, Paoliello MM, Mukhopadhyay S, Bowman AB, Aschner M. Manganese-induced parkinsonism and parkinson's disease: Shared and distinguishable features. *Int J Environ Res Public Health* 2015;12(7):7519-40. doi: 10.3390/ijerph120707519

3. Takeda A. Manganese action in brain function. *Brain Res Brain Res Rev* 2003;41(1):79-87. doi.org/10.1016/S0165-0173(02)00234-5

4. Long Z, Jiang YM, Li XR, Fadel W, Xu J, Yeh CL, et al. Vulnerability of welders to manganese exposure--a neuroimaging study. *Neurotoxicology* 2014;45:285-92. doi: 10.1016/j.neuro.2014.03.007

5. Oulhote Y, Mergler D, Barbeau B, Bellinger DC, Bouffard T, Brodeur ME, et al. Neurobehavioral function in school-age children exposed to manganese in drinking water. *Environ Health Perspect* 2014;122(12):1343-50. doi: 10.1289/ehp.1307918

6. Peres TV, Schettinger MR, Chen P, Carvalho F, Avila DS, Bowman AB, et al. Manganese-induced neurotoxicity: a review of its behavioral consequences and neuroprotective strategies. *BMC Pharmacol Toxicol* 2016;17(1):57. doi: 10.1186/s40360-016-0099-0

7. Yousefi Babadi V, Sadeghi L, Amraie E, Rezaei M, Malekirad AA, Abarghouei Nejad M. Manganese toxicity in the central nervous system: Decreeing of catecholamine in rat's brains. *Health* 2013;5(12):2146-9. doi: 10.4236/health.2013.512292

8. Belyaeva EA, Sokolova TV, Emelyanova LV, Zakharova IO. Mitochondrial electron transport chain in heavy metal-induced neurotoxicity: Effects of cadmium, mercury, and copper. *ScientificWorldJournal* 2012;2012:136063. doi: 10.1100/2012/136063

9. Safaeian L, Haghjoo Javanmard S, Ghanadian M, Seifabadi S. Cytoprotective and antioxidant effects of echium amoenum anthocyanin-rich extract in human endothelial cells (huvecs). *Avicenna J Phytomed* 2015;5(2):157-66.

10. Ranjbar A, Khorami S, Safarabadi M, Shahmoradi A, Malekirad AA, Vakilian K, et al. Antioxidant activity of iranian echium amoenum fisch & c.A. Mey flower decoction in humans: A cross-sectional before/after clinical trial. *Evid Based Complement Alternat Med* 2006;3(4):469-73. doi: 10.1093/ecam/nel031

11. Nadi F. Bioactive compound retention in Echium amoenum Fisch. & C. A. Mey. petals: Effect of fluidized bed drying conditions. *Int J Food Prot* 2017;20:2249-60. doi: 10.1080/10942912.2016.1233436

12. Abolhassani M. Antibacterial effect of borage (echium amoenum) on staphylococcus aureus. *Braz J Infect Dis* 2004;8(5):382-5. doi: 10.1590/S1413-86702004000500008

13. Rabbani M, Sajjadi SE, Vaseghi G, Jafarian A. Anxiolytic effects of echium amoenum on the elevated plus-maze model of anxiety in mice. *Fitoterapia* 2004;75(5):457-64. doi: 10.1016/j.fitote.2004.04.004

14. Hosseini N, Abolhassani M. Immunomodulatory properties of borage (Echium amoenum) on BALB/c mice infected with Leishmania major. *J Clin Immunol* 2011;31(3):465-71. doi: 10.1007/s10875-010-9502-6

15. Abed A, Minaiyan M, Ghannadi A, Mahzouni P, Babavalian MR. Effect of echium amoenum fisch. Et mey a traditional iranian herbal remedy in an experimental model of acute pancreatitis. *ISRN Gastroenterol* 2012;2012:141548. doi: 10.5402/2012/141548

16. Sayyah M, Boostani H, Pakseresht S, Malaieri A. Efficacy of aqueous extract of echium amoenum in treatment of obsessive-compulsive disorder. *Prog Neuropsychopharmacol Biol Psychiatry* 2009;33(8):1513-6. doi: 10.1016/j.pnpbp.2009.08.021

17. Munoz-Espada AC, Watkins BA. Cyanidin attenuates PGE2 production and cyclooxygenase-2 expression in LNCaP human prostate cancer cells. *J Nutr Biochem* 2006;17(9):589-96. doi: 10.1016/j.jnutbio.2005.10.007

18. Sarnyai Z, Sibille EL, Pavlides C, Fenster RJ, McEwen BS, Toth M. Impaired hippocampal-dependent learning and functional abnormalities in the hippocampus in mice lacking serotonin(1A) receptors. *Proc Natl Acad Sci U S A* 2000;97(26):14731-6. doi: 10.1073/pnas.97.26.14731

19. Robison G, Zakharova T, Fu S, Jiang W, Fulper R, Barrea R, et al. X-ray fluorescence imaging of the hippocampal formation after manganese exposure. *Metallomics* 2013;5(11):1554-65. doi: 10.1039/c3mt00133d

20. Deepa P, Kannappan N. Comparative in vitro antioxidant studies of aqueous solution of formulated poly herbal formulation with marketed preparation. *Der Pharm Lett* 2012;4(5):1515-7.

21. Yankelevitch-Yahav R, Franko M, Huly A, Doron R. The forced swim test as a model of depressive-like behavior. *J Vis Exp* 2015(97). doi: 10.3791/52587

22. Overstreet DH. Modeling depression in animal models. *Methods Mol Biol* 2012;829:125-44. doi: 10.1007/978-1-61779-458-2_7

23. Keston AS, Brandt R. The fluorometric analysis of ultramicro quantities of hydrogen peroxide. *Anal Biochem* 1965;11:1-5.

24. LeBel CP, Ischiropoulos H, Bondy SC. Evaluation of the probe 2',7'-dichlorofluorescin as an indicator of reactive oxygen species formation and oxidative stress. *Chem Res Toxicol* 1992;5(2):227-31.

25. Bradford MM. A rapid and sensitive method for the quantitation of microgram quantities of protein utilizing the principle of protein-dye binding. *Anal Biochem* 1976;72:248-54.

26. Niki E. Lipid peroxidation products as oxidative stress biomarkers. *Biofactors* 2008;34(2):171-80. doi: 10.1002/biof.5520340208.

27. Buege JA, Aust SD. Microsomal lipid, Peroxidation. In: Flesicher S, Packer L, editors. Methods in Enzymology. New-York: Academic Press; 1978.

28. Oyanagui Y. Reevaluation of assay methods and establishment of kit for superoxide dismutase activity. *Anal Biochem* 1984;142(2):290-6.

29. Mittal M, Flora SJ. Vitamin E supplementation protects oxidative stress during arsenic and fluoride antagonism in male mice. *Drug Chem Toxicol* 2007;30(3):263-81. doi:10.1080/01480540701380075

30. Felice LJ, Felice JD, Kissinger PT. Determination of catecholamines in rat brain parts by re- verse-phase ion-pair liquid chromatography. *J Neurochem* 1978;31(6):1461-5.

31. Sadeghi L, Rizvanov AA, Salafutdinov, II, Dabirmanesh B, Sayyah M, Fathollahi Y, et al. Hippocampal asymmetry: Differences in the left and right hippocampus proteome in the rat model of temporal lobe epilepsy. *J Proteomics* 2017;154:22-9. doi: 10.1016/j.jprot.2016.11.023

32. Jacquier M, Crauste F, Soulage CO, Soula HA. A predictive model of the dynamics of body weight and food intake in rats submitted to caloric restrictions. *PLoS One* 2014;9(6):e100073. doi: 10.1371/journal.pone.0100073

33. Yin N, Yao X, Zhou Q, Faiola F, Jiang G. Vitamin E attenuates silver nanoparticle-induced effects on body weight and neurotoxicity in rats. *Biochem Biophys Res Commun* 2015;458(2):405-10. doi: 10.1016/j.bbrc.2015.01.130

34. Gao L, Laude K, Cai H. Mitochondrial pathophysiology, reactive oxygen species, and cardiovascular diseases. *Vet Clin North Am Small Anim Pract* 2008;38(1):137-55, vi. doi: 10.1016/j.cvsm.2007.10.004

35. Sharma B, Singh S, Siddiqi NJ. Biomedical implications of heavy metals induced imbalances in redox systems. *Biomed Res Int* 2014;2014:640754. doi: 10.1155/2014/640754

36. Fu PP, Xia Q, Hwang HM, Ray PC, Yu H. Mechanisms of nanotoxicity: generation of reactive oxygen species. *J Food Drug Anal* 2014;22(1):64-75. doi: 10.1016/j.jfda.2014.01.005

37. Barrera G. Oxidative stress and lipid peroxidation products in cancer progression and therapy. *ISRN Oncol* 2012;2012:137289. doi: 10.5402/2012/137289

38. Pernot F, Heinrich C, Barbier L, Peinnequin A, Carpentier P, Dhote F, et al. Inflammatory changes during epileptogenesis and spontaneous seizures in a mouse model of mesiotemporal lobe epilepsy. *Epilepsia* 2011;52(12):2315-25. doi: 10.1111/j.1528-1167.2011.03273.x

39. Zhan CD, Sindhu RK, Pang J, Ehdaie A, Vaziri ND. Superoxide dismutase, catalase and glutathione peroxidase in the spontaneously hypertensive rat kidney: Effect of antioxidant-rich diet. *J Hypertens* 2004;22(10):2025-33.

40. Vermeij WP, Alia A, Backendorf C. Ros quenching potential of the epidermal cornified cell envelope. *J Invest Dermatol* 2011;131(7):1435-41. doi: 10.1038/jid.2010.433

41. Kobayashi K. Role of catecholamine signaling in brain and nervous system functions: New insights from mouse molecular genetic study. *J Investig Dermatol Symp Proc* 2001;6(1):115-21. doi: 10.1046/j.0022-202x.2001.00011.x

42. Noh JS, Kim EY, Kang JS, Kim HR, Oh YJ, Gwag BJ. Neurotoxic and neuroprotective actions of catecholamines in cortical neurons. *Exp Neurol* 1999;159(1):217-24. doi: 10.1006/exnr.1999.7144

43. Tai YK, Chew KC, Tan BW, Lim KL, Soong TW. Iron mitigates dmt1-mediated manganese cytotoxicity via the ask1-jnk signaling axis: Implications of iron supplementation for manganese toxicity. *Sci Rep* 2016;6:21113. doi: 10.1038/srep21113

44. Wang C, Youle RJ. The role of mitochondria in apoptosis. *Annu Rev Genet* 2009;43:95-118. doi: 10.1146/annurev-genet-102108-134850

45. Brentnall M, Rodriguez-Menocal L, De Guevara RL, Cepero E, Boise LH. Caspase-9, caspase-3 and caspase-7 have distinct roles during intrinsic apoptosis. *BMC Cell Biol* 2013;14:32. doi: 10.1186/1471-2121-14-32

46. Dhandapani S, Subramanian VR, Rajagopal S, Namasivayam N. Hypolipidemic effect of cuminum cyminum l. On alloxan-induced diabetic rats. *Pharmacol Res* 2002;46(3):251-5.

26

Ameliorative Activity of Ethanolic Extract of *Artocarpus heterophyllus* Stem Bark on Alloxan-induced Diabetic Rats

Basiru Olaitan Ajiboye[1]*, Oluwafemi Adeleke Ojo[1], Oluwatosin Adeyonu[1], Oluwatosin Imiere[1], Babatunji Emmanuel Oyinloye[1], Oluwafemi Ogunmodede[2]

[1]*Department of Chemical Sciences, Biochemistry Programme, Afe Babalola University, Ado-Ekiti, Ekiti State, Nigeria.*
[2]*Department of Chemical Sciences, Industrial Chemistry Programme, Afe Babalola University, Ado-Ekiti, Ekiti State, Nigeria.*

Article info

Keywords:
· *Artocarpus heterophyllus* stem bark
· Alloxan
· Serum lipid profiles
· Haematological parameters

Abstract

Purpose: Diabetes mellitus is one of the major endocrine disorders, characterized by impaired insulin action and deficiency. Traditionally, *Artocarpus heterophyllus* stem bark has been reputably used in the management of diabetes mellitus and its complications. The present study evaluates the ameliorative activity of ethanol extract of *Artocarpus heterophyllus* stem bark in alloxan-induced diabetic rats.

Methods: Diabetes mellitus was induced by single intraperitoneal injection of 150 mg/kg body weight of alloxan and the animals were orally administered with 50, 100 and 150 mg/kg body weight ethanol extract of *Artocarpus heterophyllus* stem bark once daily for 21 days.

Results: At the end of the intervention, diabetic control rats showed significant (p<0.05) weight reduction, abnormal haematological parameters, high serum lipids (except high density lipoprotein) concentrations, increased creatinine, bilirubin and urea levels with decreased in albumin level when compared with non-diabetic control rats. All these alterations were reverted to normal after administered with different doses of ethanol extract of *Artocarpus heterophyllus* stem bark most especially at 150 mg/kg body weight which exhibited no significant (p>0.05) different with non-diabetic rats.

Conclusion: The results suggest that ethanol extract of *Artocarpus heterophyllus* stem bark may be useful in ameliorating complications associated with diabetes mellitus patients.

Introduction

Diabetes mellitus is a chronic metabolic disorder characterized by derangements in carbohydrate, protein and lipid metabolisms, due to defective or deficiency in insulin secretion and action.[1] Insulin is a hormone secreted by the beta cells of the Islets of Langerhans of the pancreas, it helps in glucose uptake by the cells, thereby prevents increase in fasting blood glucose levels.[2]

Diabetes mellitus is also associated with hyperglycaemia, which promotes oxidative stress through non-enzymatic glycation and glucose auto-oxidation.[3] This oxidative stress has been implicated in the complications of diabetes mellitus, including dyslipidaemia, a major risk factor for cardiovascular disease,[4] anaemia, nephropathy, and hepatopathy.[3] It is believed that therapeutic agents (like metformin, gliberclamide etc.) normally reduces the effects of oxidative damages in diabetes mellitus patients and therefore ameliorate its complications.[3] But these drugs are characterized with some side effects such as hypoglycaemia, hypersensitivity, gastrointestinal disturbances, lactic acidosis, liver toxicity amongst others.[5,6] Furthermore, in recent years, the search for alternative therapeutic agents in the management/treatment of diabetes has been the major focus of scientific researches across the globe.[7] Added to this, the therapeutic efficacy of medicinal plant due to their believed minimal side effects and its affordability over modern synthetic drugs has been recommended. In this regards many herbal medicines and medicinal plants[7] have been used traditionally for the control and management/ treatment of diabetes mellitus in different parts of the world.[8] It has been reported that screening of medicinal plants for therapeutic purposes, is an important aspect in drug development because they may possess anti-aneamia, anti-dyslipideamia, anti-nephropathy and anti-hepatopathy which may be useful in the management of diabetes mellitus.[9]

Artocarpus heterophyllus (jack fruit) is an example of plant that may be used in this regards, it belongs to a family of *Moraceae* and grown in tropical climates. *Artocarpus heterophyllus* has been considered a rich source of carbohydrates, minerals, dietary fiber and vitamins amongst others.[10] Its stem bark has also been reported to be of great importance in the management of diabetes mellitus locally.[11] In addition, the inhibitory ability of *Artocarpus heterophyllus* stem bark on alpha-amylase and alpha-glucosidase has been documented.[12]

Therefore, the present study was designed to examine the ameliorative effects of ethanol extract of *Artocarpus*

---
*Corresponding author: Basiru Olaitan Ajiboye, Email: bash1428@yahoo.co.uk

heterophyllus stem bark on haematological parameters, serum lipid profiles, liver and kidney functions indices of alloxan-induced diabetic rats.

Materials and Methods
Chemicals
Alloxan used was a product of Sigma Aldrich (St. Louis, MO, USA). Glibenclamide used was a product of Sandoz SA (Pty) Ltd. (Gauteng, South Africa). All assay kits used were obtained from Randox while other chemicals used were purchased from Merck Chemical (Germany).

Collection of Plant Material
The fresh peeled stem bark of *Artocarpus heterophyllus* were collected at a farm in Ibadan, Oyo State, Nigeria. This was then identified and authenticated at the Department of Plant Science, Ekiti State University, Ado-Ekiti, Nigeria.

Extract preparation
The stem bark of *Artocarpus heterophyllus* was shade-dried to a constant weight. Thereafter, kitchen blender was used to blend the dried stem bark of *Artocarpus heterophyllus* into fine power and stored in air-tight containers. Thereafter, 100 grams of powdered plant sample was extracted with 1 litre of 70% ethanol for 48 hours. The extract was then filtered with Whatman filter paper and the filtrate was evaporated to dryness using a freeze dryer. The extract (SBAH) was reconstituted in distilled water and used for subsequent analysis.

Qualitative phytochemical screening
The methods described by[13-15] were employed in these determinations. These include:
(a)   Test for Tannins
1 ml of SBAH was boiled with 20 ml of distilled water in a test tube and filtered. Thereafter, a few drops of 0.1% ferric chloride was added and formation of a green or a blue–black coloration confirm the presence of tannin
(b)   Test for Phlobatannins:
Deposition of a red precipitate when 2 ml of SBAH was boiled with 1% aqueous hydrochloric acid was taken as evidence for the presence of phlobatannins.
(c)   Test for Saponin:
5 ml of the SBAH was boiled with 20 ml of distilled water in a water bath and filtered. Then 10 ml of the filtrate was mixed with another 5 ml of distilled water and shaken vigorously till formation of a stable persistent froth. The frothing was further mixed with 3 drops of olive oil and shaken vigorously until formation of emulsion which confirms the presence of saponin.
(d)   Test of Flavonoids:
In this test, 3 ml of 1 % aluminium chloride was added to 5 ml of SBAH. A yellow coloration was observed indicating the presence of flavonoids.
(e)   Test for Steroids
2 ml of acetic anhydride was added to 2 ml SBAH, thereafter, 2 ml H_2SO_4. The formation of blue or green indicate the presence of steroids.
(f)   Test for Terpenoids

5 ml of SBAH was mixed with 2 ml of chloroform, then 3 ml concentrated H_2SO_4 was added to form a layer. The formation of reddish brown coloration at the interface indicate the presence of terpenoids.
(g)   Test for Cardiac Glycosides
5 ml of SBAH was added to 2 ml of glacial acetic acid containing one drop of ferric chloride solution. Thereafter 1 ml of concentrated sulphuric acid was added. Formation of a violet-green ring appearing below the brown ring, in the acetic acid layer, indicates the presence of glycoside.
(h)   Test for Alkaloids:
1 ml of the SBAH was stirred with 5 ml of 1% aqueous HCl on a steam bath, then filtered while hot. Distilled water was added to the residue and 1 ml of the filtrate was added with a few drops of either Mayer's reagent (Potassium mercuric iodide- solution) or Wagner's reagent (solution of iodine in Potassium iodide) or Dragendorff's reagent (solution of Potassium bismuth iodide). The formation of a cream colour with Mayer's reagent and reddish-brown precipitate with Wagner's and Dragendorff's reagent confirm the presence of alkaloids.
(i)   Test for Anthraquinone
5 ml of SBAH was mixed with 10 ml of benzene, filtered and 5 ml of 10 % NH_3 solution was added to the filtrate. Thereafter, the mixture was shaken until the appearance of pink, red or violet colour.
(j)   Test for Chalcones
2 ml of ammonia solution was added to 5 ml of SBAH and formation of a reddish colour confirmed presence of chalcones.
(k)   Test for Phenol
5 ml of the SBAH was pipetted into a 30 ml test tube, then 10 ml of distilled water was added. 2 ml of ammonium hydroxide solution and 5 ml of concentrated amyl alcohol were then added to the mixture and left for 30 minutes. Formation of bluish green colour indicate the presence of phenol.

Experimental Animals
A total of 36 albino rats' weighting between 180-200 g obtained from Animal Holding Unit of Afe Babalola University, Ado-Ekiti, Ekiti State, Nigeria were used in this study. The animals were kept under standard environmental conditions for 21 days of the experimental period. Prior to this the animals were acclimatized for 7 days. All the animals had free access to food and water throughout the experimental period. All procedures followed were in accordance with the ethical standards of Afe Babalola University Animal Committee with Ethical Approval Number (ABUAD/SCI/004). Also the principle of Laboratory Animal Care were followed throughout the experimental period.

Induction of Diabetes
Freshly prepared alloxan monohydrate of 150 mg/kg body weight dissolved in 0.9% sterile NaCl of pH 7[16] was administered intraperitoneally to rats in group B to F to induce diabetes. Prior to this, their fasting blood glucose levels had been determined. Also, after 48 hours of alloxan

induction, the rats fasting blood glucose levels were assessed with the aid of Acucheck Advantage II glucometer and those that had fasting blood glucose level ≥ 200 mg/dl were considered diabetic and used for the study.[17] The rats were divided into six groups with six rats per group as follows:

Group A: Non-diabetic control rats received distilled water (3 mg/kg body weight)

Group B: Diabetic-control rats received distilled water (3 ml/kg body weight)

Group C: Diabetic rats received glibenclamide (5 mg/kg bodyweight)

Group D: Diabetic rats received 50 mg/kg body weight of SBAH

Group E: Diabetic rats received 100 mg/kg body weight of SBAH

Group F: Diabetic rats received 150 mg/kg body weight of SBAH

Collection and analysis of samples

On the 20th day of oral administration, the animals were fasted overnight for 12 hours and on the 21st day the animals were anaesthetized with halothane and then sacrificed. The animal's blood were then collected by cardiac puncture into ETDA bottles and plain sample bottles. The former were used for haematological parameters determination while the latter were allowed to clot for two hours and centrifuged at 3000 rpm for 10 minutes, after which serum was recovered for analysis.

Haematological parameters determination

The levels of packed cell volume (PCV), haemoglobin (HB), white blood cell (WBC), red blood cell (RBC), neutrophil (N), lymphocyte (L), monocyte (M), eosinophil (E), mean corpuscular haemoglobin concentration (MCHC), mean corpuscular haemoglobin (MCH) and mean corpuscular haemoglobin (MCH) were determined using automated haematology analyzer (System KX-21N[Tm], Japan).

Serum lipid profile determinations

The method[18] modified by[19] was employed for determination of cholesterol concentration. The method of[20] was employed for determination of triglycerides concentration and high density lipoprotein (HDL) concentration, while the Friedwald equation[21] was used for determining very low density lipoprotein (VLDL) concentration and low density lipoprotein (LDL) concentration. Atherogenic index (AI) and coronary artery risk index (CRI) were carried out using[22] and[23] respectively.

Determination of some liver and kidney function indices

The method of[24] was used for albumin determination, while the method described by[25] was employed for bilirubin determination. Creatinine was determined using the method described by Tietz and co-workers[26] while urea was estimated according to the method of Fawcett and Scott.[27] Alanine and aspartate aminotransferase (ALT and AST) activities were determined using the method of Reitman

and Frankel.[28] Alkaline phosphatase was determined as described by Wright et al.[29]

Statistical Analysis

The data were analysed with students' T-test and one way ANOVA. Values of $p<0.05$ were considered significant.

Results and Discussion

Ajiboye et al[30] reported that plants were endowed with series of secondary metabolites like terpenoids, phenolic, lignins, stilbenes, tannins, flavonoids, quinones, coumarins, alkaloids, amines, betalains amongst others. They were free radical scavenging, making them serve as antioxidant compounds and possess antidiabetic activity amongst others. In this study, the ethanol extract of Artocarpus heterophyllus stem bark demonstrated the presence of saponins (Table 1) which possess cholesterol and fasting blood glucose levels lowering effect making it useful for diabetes mellitus patients.[31]

Table 1. Qualitative screening of some phytochemical constituents of ethanol extract of Artocarpus heterophyllus stem bark

Parameters	Artocarpus heterophyllus stem bark
Tannin	+
Phlobatannin	+++
Saponin	+++
Flavonoid	+
Steroid	-
Terpenoid	++
Cardiac glycosides	+++
Alkaloid	+++
Anthraquinone	-
Chalcones	-
Phenol	+++

+++ = much abundant, ++ = less abundant, + = minute and - = absent

The flavonoid (Table 1) in the ethanol extract of Artocarpus heterophyllus stem bark could make it useful as antidiabetic and anticancer agents.[32] Also, Ajiboye et al[30] reported the role of flavonoid in preventing oxidation of LDL therefore reducing the risk for the development of atherosclerosis, one of diabetes mellitus complication. The presence of tannin could make the extract useful in hastening wound healing in diabetes mellitus patients.[33] The tannin, phenol and alkaloid in Table 1 also strengthen the possibility of antidiabetic activity of the extract.[33,34] Alloxan is one the chemicals that are widely used to induce diabetes in experimental animals due to its toxicity on the beta cell of pancreas islet, leading to weight reduction, anaemia, hyperlipidaemia, hepatopathy and nephropathy.[35] In this study there were significant ($p<0.05$) weight reductions in diabetic control rats when compared to non-diabetic control rats. Administration of diabetic rats with 50, 100 and 150 mg/kg body weight of Artocarpus heterophyllus stem bark significantly ($p<0.05$) increased the body weight especially at 150 mg/kg body weight (Figure 1). This is in accordance with[36] that diabetes mellitus patients were characterized by loss of body weight due to increased protein catabolism, as a result of insulin insufficiency.

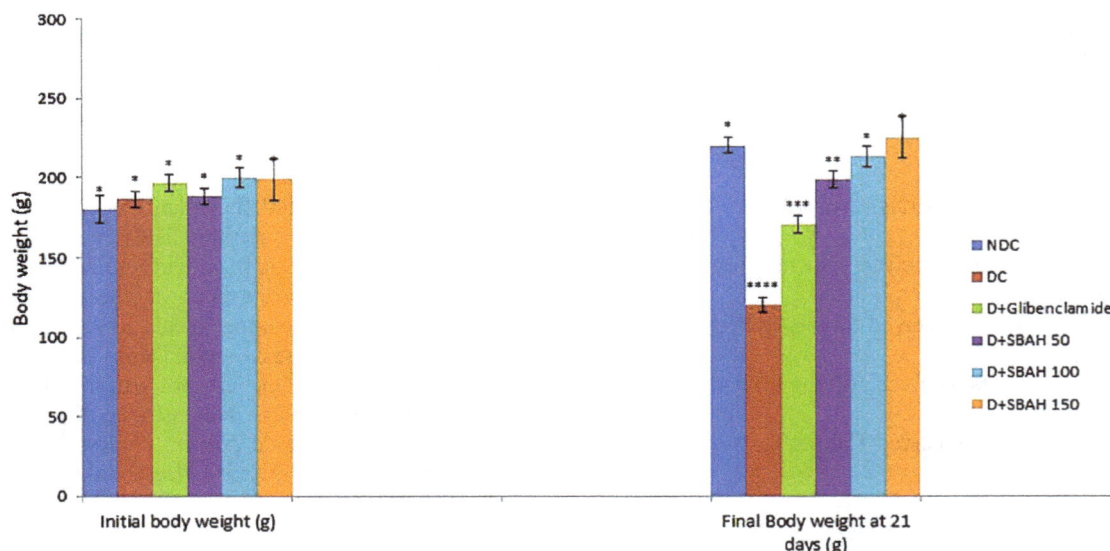

Figure 1. Effect of ethanol extract of *Artocarpus heterophyllus* stem bark on body weight of alloxan-induced diabetic rats
Bars with different superscript are significantly different at p<0.05
NDC (non-diabetic control), DC (Diabetic control), D+ SBAH 50 (Diabetic rats received 50 mg/kg body weight of *Artocarpus heterophyllus* stem bark), D + SBAH 100 (Diabetic rats received 100 mg/kg body weight of *Artocarpus heterophyllus* stem bark, and SBAH 150 (Diabetic rats received 150 mg/kg body weight of *Artocarpus heterophyllus* stem bark

Diabetes mellitus has been characterized by anaemia as reported by,[37] which is supported by the present study especially in diabetic control rats (Table 2). This might due to excess glucose in the hemoglobin, results in glycosylated hemoglobin with decrease in red blood cell (RBC) and packed cell volume (PCV), an indicator of imbalance between its synthesis and destruction.[38]

Anaemia in diabetes mellitus patients may also be attributed to damage in the synthesis of erythropoietin, hormone whose function in promoting formation of the red blood cells, probably due to excess blood glucose.[38,39] This was coupled with significant (p<0.05) decrease in MCV, MCHC and MCH

Table 2. Effect of ethanol extract of *Artocarpus heterophyllus* stem bark on haematological parameters of alloxan-induced diabetic rats

Parameters	NDC	DC	D+glibenclamide	D+ SBAH50	D+ SBAH100	D+150 SBAH
PCV (%)	46.48±0.24*	19.26±1.24****	38.16±1.40***	37.10±0.09***	42.10±0.05**	46.20±1.10*
HB (g/dl)	18.42±0.05*	8.42±0.10*****	10.21±1.15****	12.40±0.01***	15.10±1.10**	18.20±1.10*
WBC (x 10^3/µl)	3.10±1.00*	1.01±0.02***	2.80±0.03**	2.94±0.01**	3.08±0.08*	3.20±0.05*
N (%)	63.01±0.10*	42.19±1.10*****	52.10±1.20****	54.10±1.10***	59.10±0.20**	62.94±1.10*
L (%)	42.23±0.16*	26.10±1.01*****	30.10±0.02****	33.42±0.10***	38.44±1.16**	42.96±0.08*
M (%)	11.20±0.03*	6.01±0.06****	8.20±1.04**	9.60±0.89**	10.01±0.05**	11.46±0.14*
E (%)	5.10±0.01*	1.28±0.12****	3.10±0.06***	3.98±0.06***	4.22±0.10*,**	4.98±0.94*
RBC (x10^{11}/l)	5.94±0.10*	2.48±0.04****	3.28±0.13***	3.84±0.48***	4.46±0.10**	5.68±0.14*
MCHC (g/dl)	42.10±0.04*	28.40±1.10*****	32.18±0.08****	36.40±1.20***	39.20±0.08**	42.84±0.10*
MCV (fl)	96.42±0.10*	58.29±0.56****	86.30±0.94***	92.40±1.02**	93.82±0.94**	96.10±0.04*
MCH (pg)	40.44±1.16*	30.01±0.46****	34.21±0.14***	34.96±0.12***	38.41±0.12**	40.80±0.08*

Each value is a mean of six replicates ± SEM. Values with different superscript along the row are significantly different at p<0.05. PCV (packed cell volume), HB (haemoglobin), WBC (white blood cell), N (neutrophil), L (lymphocyte), M (monocyte), E (eosinophil), RBC (red blood cell), MCHC (mean corpuscular haemoglobin concentration), MCV (mean corpuscular volume), MCH (mean corpuscular haemoglobin), NDC (non-diabetic control), DC (Diabetic control), D+ SBAH 50 (Diabetic rats received 50 mg/kg body weight of *Artocarpus heterophyllus* stem bark), D + SBAH 100 (Diabetic rats received 100 mg/kg body weight of *Artocarpus heterophyllus* stem bark, and SBAH 150 (Diabetic rats received 150 mg/kg body weight of *Artocarpus heterophyllus* stem bark

In addition, the significant (p<0.05) reduction observed in WBC and its differentials (lymphocytes, neutrophil, monocytes and eosinophil) (Table 2) in diabetes control rats might suggest decrease in immune cells in mopping up free radicals generated.[40] Treatment of diabetic rats with ethanol extract of *Artocarpus heterophyllus* stem bark reversed all this haematological abnormalities especially at 150 mg/kg body weight probably due antioxidant nature of the plant.

There were significant (p<0.05) increase in serum lipid profiles and calculated atherogenic and coronary risk indices with a reduction in serum high density lipoprotein-cholesterol (HDL) in diabetic control rats when compared to non-diabetic rats (Table 3). This is in accordance with Wilson and Islam[41] that hyperlipidaemia is another factor directly linked to diabetes mellitus, also, high circulating blood lipid concentrations secrete humoral factors like resistin and adiponectin that alter insulin sensitivity. In this study, hyperlipidaemia were encouraged in diabetic control rats by increasing the levels of low density lipoprotein-cholesterol (LDL), very low density lipoprotein-cholesterol (VLDL) and total cholesterol.[42,43] Oral intervention of diabetic rats administered with 50, 100 and 150 mg/kg body weight of ethanol extract of *Artocarpus heterophyllus* stem bark as well as glibenclamide demonstrated reduction in atherogenesis and coronary artery diseases likewise augmenting the HDL-cholesterol. This is in line with the report of amongst others.[43]

Table 3. Effect of ethanol extract of *Artocarpus heterophyllus* stem bark on serum lipid Profiles, atherogenic and coronary indices of alloxan-induced diabetic rats

Groups	TC (mg/dl)	TG (mg/dl)	LDL (mg/dl)	VLDL (mg/dl)	HDL (mg/dl)	AI	CRI
NDC	80.40 ± 0.50*	64.10 ± 1.20*	23.37 ± 0.01*	12.82 ± 1.03*	44.21 ± 0.05*	0.82 ± 0.10*	1.82 ± 0.01*
DC	110.40±0.40*****	120.10±0.10*****	66.26±0.40*****	24.02±0.05***	20.12±0.18*****	4.49±0.40*****	5.49±0.04****
D+glib	92.10 ± 1.20****	84.20 ± 0.11****	43.16±1.20****	16.84±0.84**	32.10±1.10****	1.87±0.24****	2.87±0.32***
D+ SBAH 50	90.10 ±0.40***	76.20±1.10***	38.62±1.12***	15.24±1.40*, **	36.24±1.40***	1.49±0.02***	2.49±0.14***
D+ SBAH100	84.48 ±0.42**	68.10±1.12**	29.88±0.08**	13.21±1.01*	40.98±1.01**	1.06±0.02**	2.06±0.06**
D+ SBAH150	81.20±0.12*	63.89±0.14*	24.48±0.80*	12.78±1.06*	43.94±1.20*	0.85±0.05*	1.85±0.02*

Each value is a mean of six replicates ± SEM. Values with different superscript across the column are significantly different at p<0.05. D+Glib (D+glibenclamide), TC (total cholesterol), TG (Triglyceride), LDL (low density lipoprotein-cholesterol), VLDL (very low density lipoprotein-cholesterol), HDL (high density lipoprotein-cholesterol), AI (atherogenic index), CRI (coronary risk index), NDC (non-diabetic control), DC (Diabetic control), D+ SBAH 50 (Diabetic rats received 50 mg/kg body weight of *Artocarpus heterophyllus* stem bark), D + SBAH 100 (Diabetic rats received 100 mg/kg body weight of *Artocarpus heterophyllus* stem bark, and SBAH 150 (Diabetic rats received 150 mg/kg body weight of *Artocarpus heterophyllus* stem bark

Moreover, diabetes mellitus has been characterized by hepatopathy and nephropathy,[44] which is supported by the present study (Table 4). This is buttressed with high level of liver-function enzymes like AST, ALT and ALP and other biochemical parameters (urea, creatinine, albumin and bilirubin) in diabetic control rats compared to others groups. The hepato and nephro protective abilities of 50, 100 and 150 mg/kg body weight of ethanol extract of *Artocarpus heterophyllus* stem bark supported by reduction in serum AST, ALT and ALP activities, as well as urea, creatinine (breakdown of muscle mass, as result of increase in gluconeogenesis) and bilirubin levels with increase in albumin (probably due to decrease in gluconeogenesis) levels when compared to diabetic control rats.

Table 4. Effect of ethanol extract of *Artocarpus heterophyllus* stem bark on serum ALT, AST, ALP and other biochemical parameters of alloxan-induced diabetic rats

Groups	ALT (u/l)	AST (u/l)	ALP (u/l)	Albumin (g/l)	Bilirubin(mg/dl)	Creatinine(mg/dl)	Urea (mg/dl)
NC	72.02±1.20*	84.10±0.06*	143.02±1.20*	20.23±1.20*	4.20±0.12*	2.64±0.42**	34.20±1.10*
NDC	126.20±0.90****	140.11±1.30****	500.11±1.02*****	10.10±1.12*****	15.40±0.10****	6.20±1.01***	86.19±0.18*****
D+glib	84.20±1.20***	96.10±0.06***	320.14±0.11****	13.79±0.60****	8.20±1.30***	3.20±0.10**	56.24±1.12****
D+SBAH 50	83.94±1.42***	95.01±2.01***	284.01±0.42***	16.21±0.27***	6.38±0.12***	2.90±0.08*	50.12±1.10***
D+SBAH100	76.20±1.02**	88.10±1.10**	246.15±0.12**	18.53±0.80**	5.80±0.19**	2.70±0.06*	41.12±0.18**
D+SBAH150	73.40±0.41*	85.25±0.20*	153.21±2.12*	20.10±0.31*	4.64±0.18*	2.66±0.10*	34.69±1.14*

Each value is a mean of six replicates ± SEM. Values with different superscript across the column are significantly different at p<0.05. NDC (non-diabetic control), DC (Diabetic control), D+glib (D+glibenclamide), D+ SBAH 50 (Diabetic rats received 50 mg/kg body weight of *Artocarpus heterophyllus* stem bark), D + SBAH 100 (Diabetic rats received 100 mg/kg body weight of *Artocarpus heterophyllus* stem bark, and SBAH 150 (Diabetic rats received 150 mg/kg body weight of *Artocarpus heterophyllus* stem bark

Conclusion

The results of the present study show that various doses of ethanol extract of *Artocarpus heterophyllus* stem bark demonstrates the presence of different phytochemical compounds which serve as antioxidant, therefore improved weight gain, ameliorate anaemia, hyperlipidaemia to normolipidaemia, and demonstrated hepato and nephro-protective in diabetic rats.

Acknowledgments

The authors are very grateful to all the Technologists in Biochemistry Laboratory of Afe Babalola University, Ado-Ekiti.

Conflict of Interest

The authors declare no conflict of interest

References

1. Sada NM, Tanko Y, Mabrouk MA. Modulatory role of soya beans supplement on lipid profiles and liver enzymes on alloxan-induced diabetic Wistar rats. *Eur J Exp Bio* 2013; 3(2):62-7

2. Hesham ZT, Hassan NM, Khalil HI, Kerolles SY. Antidiabetic effects of dietary formulas prepared from some grains and vegetables on type 2 diabetic rats. *J Agroaliment Proc Technol* 2014;20(1):69-79.

3. Azeez OI, Oyagbemi AA, Oyeyemi MO, Odetola AA. Ameliorative effects of cnidoscolus aconitifolius on alloxan toxicity in wistar rats. *Afr Health Sci* 2010;10(3):283-91.

4. Anaelechi JO, Japhet MO, Ude T, Ubuo KA, John EO, Ifeadike C, et al. Effects of *Telfairia occidentalis* seeds on the serum lipid profile and atherogenic indices of male albino Wistar rats. *Pak J Nutr* 2015;14(9):557-62. doi: 10.3923/pjn.2015.557.562

5. Hung HY, Qian K, Morris-Natschke SL, Hsu CS, Lee KH. Recent discovery of plant-derived anti-diabetic natural products. *Nat Prod Rep* 2012;29(5):580-606. doi: 10.1039/c2np00074a

6. Visweswara Rao P, Madhavi K, Dhananjaya Naidu M, Gan SH. Rhinacanthus nasutus improves the levels of liver carbohydrate, protein, glycogen, and liver markers in streptozotocin-induced diabetic rats. *Evid Based Complement Alternat Med* 2013;2013:102901. doi: 10.1155/2013/102901

7. Patel DK, Prasad SK, Kumar R, Hemalatha S. An overview on antidiabetic medicinal plants having insulin mimetic property. *Asian Pac J Trop Biomed* 2012;2(4):320-30. doi: 10.1016/s2221-1691(12)60032-x

8. Ramachandran S, Rajasekaran A, Manisenthilkumar KT. Investigation of hypoglycemic, hypolipidemic and antioxidant activities of aqueous extract of terminalia paniculata bark in diabetic rats. *Asian Pac J Trop Biomed* 2012;2(4):262-8. doi: 10.1016/s2221-1691(12)60020-3

9. Tiwari AK, Rao JM. Diabetes mellitus and multiple therapeutic approaches of phytochemicals: present status and future prospects. *Curr Sci* 2002;83:30-8

10. Omar HS, Hesham A, El-Beshbishy HA, Moussa Z, Taha KF, Singab ANB. Antioxidant activity of *artocarpus heterophyllus* lam. (Jack Fruit) leaf extracts: remarkable attenuations of hyperglycemia and hyperlipidemia in streptozotocin-diabetic rats. *Sci World J* 2011;11:788–800. doi: 10.1100/tsw.2011.71

11. Makherjee B. Traditional medicine. New Delhi: Mohan Primalani for Oxford and IBH publishing; 1993.

12. Ajiboye BO, Ojo OA, Adeyonu O, Imiere O, Olayide I, Fadaka A, et al. Inhibitory effect on key enzymes relevant to acute type-2 diabetes and antioxidative activity of ethanolic extract of *Artocarpus heterophyllus* stem bark. *J Acute Dis* 2016;5(5):423-9. doi: 10.1016/j.joad.2016.08.011

13. Sofowora A. Medicinal Plants and Traditional Medicines in Africa. New York: Chichester John Willey & Sons; 1993.

14. Trease GE, Evans WC. A Text-book of Pharmacognosy. London: Bailliere Tindall Ltd; 1989.

15. Harborne JB. Phytochemical Methods: A Guide to Modern Techniques of Plant Analysis. London: Chapman A & Hall; 1973.

16. Ebong PE, Atangwho IJ, Eyong EU, Egbung GE. The antidiabetic efficacy of combined extracts from two continental plants: *Azadirachta indica* (A. Juss) (Neem) and *Vernonia amygdalina* (Del.) (African Bitter Leaf). *Am J Biochem Biotech* 2008;4(3):239-44. doi:10.3844/ajbbsp.2008.239.244

17. Ajiboye BO, Edobor G1, Ojo AO, Onikanni SA, Olaranwaju OI, Muhammad NO. Effect of aqueous leaf extract of *Senecio biafrae* on hyperglycaemic and serum lipid profile of alloxan-induced diabetic rats. *Inter J Dis Disor* 2014;2(1):059-64

18. Trinder P. Determination of total cholesterol. *Ann Clin Biochem* 1969;6:24–7.

19. Roeschlan P, Bernt E, Grnber W. Total cholesterol estimation by CHOD-PAP enzymatic method. *Clin Chem* 1974;12:403.

20. Tietz NW. Clinical Guide to Laboratory Tests. 3rd ed. Philadelphia, USA: Saunders Company; 1995.

21. Friedewald WT, Levy RI, Fredrickson DS. Estimation of the concentration of low-density lipoprotein cholesterol in plasma, without use of the preparative ultracentrifuge. *Clin Chem* 1972;18(6):499-502.

22. Liu CS, Lin CC, Li TC. The relation of white blood cell count and atherogenic index ratio of ldl-cholesterol to hdl-cholesterol in taiwan school children. *Acta Paediatr Taiwan* 1999;40(5):319-24.

23. Boers M, Nurmohamed MT, Doelman CJ, Lard LR, Verhoeven AC, Voskuyl AE, et al. Influence of glucocorticoids and disease activity on total and high density lipoprotein cholesterol in patients with rheumatoid arthritis. *Ann Rheum Dis* 2003;62(9):842-5.

24. Dumas BT, Watson WA, Biggs HG. Albumin standards and the measurement of serum albumin with bromcresol green. 1971. *Clin Chim Acta* 1997;258(1):21-30.

25. Sherlock S. In Liver Disease. London: CIBA Symposium; Churchill, 1951.

26. Tietz NW, Pruden EL, Siggaad-Anderson A. Tietz Textbook of clinical chemistry. London: Saunders Company; 1994.

27. Fawcett JK, Scott JE. A rapid and precise method for the determination of urea. *J Clin Pathol* 1960;13:156-9.

28. Reitman S, Frankel S. A colorimetric method for the determination of serum glutamic oxalacetic and glutamic pyruvic transaminases. *Am J Clin Pathol* 1957;28(1):56-63.

29. Wright PJ, Leathwood PD, Plummer DT. Enzymes in rat urine: Alkaline phosphatase. *Enzymologia* 1972;42(4):317-27.

30. Ajiboye BO, Ibukun EO, Edobor GI, Ojo OA, Onikanni SA. Qualitative and quantitative analysis of phytochemicals in *Senecio biafrae* leaf. *Int J Inv Pharm Sci* 2013;1(5):428-32

31. Osagie AU, Eka OU. Mineral elements in plant foods. In: Nutritional quality of Plant foods. Nigeria: Ambik press; 1998.

32. Tanko Y, Yaro HA, Isa M, Yerima M, Saleh IA, Mohammed A. Toxicological and hypoglycaemic studies on the leaves of *Cissampelos mucronata* (Menispermaceae) on blood glucose levels of streptozotocin-induced diabetic Wistar rats. *J Med Plants Res* 2007;1(5):113-6.

33. Okwu DE, Josiah C. Evaluation of the chemical composition of two Nigerian medicinal plants. *Afr J Biotechnol* 2006;5(4):357-61.

34. Adefegha SA, Oboh G. Antioxidant and inhibitory properties of *Clerodendrum volubile* leaf extracts on key enzymes relevant to non-insulin dependent diabetes mellitus and hypertension. *J Taibah Univ Sci* 2016;10(4):521-33. doi: 10.1016/j.jtusci.2015.10.008

35. Gomathi D, Kalaiselvi M, Ravikumar G, Devaki K, Uma C. Evaluation of antioxidants in the kidney of streptozotocin induced diabetic rats. *Indian J Clin Biochem* 2014;29(2):221-6. doi: 10.1007/s12291-013-0344-x

36. Moodley K, Joseph K, Naidoo Y, Islam S, Mackraj I. Antioxidant, antidiabetic and hypolipidemic effects of tulbaghia violacea harv. (wild garlic) rhizome methanolic extract in a diabetic rat model. *BMC Complement Altern Med* 2015;15:408. doi: 10.1186/s12906-015-0932-9

37. Aladodo RA, Muhammad, NO, Balogun EA. Effects of aqueous root extract of *Jatropha curcas* on hyperglyceamic and haematological indices in alloxan-induced diabetic rats. *Fount J Nat Appl Sci* 2013;2(1):52-8.

38. Ojo OA, Ajiboye BO, Oyinloye BE, Ojo AB. Hematological Properties of *Irvingia gabonensis* in Male Adult Rats. *J Pharm Sci Innov* 2014;8(18):599-602. doi: 10.7897/2277-4572.035190

39. Horiguchi H, Sato M, Konno N, Fukishima, M. Long-term cadmium exposure induces anemia in rats through hypoproduction of erythropoietin in the kidneys. *Arch Toxicol* 1996;71(1-2):11-9.

40. Ajiboye BO, Muhammad NO. Investigation into the haematological parameters of albino rats fed with *Rana galamensis*–based diet as an alternative source of protein in animal feed. *J Global Agric Ecology* 2015;2(4):112-6.

41. Wilson RD, Islam MS. Fructose-fed streptozotocin-injected rat: An alternative model for type 2 diabetes. *Pharmacol Rep* 2012;64(1):129-39.

42. Ajiboye BO, Muhammad NO, Oloyede HOB. Serum Lipid Profile of Alloxan-induced Diabetic Rats Fed *Triticum aestivum*-based Diet. *Int J Trop Dis Health* 2015;5(4):260-8. doi: 10.9734/IJTDH/2015/12877

43. Mohammed A, Koorbanally NA, Islam MS. Ethyl acetate fraction of aframomum melegueta fruit ameliorates pancreatic beta-cell dysfunction and major diabetes-related parameters in a type 2 diabetes model of rats. *J Ethnopharmacol* 2015;175:518-27. doi: 10.1016/j.jep.2015.10.011

44. Kokou I, Damintoti KS, Amegnona A, Yao A, Messanvi G. Effect of *Aframomum melegueta* on carbon tetrachloride induced liver injury. *J Appl Pharm Sci* 2013;3(9):98-102. doi:10.7324/JAPS.2013.3918

27

Chemical Profile and Biological Activity of *Casimiroa Edulis* Non-Edible Fruit's Parts

Wafaa Mostafa Elkady[1]*, **Eman Ahmed Ibrahim**[2], **Mariam Hussein Gonaid**[1], **Farouk Kamel El Baz**[2]

[1] *Pharmacognosy Department, Faculty of Pharmaceutical Sciences & Pharmaceutical Industries, Future University in Egypt, New Cairo, Egypt.*
[2] *Plant Biochemistry Department, National Research Centre, Dokki, Cairo, Egypt.*

Article info

Keywords:
· *Casimiroa edulis*
· Fatty acids
· Phenolic contents
· Antioxidant
· Anti-inflammatory
· Caco-2

Abstract

Purpose: the non-edible fruit parts of *Casimiroa edulis* Llave et were evaluated for their active constituents and their potential as antioxidants, anti-inflammatory and antitumor activity.

Methods: Fruits peel (FP) and seeds kernel (SK) of *Casimiroa edulis* Llave et Lex. were extracted successively with hexane and then methanol. Fatty acids were prepared from hexane extracts and identified by GC. Total flavonoid, phenolic acids and tannins contents in methanol extracts were determined by UV spectrophotometer and identified by HPLC. Antioxidant, in-vitro anti-inflammatory activity and antitumor effect against Caco-2 cell line were determined .

Results: GC analysis of hexane extracts showed that oleic acid (47.00%) was the major unsaturated fatty acids in both extracts while lignoceric acid (15.49%) is the most abundant saturated fatty acid in (FP). Total phenolic, flavonoid and tannin contents in (FP) & (SK) methanol extracts were; 37.5±1.5, 10.79±0.66 and 22.28±0.23 for (FP); 53.5±1.5mg/g, 14.44±0.32 mg/g; and 53.73±3.58 mg/g for (SK) respectively. HPLC analysis of methanol extract revealed that; the major phenolic compound was pyrogallol in (FP) and p-hydroxybenzoic acid in (SK), the major flavonoid was luteolin 6-arabinose-8-glucose in (FP) and acacetin in (SK).

Conclusion: This study showed that non-edible parts of C. edulis fruit is a rich source of different phenolic compounds and fatty acids which has great antioxidant, anti-inflammatory and antitumor activities; that could be used as a natural source in pharmaceutical industry.

Introduction

Family Rutaceae; is a small family made up of cultivated fruiting trees and medicinal herbs frequently called citrus family, it has a great economic importance because of its several edible Citrus fruits as orange, lemon, etc. Family Rutaceae is dispersed all over the world, particularly in warm climate and tropical areas, mostly found in Africa and Australia.[1]

Casimiroa edulis Llaveet Lex. is a non-citrus fruit belongs to this family, it is commonly known as Zapote blanco or white sapota and mainly cultivated in Mexico and Central America. *C. edulis* is widely consumed in different parts of the world for its valuable fruit;[2] as it is a rich source of sugar, protein, ascorbic acid, phenols, carotenoids, polyunsaturated fatty acids and minerals like Fe, Cu, Zn, Ca and K.[3] It is traditionally used in many countries as a sleep inducer as it has interesting sedative-like effects.[2] *C. edulis* leaves and seeds were found to affect blood pressure, cardiac activity aortic muscular tone,[4] and to possess anticonvulsant activity.[5] Methanol extract *of C. edulis* leaves also showed strong antioxidant activity.[3]

Different classes of compounds were previously separated from different parts of *C. edulis*; furocoumarins and polymethoxyflavones were isolated from the leaves that exhibited adipogenesis activity.[6] Moreover the leaves essential oil had promising antimicrobial activity and

mainly contain sesquiterpene hydrocarbons as major constituents.[7] Zapotin; a flavanoidal compound which considered as chemo-preventive agent was isolated from the seeds; it was also chemically synthesized because of its great anticancer activity.[8] Different compounds were also isolated from the seeds methanolic extract and showed great cardiovascular activity. [9]

Several studies reported that; *C. edulis* can be considered as valuable plant, so the aim of this study is to evaluate the importance of the non-edible parts of *C. edulis* fruit to evaluate its chemical composition as well as antioxidant, anti-inflammatory and antitumor potential.

Materials and Methods

Plant material

The fruit of *C. edulis* was collected from a public garden in Helwan, Cairo, Egypt and identified by taxonomist Therese Labib, consultant in the central gardening administration, Orman garden, Giza, Egypt. Fruits were peeled (FP), seeds were separated from the fruit and the kernel was obtained after removing the seed testa (SK). Both were separately dried at room temperature. A voucher specimen (PHG-8) has been deposited in the Pharmacognosy Department, Faculty of Pharmacy, Future University in Egypt (FUE), New Cairo, Egypt.

Corresponding author: Wafaa Mostafa Elkady, Email: welkady@fue.edu.eg

Preparation of plant extract

100 gm fruit peel (FP) and 100 gm seed kernel (SK) of *C. edulis* were separately coarsely powdered and extracted with n-hexane then by methanol for 72 h using a Soxhlet extractor at 60°C. All the extracts were dried separately under reduced pressure.

Chemical composition

GC analysis of the Fatty Acids composition of hexane extract
Hexane extracts of (FP)He and (SK)He were subjected separately to direct methylation in 1.5% sulfuric acid – methanol at 95°C for 2 h.[10]

Total Flavonoid, Phenolic acids &Tannins content in methanol extract of C. edulis
This was determined for the methanol extracts of (FP)Me and (SK)Me according to methods described previously.[11,12]

HPLC Analysis of the methanol extracts
The phenolic and flavonoid compounds of (FP)Me and (SK)Me of *C. edulis* were extracted according to the method described by Mattila *et al.*[13]

Biological activity for methanol and hexane extracts

Antioxidant activity of C. edulis extracts using ABTS, DPPH and Total antioxidant activity
It was carried out according to Arnao *et al.*,[14] Ye *et al.* method.[15,16]

In vitro Antitumor activity
The activity was tested on Caco-2 cell line using sulforhodamin B assay.[17]

In vitro Anti-inflammatory activity using bovine albumin serum
This was tested using the method of Rahman *et al.*[18]

Statistical analysis

All result is expressed as mean value of three replicate. Data were statistically analyzed through analysis of variance (ANOVA) and Duncans test at P>0.01 using CoStat Statistics Software.

Results and Discussion
Chemical composition

Fatty acids composition of C. edulis hexane extracts
"Table 1" showed that Both (FP)He and (SK)He extracts revealed high percentage of total unsaturated fatty acids 71.15% and 94.20% respectively. The monounsaturated fatty acids oleic acid (omega-9) is the most abundant in both extracts; (36%) in (FP)He and (47%) in (SK)He; Also palmitoleic acid was found in (FP)He (20%) and (SK)He (21%). Furthermore, the hexane extracts showed the presence of different long chain mono and poly unsaturated fatty acids. The unsaturated fatty acids have a great role in decreasing the risk of certain cancers, as colon cancers, breast and prostate.[19]

(FP)He has higher percent of total saturated fatty acid 28.85% than that in (SK)He 5.8%; lignoceric acid 15.49% was the major in (FP)He while palmitic acid 3.01% was the highest in (SK)He; these fatty acids play important role in increasing LDL cholesterol level.[20]

Table 1. GC analysis of unsaturated fatty acid% in hexane extracts

Unsaturated fatty acid		Fatty acid %	
		(FP)He extract	(SK)He extract
$C_{14:1}$	Myristoleic	1.64	0.5
$C_{15:1}$	Pentadecanoic acid	1.29	0.32
$C_{16:1}$	Palmitoleic acid	20.00	21.00
$C_{17:1}$	Heptadecanoic acid	0.35	0.63
$C_{18:1}$	Oleic acid	36.00	47.00
$C_{18:1}$	Vaccenic acid	0.3	ND
$C_{18:2}$	Linoleic acid	2.18	9.00
$C_{18:3}$	α-Linolenic acid	2.56	1.09
$C_{18:3}$	γ-Linolenic acid	ND	9.01
$C_{20:2}$	Eicosadienoic acid	1.09	2.20
$C_{20:3}$	Eicosatrienoic acid	1.28	1.9
$C_{22:1}$	Erucic acid	1.89	ND
$C_{24:1}$	Nervonic acid	2.57	1.55
Saturated fatty acid		(FP)He extract	(SK)He extract
$C_{6:0}$	Caproic acid	0.77	ND
$C_{8:0}$	Caprylic acid	0.60	ND
$C_{10:0}$	Capric acid	0.13	ND
$C_{11:0}$	Undecylic acid	0.2	ND
$C_{12:0}$	Lauric acid	0.67	0.15
$C_{13:0}$	Tridecylic acid	2.47	ND
$C_{14:0}$	Myristic acid	3.4	0.2
$C_{15:0}$	Pentadecylic acid	2.06	0.63
$C_{16:0}$	Palmitic acid	1.23	3.01
$C_{17:0}$	Heptadecanoic acid	ND	1.30
$C_{21:0}$	Heneicosylic acid	0.45	ND
$C_{22:0}$	Behenic acid	1.28	0.3
$C_{23:0}$	Tricosylic acid	0.1	0.21
$C_{24:0}$	Lignoceric acid	15.49	ND
Total mono-unsaturated fatty acid%		64.04	71
Total poly-unsaturated fatty acid %		7.11	23.2
Total saturated fatty acid %		28.85	5.8

ND: not detectable (FP)He: fruit peel hexane extract (SK)He: seed kernel hexane extract

Lipid profile presented in "Table 1" showed that both (FP)He and (SK)He extracts have great percentage of unsaturated fatty acids more than the saturated one; this indicate that the non-edible parts of *C. edulis* can be considered as a valuable natural source that offer a way of increasing the availability of unsaturated fatty acids especially oleic, palmiotleic, linoleic and γ-linolenic acid. Previous studies proved that those acids have a role in inflammation suppression.[20]

Total Flavonoid, Phenolic acids & Tannins contents in C. edulis methanol extract

The results of qualitative analysis of both extracts (FP)Me & (SK)Me revealed the presence of considerable amount of secondary metabolites which could be an indication for their pharmaceutical

potential. The results in "Table 2" showed that they are more abundant in (SK)Me than that in (FP)Me.

HPLC Analysis of phenolic compounds and flavonoid contents in C. edulis methanol extracts

"Table 3" recorded that the (FP)Me and (SK)Me extracts contained different phenolic and flavonoid compounds.

Table 2. Total phenolic acid, flavonoid and tannin contents in *C. edulis* methanol extracts

Methanol extract	Phenolic (mg/g) DW	Flavonoids (mg/g) DW	Tannins (mg/g) DW
(FP)Me	37.5±1.5[b]	10.79±0.66[b]	22.28±0.23[b]
(SK)Me	53.5±1.5[a]	14.44±0.32[a]	53.73±3. 58[a]
LSD	1.9	5.6	9.5

DW: dry weight, (FP)Me: fruit peel methanol extract, (SK)Me: seed kernel hexane extract

Table 3. HPLC analysis of the phenolic and flavonoids compounds in *C. edulis* methanol extracts

Phenolic compounds	(FP)Me (mg/100g) DW	(SK)Me (mg/100g) DW
3,4,5-methoxycinnamic acid	3.43	37.34
4-amino benzoic acid	79.86	4.86
Benzoic acid	252.60	251.11
Caffeic acid	15.38	48.76
Catechein	169.77	240.81
Catechol	230.60	190.87
Chlorogenic acid	175.36	410.98
Cinnamic acid	6.36	24.44
Ellagic acid	52.37	133.42
Epicatechein	176.30	60.97
e-vanillic acid	457.57	344.81
Ferulic acid	53.20	58.32
Gallic acid	21.56	28.94
Iso-ferulic acid	100.11	22.34
p-coumaric acid	52.04	55.63
P-hydroxy benzoic acid	185.72	1571.13
Protocatechuic acid	79.86	89.72
Pyrogallol	1846.16	695.98
Reversetrol	7.00	14.45
Rosmarinic acid	30.37	11.27
Salycilic acid	18.39	60.80
Vanillic acid	53.48	49.70
α- coumaric acid	7.75	36.95
Flavonoids compounds	**(FP)Me (mg/100g) DW**	**(SK)Me (mg/100g) DW**
Luteolin-6-arabinose-8-glucose	1907.92	1242.72
Luteolin-6-glucose-8-arabinose	537.94	561.91
Apigenin-6-arabinose-8-galactose	97.63	41.01
Apigenin-6-rhamnose-8-glucose	322.24	592.74
Apigenin-6-glucose-8-rhamnose	823.66	129.61
Apigenin-7-*O*-neohespiroside	-	17.94
Apigenin-7-*O*-glucose	-	54.66
Luteolin-7-*O*-glucose	-	26.09
Kampferol-3,7-dirhamoside	-	47.02
Luteolin	1103.24	150.63
Acacetin	103.93	2560.78
Naringin	3.48	291.92
Rutin	238.18	181.26
Hespirdin	196.86	-
Quercetrin	25.10	37.75
Quercetin	35.92	298.65
Kampferol	6.66	14.70
Hespirtin	10.45	26.26
Apigenin	0.48	87.31
Rhamnetin	2.58	66.26
Total identified compounds	16	19

Twenty three phenolic compounds were identified in both (FP)Me and (SK)Me by comparison with authentic reference compounds. In (FP)Me pyrogallol is the most abundant phenolic compound 1846.16 mg/100g followed by e-vanillic acid 457.57 mg/100g, benzoic acid 252.6 mg/100g and catechol tannins 230.6 mg/100g. The major phenolic compound in (SK)Me was *P*-hydroxy benzoic acid 1571.13 mg/100g followed by pyrogallol 695.98 mg/100g then cholinergic acid 410.98 mg/100g and e-vanillic acid 344.81 mg/100g.

The total flavonoid compounds identified in (FP)Me extract was 16 compounds the major compound was luteolin 6-arabinose-8-glucose 1907.92 mg/100g.

Biological activity
Antioxidant activity of C. edulis extracts
The antioxidant activity of the methanol and hexane extracts of both (FP) and (SK) was evaluated using the ABTS and DPPH free radical-scavenging assay; "Figure 1a and 1b" showed that the (SK) extracts has higher antioxidant activity than the (FP) extracts, this may be attributed to the higher unsaturated fatty acid, phenolic & flavonoid contents.

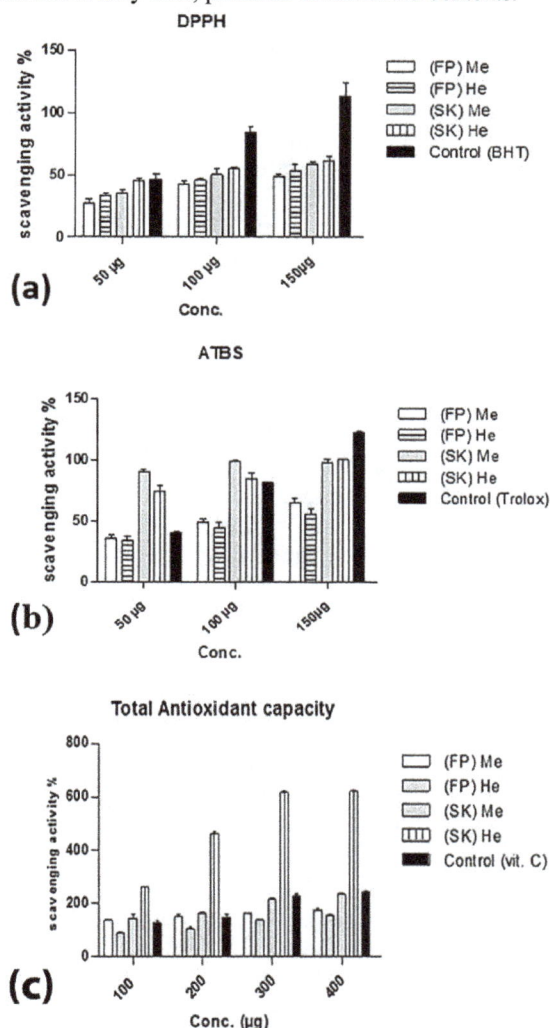

(a)

(b)

(c)

Figure 1. Antioxidant activity of *C. edulis* extracts(FP) Me: fruit peel methanol extract, (SK) Me: seed kernel hexane extract, (FP) He: fruit peel hexane extract, (SK) He: seed kernel hexane extract

On the other hand the results showed that most powerful antioxidant activity is presented in the (SK)He extract "Figure 1c"; this could be due to the high percentage of the unsaturated fatty acids 94.2% "Table 1" especially oleic acid which has great role in protection of cell membranes from free radicals.[21]

The antioxidant activity was also previously reported in the edible parts and leaves methanol extract of *C. edulis*.[3]

In vitro Anti-inflammatory activity
Results in "Figure 2" showed that the (SK)He extract at different doses (50, 100 and 150µg/ml) has the most potent anti-inflammatory activity compared with (Diclofenac) as control drug. This effect may be due to the high percentage of the unsaturated fatty acids in (SK)He extract;[22] the potential anti-inflammatory activity of the methanol extracts can be also attributed to the presence of higher percentage of phenolic contents.

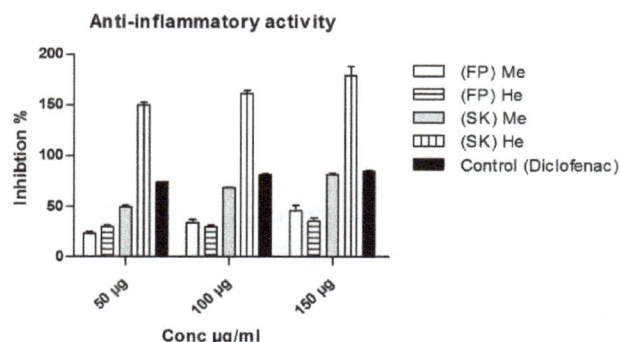

Figure 2. Anti-inflammatory activity of *C. edulis* extracts (FP) Me: fruit peel methanol extract, (SK) Me: seed kernel hexane extract, (FP) He: fruit peel hexane extract ,(SK) He: seed kernel hexane extract

Antitumor activity of C. edulis extracts
"Figure 3" reveled that (FP) and (SK) extracts have certain inhibition effect against the Caco-2 cell line but the most active extract is the (FP)He extract when compared with reference drug doxorubicin, where the IC_{50} is 45 µg/ml.

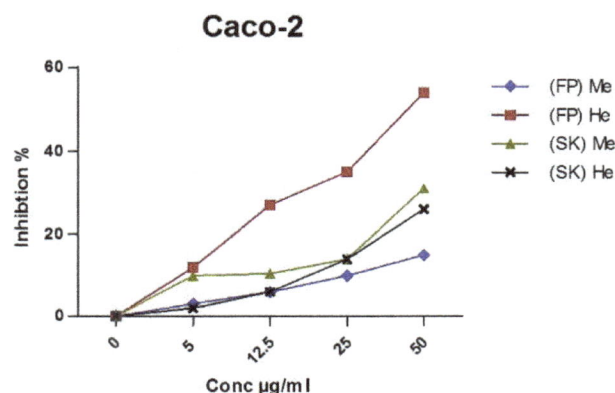

Figure 3. Antitumor activity of *C. edulis* extracts (FP) Me: fruit peel methanol extract, (SK) Me: seed kernel hexane extract, (FP) He: fruit peel hexane extract, (SK) He: seed kernel hexane extract

Conclusion
C. edulis non edible fruit parts could be considered as a valuable source for different useful metabolites as unsaturated fatty acid in the hexane extract and poly-phenolic, flavonoids and tannins in methanol extract; both extracts revealed great importance as antioxidant, anticancer and anti-inflammatory activities. Thus the non-edible part of fruit which is considered as waste product may be phyto-therapeutically used. However; further *in vivo* studies are required to authenticate such biological activities in order to formulate safe effective pharmaceutical herbal product.

Conflict of Interest
The authors declare no conflict of interests.

References
1. Pollio A, De Natale A, Appetiti E, Aliotta G, Touwaide A. Continuity and change in the mediterranean medical tradition: Ruta spp. (rutaceae) in hippocratic medicine and present practices. *J Ethnopharmacol* 2008;116(3):469-82. doi: 10.1016/j.jep.2007.12.013
2. Romero ML, Escobar LI, Lozoya X, Eniquez RG. High-performance liquid chromatographic study of casimiroa edulis: I. Determination of imidazole derivatives and rutin in aqueous and organic extracts. *J Chromatogr A* 1983(281):245-51. doi: 10.1016/S0021-9673(01)87882-1
3. Moo-Huchin VM, Estrada-Mota I, Estrada-Leon R, Cuevas-Glory L, Ortiz-Vazquez E, Vargas y Vargas Mde L, et al. Determination of some physicochemical characteristics, bioactive compounds and antioxidant activity of tropical fruits from yucatan, mexico. *Food Chem* 2014;152:508-15. doi: 10.1016/j.foodchem.2013.12.013
4. Magos GA, Vidrio H. Pharmacology of *casimiroa edulis*; part i. Blood pressure and heart rate effects in the anesthetized rat. *Planta Med* 1991;57(1):20-4. doi: 10.1055/s-2006-960008
5. Garzon-De la Mora P, Garcia-Lopez PM, Garcia-Estrada J, Navarro-Ruiz A, Villanueva-Michel T, Villarreal-de Puga LM, et al. *Casimiroa edulis* seed extracts show anticonvulsive properties in rats. *J Ethnopharmacol* 1999;68(1-3):275-82.
6. Nagai H, Tanaka T, Goto T, Kusudo T, Takahashi N, Kawada T. Phenolic compounds from leaves of *casimiroa edulis* showed adipogenesis activity. *Biosci Biotechnol Biochem* 2014;78(2):296-300. doi: 10.1080/09168451.2014.877821
7. Awaad AS, Al-Jaber NA, Soliman GA, Al-Outhman MR, Zain ME, Moses JE, et al. New biological activities of *casimiroa edulis* leaf extract and isolated compounds. *Phytother Res* 2012;26(3):452-7. doi: 10.1002/ptr.3690
8. Toton E, Romaniuk A, Budzianowski J, Hofmann J, Rybczynska M. Zapotin (5,6,2',6'-tetramethoxyflavone) modulates the crosstalk between autophagy and apoptosis pathways in cancer cells with overexpressed constitutively active pkc. *Nutr Cancer* 2016;68(2):290-304. doi: 10.1080/01635581.2016.1134595
9. Magos GA, Vidrio H, Reynolds WF, Enriquez RG. Pharmacology of *casimiroa edulis* iv. Hypotensive effects of compounds isolated from methanolic extracts in rats and guinea pigs. *J Ethnopharmacol* 1999;64(1):35-44.
10. Barnsteiner A, Lubinus T, di Gianvito A, Schmid W, Engel KH. Gc-based analysis of plant stanyl fatty acid esters in enriched foods. *J Agric Food Chem* 2011;59(10):5204-14. doi: 10.1021/jf104930z
11. Saenkod C, Liu Z, Huang JYG. Antioxidative biochemical properties of extracts from some chinese and thai rice varieties. *Afr J Food Sci* 2013;9(7):300-5. doi: 10.5897/AJFS2013.1010
12. Singleton VL, Orthofer R, Lamuela-Raventos RM. Analysis of total phenols and other oxidation substrates and antioxidant by means of folin-ciocalteu reagent. *Method Enzymol* 1999;299:152-78. doi: 10.1016/S0076-6879(99)99017-1
13. Mattila P, Astola J, Kumpulainen J. Determination of flavonoids in plant material by hplc with diode-array and electro-array detections. *J Agric Food Chem* 2000;48(12):5834-41.
14. Arnao MB, Cano A, Acosta M. The hydrophilic and lipophilic contribution to total antioxidant activity. *Food Chem* 2001;73(2):239-44. doi: 10.1016/S0308-8146(00)00324-1
15. Ye H, Zhou C, Sun Y, Zhang X, Liu J, Hu Q, et al. Antioxidant activities of ethanol extracts from brown seaweed *sargassum pallidum*. *Eur Food Res Technol* 2009;230:101-9. doi: 10.1007/s00217-009-1147-4
16. Prieto P, Pineda M, Aguilar M. Spectrophotometric quantitation of antioxidant capacity through the formation of a phosphomolybdenum complex: Specific application to the determination of vitamin e. *Anal Biochem* 1999;269(2):337-41. doi: 10.1006/abio.1999.4019
17. Tsai AC, Pai HC, Wang CY, Liou JP, Teng CM, Wang JC, et al. In vitro and in vivo anti-tumour effects of mpt0b014, a novel derivative aroylquinoline, and in combination with erlotinib in human non-small-cell lung cancer cells. *Br J Pharmacol* 2014;171(1):122-33. doi: 10.1111/bph.12427
18. Rahman H, Eswaraiah CM, Dutta AM. In-vitro anti-inflammatory and anti-arthritic activity of *oryza sativa* var. Joha rice (an aromatic indigenous rice of assam). *American Eurasian J Agric Environ Sci* 2015;15(1):115-21. doi: 10.5829/idosi.aejaes.2015.115.121
19. Lunn J, Theobald HE. The health effects of dietary unsaturated fatty acids. *Brit Nutr Bull* 2006;31(3):178-224. doi: 10.1111/j.1467-3010.2006.00571.x

20. Bernstein AM, Roizen MF, Martinez L. Purified palmitoleic acid for the reduction of high-sensitivity c-reactive protein and serum lipids: A double-blinded, randomized, placebo controlled study. *J Clin Lipidol* 2014;8(6):612-7. doi: 10.1016/j.jacl.2014.08.001

21. Haug A, Hostmark AT, Harstad OM. Bovine milk in human nutrition--a review. *Lipids Health Dis* 2007;6:25. doi: 10.1186/1476-511x-6-25

22. Ugur G, Chris S. N-3 omega fatty acids: A review of current knowledge. *Int J Food Sci Tech* 2010;45:417-36. doi: 10.1111/j.1365-2621.2009.02151.x

28

Antimicrobial Activity of Carbon-Based Nanoparticles

Solmaz Maleki Dizaj[1], Afsaneh Mennati[2], Samira Jafari[1], Khadejeh Khezri[2], Khosro Adibkia[3]*

[1] *Biotechnology Research Center and Faculty of Pharmacy, Tabriz University of Medical Sciences, Tabriz, Iran.*
[2] *Faculty of Science, Physical Chemistry Group, Uremia Payam Noor University, Uremia, Iran.*
[3] *Drug Applied Research Center and Faculty of Pharmacy, Tabriz University of Medical Sciences, Tabriz, Iran.*

Article info

Keywords:
· Carbon nanotubes
· Fullerene
· Graphene oxide
· Antimicrobial activity
· Antimicrobial mechanism
· Metal-carbon nanocomposites

Abstract

Due to the vast and inappropriate use of the antibiotics, microorganisms have begun to develop resistance to the commonly used antimicrobial agents. So therefore, development of the new and effective antimicrobial agents seems to be necessary. According to some recent reports, carbon-based nanomaterials such as fullerenes, carbon nanotubes (CNTs) (especially single-walled carbon nanotubes (SWCNTs)) and graphene oxide (GO) nanoparticles show potent antimicrobial properties. In present review, we have briefly summarized the antimicrobial activity of carbon-based nanoparticles together with their mechanism of action. Reviewed literature show that the size of carbon nanoparticles plays an important role in the inactivation of the microorganisms. As major mechanism, direct contact of microorganisms with carbon nanostructures seriously affects their cellular membrane integrity, metabolic processes and morphology. The antimicrobial activity of carbon-based nanostructures may interestingly be investigated in the near future owing to their high surface/volume ratio, large inner volume and other unique chemical and physical properties. In addition, application of functionalized carbon nanomaterials as carriers for the ordinary antibiotics possibly will decrease the associated resistance, enhance their bioavailability and provide their targeted delivery.

Introduction

The increasing resistance of the microorganisms towards antibiotics has been led to serious health problems in the recent years. Most infection-causing bacteria are resistant to at least one of the antibiotics that are generally used to eradicate the infection.[1] This problem encourages the researchers to study the new agents which can effectively inhibit microbial growth.

Nanomaterials have been considered for use in the optical devices, superconductors, fuel cells, catalysts, biosensors, drug and gene delivery and so on.[2-5] Nanomaterials as the novel drug delivery systems have been also applied to improve the physicochemical and therapeutic effectiveness of the drugs.[6-8] Likewise, nanotechnology in pharmaceuticals and microbiology showed promising applications to overcome the problem of antibiotic resistance.[2,9-11] Over the past few years, various nano-sized antibacterial agents such as metal and metal oxide nanoparticles have been evaluated by researchers. Several types of metal and metal oxide nanoparticles such as silver (Ag), silver oxide (Ag$_2$O), titanium dioxide (TiO$_2$), zinc oxide (ZnO), gold (Au), calcium oxide (CaO), silica (Si), copper oxide (CuO), and magnesium oxide (MgO) have been known to show antimicrobial activity.[12-18]

It has been known that carbon-based nanoparticles exhibit high antimicrobial activity as well. Early studies indicated that fullerenes, single-walled carbon nanotubes (SWCNTs) and graphene oxide (GO) nanoparticles showed potent microcidal properties. These new allotropic types of carbon have been discovered in the last two decades, and, since then, they have used in many field of science.[19-21]

It has also been revealed that, the size and surface area of carbon nanomaterials are important parameters affecting their antibacterial activity; that is, increasing the nanoparticles surface area by decreasing their size lead to improving their activity for interaction with bacteria.[22,23] Generally, the antimicrobial activity of the nanoparticles depend on their composition, surface modification, intrinsic properties, and the type of microorganism.[23, 24] It has been proposed that carbon-based nanomaterials cause membrane damage in bacteria due to an oxidative stress.[25-29] According to recent studies the physical interaction of carbon-based nanomaterials with bacteria, rather than oxidative stress, is the primary antimicrobial activity of these nanostructures.[28,30] In fact, the interactions between bacterial cells and carbon-based nanomaterials play an important role in their antimicrobial mechanism.[31] There is some evidence in the literature that the aggregation between bacterial cells and carbon nanomaterials cause direct contact between the cells and carbon nanomaterials which in turn lead to cell death.[30-32]

It is clear that, prior to biomedical application of the carbon-based nanostructures; some important issues related to their toxicity should be clearly elucidated. In

*Corresponding author: Khosro Adibkia, E-mail: adibkia@tbzmed.ac.ir

point of fact, they need to be purified and functionalized[23,33] and their solubility in physiological media should be improved as well.[34,35] In this article the antimicrobial activity of carbon-based nanoparticles and their mechanism of action were briefly reviewed.

Carbon nanotubes

CNTs are nano-sized hollow cylindrical form of carbon which has been synthesized by Lijima in 1991.[36] Since then, CNTs have been applied in many fields of science and technology. Kang et al (2007) provided the first document that showed SWCNTs had strong antimicrobial activity on *Escherichia coli* (*E. coli*). They demonstrated that SWCNTs could cause severe membrane damage and subsequent cell death.[30] In other study (2008) they presented the first evidence that the size of carbon nanotubes was an important factor affecting their antibacterial activity. They prepared SWCNTs and multi-walled carbon nanotubes (MWCNTs) and investigated their antibacterial effect against *E. coli*. Their results indicated that SWCNTs were much more toxic to bacteria than MWCNTs. The authors also reported that, direct cell contact with CNTs influenced the cellular membrane integrity, metabolism processes and morphology of *E. coli*. According to the authors, SWCNTs could penetrate into the cell wall better than MWCNTs due to their smaller nanotube diameter. Furthermore, the superior surface area of SWCNTs initiated better interaction with the cell surface.[22]

Arias and Yang (2009) investigated the antimicrobial activities of SWCNTs and MWCNTs with different surface groups towards rod-shaped or round-shaped gram-negative and gram-positive bacteria. According to their results, SWCNTs with surface groups of -OH and -COOH indicated improved antimicrobial activity to both gram-positive and gram-negative bacteria while MWCNTs with the same surface groups did not exhibit any significant antimicrobial effect. Their results showed that, formation of cell-CNTs aggregates caused to damage the cell wall of bacteria and then release of their DNA content.[37]

In a study by Yang et al (2010), the effect of SWCNTs length on their antimicrobial activity was investigated. Upon their findings the longer SWCNTs indicated stronger antimicrobial activity due to their improved aggregation with bacterial cells.[31]

Dong et al (2012) investigated the antibacterial properties of SWCNTs dispersed in different surfactant solutions (sodium holate, sodium dodecyl benzenesulfonate, and sodium dodecyl sulfate) against *Salmonella enteric (S. enteric)*, *E. coli*, and *Enterococcus faecium*. According to their results, SWCNTs exhibited antibacterial activity against both *S. enterica* and *E. coli* which was improved with the increase of nanotube concentrations. The combination of SWCNTs with surfactant solutions was also found to be low toxic to 1321N1 human astrocytoma cells, so they can be employed in biomedical applications especially for drug-resistant and multidrug-resistant microorganisms.[38] Figure 1 shows the schematic mechanism of antimicrobial activity of carbon nanotubes.

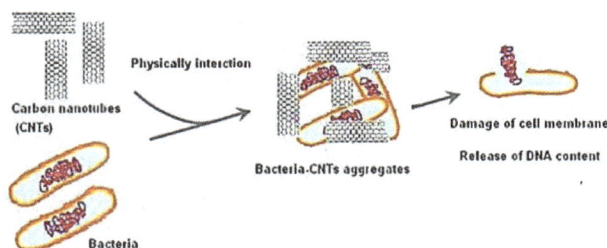

Figure 1. Mechanism of antimicrobial activity of carbon nanotubes.

Fullerenes

Fullerenes are soccer ball-shaped molecules composed of carbon atoms.[39] Fullerenes showed antimicrobial activity against various bacteria, such as *E. coli*, *Salmonella* and *Streptococcus spp*.[39] The antibacterial effect was probably due to inhibition of energy metabolism after internalization of the nanoparticles into the bacteria.[26,33] It has also been suggested that fullerene derivatives can inhibit bacterial growth by impairing the respiratory chain.[19,40] In the beginning, a decrease of oxygen uptake (at low fullerene derivative concentration) and then an increase of oxygen uptake (followed by an enhancement of hydrogen peroxide production) are occurred.[19,40] Another bactericidal mechanism which has been proposed was the induction of cell membrane disruption.[19] As stated by the literature, the hydrophobic surface of the fullerenes can easily interact with membrane lipids and intercalate into them.[19,39,40] The discovery of fullerenes ability to interact with biological membranes has encouraged many researchers to evaluate their antimicrobials applications.[41]

Among three different classes of fullerene compounds (positively charged, neutral, and negatively charged), cationic derivatives showed the maximum antibacterial effect on *E. coli* and *Shewanella oneidensis*; while the anionic derivatives were almost ineffective.[19,42] This could be owing to the strong interactions of negatively charged bacteria with the cationic fullerenes.[42]

Deryabin et al (2014) compared the antibacterial activity of two water-soluble derivatives of the fullerene. In their work, protonated amine (AF) and deprotonated carboxylic (CF) groups were added to the fullerene cage via organic linkers. The former positively charged derivative bounded effectively to the *E. coli* cells; however, the later negatively charged one did not exhibit any significant antibacterial activity. They concluded that the water-soluble cationic fullerene derivative could be used in the preparation of chemical disinfectants.[40]

Fullerenes can also be applied as photosensitizers in photodynamic therapy (PDT) when their solubility is increased via functionalizing with hydrophilic groups.[39] In fact, water soluble fullerenes in the presence of biological reducing agents produce superoxide and this process is relatively more cytotoxic towards microbial cells than mammalian cells.[43,44] Tegos et al (2005) tested antibacterial activity of fulleropyrrolidinium salts after photoirradiation and their results showed that more than 99.9% of bacterial and fungal cells were killed.

In the other study, Yu et al (2005) evaluated the antibacterial activity of a sulfobutyl fullerene derivative on environmental bacteria. They found that, the employed derivative was able to inhibit environmental bacteria after photoirradiation.[19] Moreover, Mizuno and et al (2011) reported that cationic-substituted fullerene derivative were highly effective in killing a broad spectrum of microbial cells after irradiation with white light. They evaluated a new group of synthetic fullerene derivatives, which possessed either basic or quaternary amino groups, against gram-positive (Staphylococcus aureus (S. aureus)), gram-negative bacteria (E. coli) and fungi (Candida albicans (C. albicans)). They reported that the most important affecting factor was an increased number of quaternary cationic groups that were widely dispersed around the fullerene cage to minimize aggregation. According to their results, S. aureus was found to be most susceptible; E. coli was intermediate, while C. albicans was the most resistant species. The authors suggested that, the quaternized fullerenes could effectively be applied in treatment of superficial infections, e.g. in wounds and burns, where light penetration into tissue is not problematic.[45]

Graphene oxide (GO)

A monolayer of carbon atoms which are tightly packed into a two-dimensional crystal is normally called Graphene.[44] GO nanosheets which could be readily dispersed in water are produced by chemically modification of the graphene with suspended hydroxyl, epoxyl, and carboxyl groups. It is documented that, membrane stress resulted from direct contact with sharp nanosheets is the major antimicrobial mechanism of GO.[46]
Both graphene and GO were shown inhibitory effect on the growth of E. coli. Akhavan and Ghaderi (2010) tested the antibacterial activity of graphene sheets and verified that direct interaction of the related extremely sharp edges with bacteria caused RNA effluxes through the damaged cell membranes of both gram-negative (E.) and gram-positive (S. aureus) bacteria.[47] Gurunathan et al (2012) also studied the antimicrobial activity of GO and reduced graphene oxide nanowalls. Their results proved that the direct contact of bacteria (S. aureus) with the very sharp edge of the applied nanowalls led to the cell membrane damage. According to the authors, the antibacterial effect of the reduced graphene nanowires was comparable with SWCNTs.[34] The similar antibacterial activity against E. coli were reported by Hu et al (2010) for GO and reduced graphene oxide nanosheets.[44]

In another work, Azimi et al (2014) testified the antimicrobial effect of two functionalized GO nanostructures (grapheme oxide-chlorophyllin and graphene oxide-chlorophyllin-Zn) against E. coli. The authors proposed that the functionalized GO led to cell membrane damage of E. coli. Furthermore, their results signified that the surface chemistry and metal toxicity played a major role in antibacterial activity of graphene oxide-chlorophyllin-Zn. The physical interaction of GO with the cell membrane, hydrogen bonding of colorless tetrapyrroles with a specific outer cellular component and generation of intercellular hydroxyl radicals through aqueous leaching of Zn^{2+} were suggested as the possible antibacterial mechanisms.[46]

Carbon nanocomposites composed of carbon nanostructures and metal nanoparticles (e.g. CNT-Ag and GO-Ag nanocomposites) have recently been revealed the appropriate antibacterial activity against both gram-negative and positive bacteria. However, the antibacterial activity of CNT-Ag was superior to GO-Ag nanocomposites which could be due to good dispersion of the Ag nanoparticles into the CNT.[48]

Ag-carbon nanocomplexes also showed efficient inhibitory activity against some important pathogens such as *Burkholderia cepacia*, methicillin-resistant *S. aureus*, multidrug-resistant *Acinetobacter baumannii* and *Klebsiella pneumoniae*. These nanostructures could inhibit the growth of bio-defense bacteria such as *Yersinia pestis* as well.[49]

Different types of carbon-based nanoparticles used as antimicrobial agent; their mechanisms of action as well as the associated characteristics have been summarized in Table 1.

Table 1. Types of carbon-based nanoparticles as antimicrobial agent, their mechanisms of action and characteristics

Type of nanoparticles	Proposed mechanism of antimicrobial action	Main characteristics as antimicrobial agent	The main factors that influence antimicrobial activity	References
Fullerene	Inhibit bacterial growth by impairing the respiratory chain; inhibition of energy metabolism.	Stability; Photodynamic therapy activity; high ability to functionalization; high surface/volume ratio; large inner volume	Particle size; type of functional group; surface charge.	19, 21, 39-41, 44
SWTNs	Physical interaction with cell membrane; formation of cell-CNTs aggregates; induction the cell membrane disruption.	Stability; high ability to functionalization; high surface/volume ratio; large inner volume	Particle size; particle length; type of functional group; type of buffer; concentration; surface charge.	27, 30, 31, 38
GO	Physical interaction with cell membrane; formation of cell-GO aggregates; induction the cell membrane disruption.	Stability; high ability to functionalization, high surface/volume ratio; sharp edges of nanowalles.	Particle size; type of functional group.	25, 34, 35, 44, 46

Conclusion

A number of studies have reported effective antimicrobial activity of the carbon nanostructures. The size of these nanoparticles plays an important role in the inactivation of microorganisms. Among carbon nanostructures, fullerenes, SWCNTs and GO nanoparticles and their derivatives were found to be more efficient as antibacterial agents. The probable mechanisms of their antibacterial activity were proposed as follow: inhibition of bacterial growth by impairing the respiratory chain; inhibition of energy metabolism; physical interaction with cell membrane; formation of cell-CNTs/ cell-GO aggregates; induction the cell membrane disruption. In order to biological and medicinal applications, carbon nanostructures should be purified and functionalized. Their solubility should also be enhanced in physiological media. Finally, application of carbon nanocomposites composed of carbon nanostructures and metal nanoparticles could be considered as a hopeful approach for disinfection purposes. However, further studies are necessary to understand the exact mechanisms of the antimicrobial activity of carbon nanostructures.

Conflict of Interest

The authors report no conflicts of interest.

References

1. Allahverdiyev AM, Abamor ES, Bagirova M, Rafailovich M. Antimicrobial effects of TiO(2) and Ag(2)O nanoparticles against drug-resistant bacteria and leishmania parasites. *Future Microbiol* 2011;6(8):933-40.
2. Adibkia K, Omidi Y, Siahi MR, Javadzadeh AR, Barzegar-Jalali M, Barar J, et al. Inhibition of endotoxin-induced uveitis by methylprednisolone acetate nanosuspension in rabbits. *J Ocul Pharmacol Ther* 2007;23(5):421-32.
3. Tiwari PM, Vig K, Dennis VA, Singh SR. Functionalized gold nanoparticles and their biomedical applications. *Nanomater* 2011;1(1):31-63.
4. Zinjarde SS. Bio-inspired nanomaterials and their applications as antimicrobial agents. *Chronic Young Sci* 2012;3(1):74-81.
5. Bahrami K, Nazari P, Nabavi M, Golkar M, Almasirad A, Shahverdi AR. Hydroxyl capped silver-gold alloy nanoparticles: characterization and their combination effect with different antibiotics against Staphylococcus aureus. *Nanomed J* 2014;1(3):155-61.
6. Ravishankar Rai V, Jamuna Bai A. Nanoparticles and their potential application as antimicrobials. A Méndez-Vilas A, editor. Mysore: Formatex; 2011.
7. Marambio-Jones C, Hoek EM. A review of the antibacterial effects of silver nanomaterials and potential implications for human health and the environment. *J Nanopart Res* 2010;12(5):1531-51.
8. Adibkia K, Barzegar-Jalali M, Nokhodchi A, Siahi Shadbad M, Omidi Y, Javadzadeh Y, et al. A review on the methods of preparation of pharmaceutical nanoparticles. *Pharm Sci* 2010;15(4):303-14.
9. Adibkia K, Javadzadeh Y, Dastmalchi S, Mohammadi G, Niri FK, Alaei-Beirami M. Naproxen-eudragit RS100 nanoparticles: preparation and physicochemical characterization. *Colloids Surf B Biointerfaces* 2011;83(1):155-9.
10. Mohammadi G, Nokhodchi A, Barzegar-Jalali M, Lotfipour F, Adibkia K, Ehyaei N, et al. Physicochemical and anti-bacterial performance characterization of clarithromycin nanoparticles as colloidal drug delivery system. *Colloids Surf B Biointerfaces* 2011;88(1):39-44.
11. Kannan RR, Jerley AJA, Ranjani M, Prakash VSG. Antimicrobial silver nanoparticle induces organ deformities in the developing Zebrafish (*Danio rerio*) embryos. *J Biomed Sci Engine* 2011;4;248-54.
12. Azam A, Ahmed AS, Oves M, Khan MS, Habib SS, Memic A. Antimicrobial activity of metal oxide nanoparticles against Gram-positive and Gram-negative bacteria: a comparative study. *Int J Nanomedicine* 2012;7:6003-9.
13. Besinis A, De Peralta T, Handy RD. The antibacterial effects of silver, titanium dioxide and silica dioxide nanoparticles compared to the dental disinfectant chlorhexidine on Streptococcus mutans using a suite of bioassays. *Nanotoxicology* 2014;8(1):1-16.
14. Emami-Karvani Z, Chehrazi P. Antibacterial activity of ZnO nanoparticle on grampositive and gram-negative bacteria. *Afr J Microbiol Res* 2011;5(12):1368-73.
15. Usman MS, El Zowalaty ME, Shameli K, Zainuddin N, Salama M, Ibrahim NA. Synthesis, characterization, and antimicrobial properties of copper nanoparticles. *Int J Nanomedicine* 2013;8:4467-79.
16. Chen Q, Xue Y, Sun J. Kupfer cell-mediated hepatic injury induced by silica nanoparticles in vitro and in vivo. *Int J Nanomedicine* 2013;8:1129-40.
17. Pal S, Tak YK, Song JM. Does the antibacterial activity of silver nanoparticles depend on the shape of the nanoparticle? A study of the gram-negative bacterium Escherichia coli. *Appl Environ Microb* 2007;73(6):1712-20.
18. Zarei M, Jamnejad A, Khajehali E. Antibacterial Effect of Silver Nanoparticles Against Four Foodborne Pathogens. *Jundishapur J Microb* 2014;7(1):E8720.
19. Cataldo F, Da Ros T. Medicinal chemistry and pharmacological potential of fullerenes and carbon nanotubes. Trieste: Springer; 2008.
20. Wang JT, Chen C, Wang E, Kawazoe Y. A new carbon allotrope with six-fold helical chains in all-sp2 bonding networks. *Sci Rep* 2014;4:4339.

21. Sokolov VI, Stankevich IV. The fullerenes-new allotropic forms of carbon: molecular and electronic structure, and chemical properties. *Russ Chem Rev* 1993;62(5):419.

22. Kang S, Herzberg M, Rodrigues DF, Elimelech M. Antibacterial effects of carbon nanotubes: size does matter! *Langmuir* 2008;24(13):6409-13.

23. Buzea C, Pacheco, Ii, Robbie K. Nanomaterials and nanoparticles: sources and toxicity. *Biointerphases* 2007;2(4):MR17-71.

24. Hajipour MJ, Fromm KM, Ashkarran AA, Jimenez De Aberasturi D, De Larramendi IR, Rojo T, et al. Antibacterial properties of nanoparticles. *Trends Biotechnol* 2012;30(10):499-511.

25. Gurunathan S, Han JW, Dayem AA, Eppakayala V, Kim JH. Oxidative stress-mediated antibacterial activity of graphene oxide and reduced graphene oxide in Pseudomonas aeruginosa. *Int J Nanomedicine* 2012;7:5901-14.

26. Shvedova AA, Pietroiusti A, Fadeel B, Kagan VE. Mechanisms of carbon nanotube-induced toxicity: focus on oxidative stress. *Toxicol Appl Pharmacol* 2012;261(2):121-33.

27. Vecitis CD, Zodrow KR, Kang S, Elimelech M. Electronic-structure-dependent bacterial cytotoxicity of single-walled carbon nanotubes. *ACS nano* 2010;4(9):5471-9.

28. Manke A, Wang L, Rojanasakul Y. Mechanisms of nanoparticle-induced oxidative stress and toxicity. *Biomed Res Int* 2013;2013:942916.

29. Pacurar M, Qian Y, Fu W, Schwegler-Berry D, Ding M, Castranova V, Guo NL. Cell permeability, migration, and reactive oxygen species induced by multiwalled carbon nanotubes in humanmicrovascular endothelial cells. *J Toxicol Environ Health A* 2012;75(3):129-47.

30. Kang S, Pinault M, Pfefferle LD, Elimelech M. Single-walled carbon nanotubes exhibit strong antimicrobial activity. *Langmuir* 2007;23(17):8670-3.

31. Yang C, Mamouni J, Tang Y, Yang L. Antimicrobial activity of single-walled carbon nanotubes: length effect. *Langmuir* 2010;26(20):16013-9.

32. Murray AR, Kisin ER, Tkach AV, Yanamala N, Mercer R, Young SH, et al. Factoring-in agglomeration of carbon nanotubes and nanofibers for better prediction of their toxicity versus asbestos. *Part Fibre Toxicol* 2012;9:10.

33. Bellucci S. Nanoparticles and Nanodevices in Biological Applications. Germany: Springer-Verlag, Berlin-Heidelberg; 2009.

34. Dinadayalane TC, Leszczynska D, Leszczynski J. Towards Efficient Designing of Safe Nanomaterials. Leszczynski J, Puzyn T, Kroto H, editors. Cambridge, UK: Royal society of chemistry; 2012.

35. Yang K, Wan J, Zhang S, Zhang Y, Lee ST, Liu Z. In vivo pharmacokinetics, long-term biodistribution, and toxicology of PEGylated graphene in mice. *ACS nano* 2011;5(1):516-22.

36. Han J. Carbon Nanotubes: Science and Application. Meyyappan M, editor. Boca Raton: CRC Press LLC; 2005.

37. Arias LR, Yang L. Inactivation of bacterial pathogens by carbon nanotubes in suspensions. *Langmuir* 2009;25(5):3003-12.

38. Dong L, Henderson A, Field C. Antimicrobial activity of single-walled carbon nanotubes suspended in different surfactants. *J Nanotechnol* 2012;2012:1-7.

39. Tegos GP, Demidova TN, Arcila-Lopez D, Lee H, Wharton T, Gali H, et al. Cationic fullerenes are effective and selective antimicrobial photosensitizers. *Chem Biol* 2005;12(10):1127-35.

40. Deryabin DG, Davydova OK, Yankina ZZ, Vasilchenko AS, Miroshnikov SA, Kornev AB, et al. The Activity of [60] Fullerene Derivatives Bearing Amine and Carboxylic Solubilizing Groups against Escherichia coli: A Comparative Study. *J Nanomater* 2014;2014:1-9.

41. Yang X, Ebrahimi A, Li J, Cui Q. Fullerene-biomolecule conjugates and their biomedicinal applications. *Int J Nanomedicine* 2014;9:77-92.

42. Nakamura S, Mashino T. Biological activities of water-soluble fullerene derivatives. *J Phys Conf Ser* 2009;159:012003.

43. Sharma SK, Chiang LY, Hamblin MR. Photodynamic therapy with fullerenes in vivo: reality or a dream? *Nanomedicine (Lond)* 2011;6(10):1813-25.

44. Lu Z, Dai T, Huang L, Kurup DB, Tegos GP, Jahnke A, et al. Photodynamic therapy with a cationic functionalized fullerene rescues mice from fatal wound infections. *Nanomedicine (Lond)* 2010;5(10):1525-33.

45. Mizuno K, Zhiyentayev T, Huang L, Khalil S, Nasim F, Tegos GP, et al. Antimicrobial Photodynamic Therapy with Functionalized Fullerenes: Quantitative Structure-activity Relationships. *J Nanomed Nanotechnol* 2011;2(2):1-9.

46. Azimi S, Behin J, Abiri R, Rajabi L, Derakhshan AA, Karimnezhad H. Synthesis, Characterization and Antibacterial Activity of Chlorophyllin Functionalized Graphene Oxide Nanostructures. *Sci Adv Mater* 2014;6(4):771-81.

47. Akhavan O, Ghaderi E. Toxicity of Graphene and Graphene Oxide Nanowalls Against Bacteria. *Acs nano* 2010;4:5731.

48. Yun H, Kim JD, Choi HC, Lee CW. Antibacterial Activity of CNT-Ag and GO-Ag Nanocomposites Against Gram-negative and Gram-positive Bacteria. *Bull Korean Chem Soc* 2013;34(11):3261.

49. Leid J, Ditto A, Knapp A, Shah P, Wright B, Blust R, et al. In vitro antimicrobial studies of silver carbine complexes: activity of free and nanoparticle carbene formulations against clinical isolates of pathogenic bacteria. *J Antimicrob Chemother* 2012;67:138-48.

Permissions

All chapters in this book were first published in APB, by Tabriz University of Medical Sciences; hereby published with permission under the Creative Commons Attribution License or equivalent. Every chapter published in this book has been scrutinized by our experts. Their significance has been extensively debated. The topics covered herein carry significant findings which will fuel the growth of the discipline. They may even be implemented as practical applications or may be referred to as a beginning point for another development.

The contributors of this book come from diverse backgrounds, making this book a truly international effort. This book will bring forth new frontiers with its revolutionizing research information and detailed analysis of the nascent developments around the world.

We would like to thank all the contributing authors for lending their expertise to make the book truly unique. They have played a crucial role in the development of this book. Without their invaluable contributions this book wouldn't have been possible. They have made vital efforts to compile up to date information on the varied aspects of this subject to make this book a valuable addition to the collection of many professionals and students.

This book was conceptualized with the vision of imparting up-to-date information and advanced data in this field. To ensure the same, a matchless editorial board was set up. Every individual on the board went through rigorous rounds of assessment to prove their worth. After which they invested a large part of their time researching and compiling the most relevant data for our readers.

The editorial board has been involved in producing this book since its inception. They have spent rigorous hours researching and exploring the diverse topics which have resulted in the successful publishing of this book. They have passed on their knowledge of decades through this book. To expedite this challenging task, the publisher supported the team at every step. A small team of assistant editors was also appointed to further simplify the editing procedure and attain best results for the readers.

Apart from the editorial board, the designing team has also invested a significant amount of their time in understanding the subject and creating the most relevant covers. They scrutinized every image to scout for the most suitable representation of the subject and create an appropriate cover for the book.

The publishing team has been an ardent support to the editorial, designing and production team. Their endless efforts to recruit the best for this project, has resulted in the accomplishment of this book. They are a veteran in the field of academics and their pool of knowledge is as vast as their experience in printing. Their expertise and guidance has proved useful at every step. Their uncompromising quality standards have made this book an exceptional effort. Their encouragement from time to time has been an inspiration for everyone.

The publisher and the editorial board hope that this book will prove to be a valuable piece of knowledge for researchers, students, practitioners and scholars across the globe.

List of Contributors

Sridharan Badrinathan, Micheal Thomas Shiju, Ramachandran Arya and Pragasam Viswanathan
Renal Research Lab, Centre for Bio Medical Research, School of Biosciences and Technology, VIT University, Vellore, Tamil Nadu, India

Ganesh Nachiappa Rajesh
Department of Pathology, Jawaharlal Institute of Postgraduate Medical Education and Research (JIPMER), Dhanvantrinagar, Puducherry, India

Edson Hideaki Yoshida, Natália Tribuiani, Giovana Sabadim, Débora Antunes Neto Moreno and Yoko Oshima-Franco
Post-Graduate Program in Pharmaceutical Sciences, University of Sorocaba (UNISO), Sorocaba, SP, Brazil

Eliana Aparecida Varanda
Pharmaceutical Sciences Faculty of Araraquara, São Paulo State University (UNESP), Rodovia Araraquara-Jau, Km 1, CEP 14801-902, Araraquara, São Paulo, Brazil

Keyvan Yousefi
Department of Pharmacology, Faculty of pharmacy, Tabriz University of Medical Sciences, Tabriz, Iran

Sanaz Hamedeyazdan and Fatemeh Fathiazad
Department of Pharmacognosy, Faculty of pharmacy, Tabriz University of Medical Sciences, Tabriz, Iran

Mohammadali Torbati
Department of Traditional Pharmacy, Faculty of Traditional Medicine, Tabriz University of Medical Sciences, Tabriz, Iran

Uliana Vladimirovna Karpiuk, Irina Cholak and Oksana Yemelianova
Bogomolets National Medical University, Kiev, Ukraine

Khaldun Mohammad Al Azzam
Department of Pharmaceutical Chemistry, Pharmacy Program, Batterjee Medical College for Sciences and Technology (BMC), 21442 Jeddah, Kingdom of Saudi Arabia

Zead Helmi Mahmoud Abudayeh and Ahmad Naddaf
Faculty of Pharmacy, Isra University, 11622 Amman, Jordan

Viktoria Kislichenko
National University of Pharmacy, Kharkiv, Ukraine

Abolfazl Aslani
Department of Pharmaceutics, School of Pharmacy and Novel Drug Delivery Systems Research Center, Isfahan University of Medical Sciences, Isfahan, Iran

Behzad Zolfaghari
Department of Pharmacognosy, School of Pharmacy and Isfahan Pharmaceutical Sciences Research Center, Isfahan University of Medical Sciences, Isfahan, Iran

Fatemeh Davoodvandi
Novel Drug Delivery Systems Research Center, Isfahan University of Medical Sciences, Isfahan, Iran

Mohammad Sina
Department of Medical Biotechnology, Faculty of Advanced Medical Sciences, Tabriz University of Medical Sciences, Tabriz, Iran
Biotechnology Research Center, Tabriz University of Medical Sciences, Tabriz, Iran

Davoud Farajzadeh
Biotechnology Research Center, Tabriz University of Medical Sciences, Tabriz, Iran
Department of Cellular and Molecular Biology, Faculty of Biological Sciences, Azarbaijan Shahid Madani University, Tabriz, Iran

Siavoush Dastmalchi
Biotechnology Research Center, Tabriz University of Medical Sciences, Tabriz, Iran
Department of Medicinal Chemistry, School of Pharmacy, Tabriz University of Medical Sciences, Tabriz, Iran

Farideh Doostan
Physiology Research Center, Kerman University of Medical Sciences, Kerman, Iran

Roxana Vafafar
Department of Biology, Faculty of Science, Islamic Azad University, Ahar Branch, Ahar, Iran

Parvin Zakeri-Milani and Aliasghar Pouri
Liver and Gastrointestinal Diseases Research Center, Tabriz University of Medical Sciences, Tabriz, Iran

Rogayeh Amini Afshar
Faculty of Sciences, Urmia University, Urmia, Iran

Mehran Mesgari Abbasi
Student Research Committee, Drug Applied Research Center, Tabriz University of Medical Sciences, Tabriz, Iran

Jaleh Esmaeilzadeh, Hossein Nazemiyeh and Maryam Maghsoodi
Faculty of Pharmacy, Tabriz University of Medical Sciences, Tabriz, Iran

Farzaneh Lotfipour
Faculty of Pharmacy, Tabriz University of Medical Sciences, Tabriz, Iran
Gastrointestinal and Liver Disease Research Center, Tabriz University of Medical Sciences, Tabriz, Iran

Kanchanapa Sathirachawan
School of Cosmetic Science, Mae Fah Luang University, Chiang Rai 57100, Thailand

Puxvadee Chaikul, Tawanun Sripisut, Setinee Chanpirom and Naphatsorn Ditthawuthikul
School of Cosmetic Science, Mae Fah Luang University, Chiang Rai 57100, Thailand
Phytocosmetics and Cosmeceuticals Research Group, Mae Fah Luang University, Chiang Rai 57100, Thailand

Tingting Wang, Huajuan Lin, Qian Tu, Jingjing Liu and Xican Li
School of Chinese Herbal Medicine, Guangzhou University of Chinese Medicine, Waihuang East Road No.232, Guangzhou Higher Education Mega Center, 510006, Guangzhou, China

Abbas Azadmehr
Immunology Department, Qazvin University of Medical Sciences, Qazvin, Iran
Immunology Department, Babol University of Medical Sciences, Babol, Iran

Reza Hajiaghaee
Pharmacognosy and Pharmaceutics Department of Medicinal Plants Research Center, Institute of Medicinal Plants, ACECR, Karaj, Iran

Behzad Baradaran
Immunology Research Center, Tabriz University of Medical Sciences, Tabriz, Iran

Hashem Haghdoost-Yazdi
Physiology Department, Qazvin University of Medical Sciences, Qazvin, Iran

Niloofar Bazazzadegan, Mehdi Banan and Hamid Reza Khorram Khorshid
Genetics Research Center, University of Social Welfare and Rehabilitation Sciences, Tehran, Iran

Marzieh Dehghan Shasaltaneh
Laboratory of Neuro-organic Chemistry, Institute of Biochemistry and Biophysics (IBB), University of Tehran, Tehran, Iran

Kioomars Saliminejad and Koorosh Kamali
Reproductive Biotechnology Research Center, Avicenna Research Institute, ACECR, Tehran, Iran

Md. Afjalus Siraj
Department of Pharmaceutical Science, Daniel K. Inouye College of Pharmacy, University of Hawaii at Hilo, Hilo, HI 96720, USA

Jamil A. Shilpi, Md. Golam Hossain and Shaikh Jamal Uddin
Faculty of Pharmacy Discipline, Life Science School, Khulna University, Khulna 9208, Bangladesh

Md. Khirul Islam
Department of Biochemistry, Faculty of Mathematics and Natural Sciences, University of Turku, FI-20500, Finland

Ismet Ara Jahan and Hemayet Hossain
BCSIR Laboratories, Bangladesh Council of Scientific and Industrial Research (BCSIR), Dhaka 1205, Bangladesh

Solmaz Asnaashari and Sedigheh Bamdad Moghaddam
Drug Applied Research Center, Tabriz University of Medical Sciences, Tabriz, Iran

Parina Asgharian and Abbas Delazar
Drug Applied Research Center, Tabriz University of Medical Sciences, Tabriz, Iran
Department of Pharmacognosy, Faculty of Pharmacy, Tabriz University of Medical Sciences, Tabriz, Iran

Fariba Heshmati Afshar
Drug Applied Research Center, Tabriz University of Medical Sciences, Tabriz, Iran
Faculty of Traditional Medicine, Tabriz University of Medical Sciences, Tabriz, Iran

Atefeh Ebrahimi
Department of Pharmacognosy, Faculty of Pharmacy, Tabriz University of Medical Sciences, Tabriz, Iran

Nasser Razmaraii
Drug Applied Research Center, Tabriz University of Medical Sciences, Tabriz, 5165665811, Iran
Student Research Committee, Tabriz University of Medical Sciences, Tabriz, 5166614756, Iran

Hossein Babaei
Drug Applied Research Center, Tabriz University of Medical Sciences, Tabriz, 5165665811, Iran
School of Pharmacy, Tabriz University of Medical Sciences, Tabriz, 5166414766, Iran

Alireza Mohajjel Nayebi and Yadollah Azarmi
School of Pharmacy, Tabriz University of Medical Sciences, Tabriz, 5166414766, Iran

Gholamreza Assadnassab
Department of Clinical Sciences, Tabriz Branch, Islamic Azad University, Tabriz, 5157944533, Iran

Javad Ashrafi Helan
Department of Pathobiology, Faculty of Veterinary Medicine, University of Tabriz, Tabriz, 5166617564, Iran

Zead Helmi Mahmoud Abudayeh and Ahmad Naddaf
Faculty of Pharmacy, Isra University, 11622 Amman, Jordan

Khaldun Mohammad Al Azzam
Department of Pharmaceutical Chemistry, Pharmacy Program, Batterjee Medical College for Sciences and Technology (BMC), 21442 Jeddah, Kingdom of Saudi Arabia

Uliana Vladimirovna Karpiuk
Department of pharmacognosy and botany, National Medical University is the name of O.O.Bogomolets, Ukraine

Viktoria Sergeevna Kislichenko
National University of Pharmacy, Kharkiv, Ukraine

Mahmood Sadeghi Ataabadi and Sanaz Alaee
Department of Reproductive Biology, School of Advanced Medical Sciences and Technologies, Shiraz University of Medical Sciences, Shiraz, Iran

Mohammad Jafar Bagheri and Soghra Bahmanpoor
Department of Anatomy, School of Medicine, Shiraz University of Medical Sciences, Shiraz, Iran

Amir Hooshang Mohammadpour and Sepideh Elyasi
Pharmaceutical Research Center, Mashhad University of Medical Sciences, Mashhad, Iran
Department of Clinical Pharmacy, School of Pharmacy, Mashhad University of Medical Sciences, Mashhad, Iran

Fatemeh Mashhadi, Atefeh Rezapour, Saeed Falahaty and Azadeh Zayerzadeh
Department of Clinical Pharmacy, School of Pharmacy, Mashhad University of Medical Sciences, Mashhad, Iran

Saeed Nazemi, Sepideh Afzalnia and Afsaneh Mohammadi
Research and Education Department, Razavi Hospital, Mashhad, Iran

Mohammad Afshar
Department of Anatomy, Birjand University of Medical Sciences, Birjand, Iran
Medical Toxicology Research Center, Mashhad University of Medical Sciences, Mashhad, Iran

Hamid Reza Mashreghi Moghadam
Birjand Cardiovascular Disease Research Center; Department of Cardiology, Birjand University of Medical Sciences, Birjand, Iran

Maryam Moradian
Department of Pediatric Cardiology, Rajaie Cardiovascular Medical and Research Center, Tehran, Iran

Seyed Mohammad Hasan Moallem
School of Medicine, Mashhad University of Medical Sciences, Mashhad, Iran

Mohammad Alizadeh and Elham Mirtaheri
Nutrition Research Center, Faculty of Nutrition, Tabriz University of Medical Sciences, Tabriz, Iran

Nazli Namazi
Nutrition Research Center, Faculty of Nutrition, Tabriz University of Medical Sciences, Tabriz, Iran
Diabetes Research Center, Endocrinology and Metabolism Clinical Sciences Institute, Tehran University of Medical Sciences, Tehran, Iran

Nafiseh Sargheini
Molecular Biomedicine, University of Bonn, Bonn, Germany

Sorayya Kheirouri
Department of Nutrition, Tabriz University of Medical Sciences, Tabriz, Iran

Elham Arkan and Ali barati
Nano Drug Delivery Research Center, Kermanshah University of Medical Sciences, Kermanshah, Iran

Mohsen Rahmanpanah, Leila Hosseinzadeh, Samaneh Moradi and Marziyeh Hajialyani
Pharmaceutical Sciences Research Center, Faculty of Pharmacy, Kermanshah University of Medical Sciences, Kermanshah, Iran

Behzad Mansoori, Dariush Shanehbandi and Behzad Baradaran
Immunology Research Center, Tabriz University of Medical Sciences, Tabriz, Iran

Hamed Mohammadi and Farhad Babaie
Immunology Research Center, Tabriz University of Medical Sciences, Tabriz, Iran
Department of Immunology, School of Medicine, Tabriz University of Medical Sciences, Tabriz, Iran

Maryam Hemmatzadeh
Immunology Research Center, Tabriz University of Medical Sciences, Tabriz, Iran

Mehdi Yousefi
Department of Immunology, School of Medicine, Tabriz University of Medical Sciences, Tabriz, Iran

Mehrdad Ebrazeh
Department of Laboratory Medicine, Shahid Motahari Hospital, Urmia University of Medical Sciences, Urmia, Iran

Farshid Rezaei, Rashid Jamei and Reza Heidari
Department of Biology, Faculty of Science, University of Urmia, West Azerbaijan, Iran

Sina Mojaverrostami
Young Researchers and Elite Club, Behshahr Branch, Islamic Azad University, Behshahr, Iran

Maryam Nazm Bojnordi
Department of Anatomy & Cell Biology, Faculty of Medicine, Mazandaran University of Medical Sciences, Sari, Iran

Hatef Ghasemi Hamidabadi
Immunogenetic Research Center, Department of Anatomy & Cell Biology, Faculty of Medicine, Mazandaran University of Medical Sciences, Sari, Iran

Maryam Ghasemi-Kasman
Cellular and Molecular Biology Research Center, Health Research Institute, Babol University of Medical Sciences, Babol, Iran

Mohammad Ali Ebrahimzadeh
Pharmaceutical Sciences Research Center, School of Pharmacy, Mazandaran University of Medical Sciences, Sari, Iran

Ata Mahmoodpoor
Department of Anesthesiology, Tabriz University of Medical Sciences, Tabriz, Iran

Hossein Nazemiyeh
Research Center for Pharmaceutical Nanotechnology, Tabriz University of Medical Sciences, Tabriz, Iran
Department of Pharmacognosy, Faculty of Pharmacy, Tabriz University of Medical Sciences, Tabriz, Iran

Parina Asgharian
Department of Pharmacognosy, Faculty of Pharmacy, Tabriz University of Medical Sciences, Tabriz, Iran
Student Research Committee, Tabriz University of Medical Sciences, Tabriz, Iran

Kamran Shadvar
Cardiovascular Research Center, Tabriz University of Medical Sciences, Tabriz, Iran

Hadi Hamishehkar
Drug Applied Research Center, Tabriz University of Medical Sciences, Tabriz, Iran
Sciences, Tabriz, Iran

Leila Sadeghi
Department of Animal Biology, Faculty of Natural Sciences, University of Tabriz, Tabriz, Iran

Farzeen Tanwir
Matrix Dynamics Group, University of Toronto, Canada

Vahid Yousefi Babadi
Department of Physiology, Payam Noor University of Iran, Iran

Basiru Olaitan Ajiboye, Oluwafemi Adeleke Ojo, Oluwatosin Adeyonu, Oluwatosin Imiere and Babatunji Emmanuel Oyinloye
Department of Chemical Sciences, Biochemistry Programme, Afe Babalola University, Ado-Ekiti, Ekiti State, Nigeria

Oluwafemi Ogunmodede
Department of Chemical Sciences, Industrial Chemistry Programme, Afe Babalola University, Ado-Ekiti, Ekiti State, Nigeria

Wafaa Mostafa Elkady and Mariam Hussein Gonaid
Pharmacognosy Department, Faculty of Pharmaceutical Sciences & Pharmaceutical Industries, Future University in Egypt, New Cairo, Egypt

Eman Ahmed Ibrahim and Farouk Kamel El Baz
Plant Biochemistry Department, National Research Centre, Dokki, Cairo, Egypt

Solmaz Maleki Dizaj and Samira Jafari
Biotechnology Research Center and Faculty of Pharmacy, Tabriz University of Medical Sciences, Tabriz, Iran

Afsaneh Mennati and Khadejeh Khezri
Faculty of Science, Physical Chemistry Group, Uremia Payam Noor University, Uremia, Iran

Index